Clinical Manual of
Eating Disorders

D0933249

Clinical Manual of Eating Disorders

Edited by

Joel Yager, M.D.

Professor and Vice-Chair for Education and Academic Affairs
University of New Mexico School of Medicine
Albuquerque, New Mexico
Professor Emeritus, Department of Psychiatry and Biobehavioral Sciences
David Geffen School of Medicine
University of California at Los Angeles

Pauline S. Powers, M.D.

Professor of Psychiatry and Behavioral Medicine
Department of Psychiatry and Behavioral Medicine
College of Medicine, Health Sciences Center
University of South Florida
Tampa, Florida

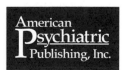

American
Psychiatric
Publishing, Inc.

Washington, DC
London, England

If you would like to buy between 25 and 99 copies of this or any other APPI title, you are eligible for a 20% discount; please contact APPI Customer Service at appi@psych.org or 800-368-5777. If you wish to buy 100 or more copies of the same title, please e-mail us at bulksales@psych.org for a price quote.

Copyright © 2007 American Psychiatric Publishing, Inc.
ALL RIGHTS RESERVED

Manufactured in the United States of America on acid-free paper
11   10   09   08   07   5   4   3   2   1
First Edition

Typeset in Adobe's Formata and AGaramond.

American Psychiatric Publishing, Inc.
1000 Wilson Boulevard
Arlington, VA 22209-3901
www.appi.org

Library of Congress Cataloging-in-Publication Data
Clinical manual of eating disorders / edited by Joel Yager, Pauline S. Powers. — 1st ed.
    p. ; cm.
    Includes bibliographical references and index.
    ISBN 978-1-58562-270-2 (pbk. : alk. paper)
    1. Eating disorders—Handbooks, manuals, etc. I. Yager, Joel. II. Powers, Pauline S.
[DNLM: 1. Eating Disorders—therapy. 2. Eating Disorders—diagnosis.
3. Psychotherapy—methods. WM 175 C641m 2007]
    RC552.E18C5559 2007
    616.85'26—dc22

                                                                                   2007006645

British Library Cataloguing in Publication Data
A CIP record is available from the British Library.

To our families, our patients, and their families.

Contents

Contributors xiii

Preface xix

1   Diagnosis, Epidemiology, and
Clinical Course of Eating Disorders 1
David B. Herzog, M.D., and Kamryn T. Eddy, M.A.
Anorexia Nervosa 2
Bulimia Nervosa 11
Eating Disorder Not Otherwise Specified 19
Conclusion. 26
References. 26

2   Assessment and Determination of Initial
Treatment Approaches for Patients
With Eating Disorders 31
Joel Yager, M.D.
Assessing The Patient. 32
Assessing the Family. 43
Choosing Initial Treatment Approaches and
the Initial Site of Treatment. 44
References. 57
Appendix: Eating Disorders Questionnaire (EDQ),
Version 9.0 60

3   Eating Disorders and Psychiatric Comorbidity:
Prevalence and Treatment Modifications 79
Randy A. Sansone, M.D., and Lori A. Sansone, M.D.
Prevalence of Axis I and Axis II Disorders in
Patients With Eating Disorders 80
Treatment Modifications for Comorbid
Psychiatric Disorders and Eating Disorders 84

Conclusion. 106
References. 107

4   **Management of Anorexia Nervosa in**
    Inpatient and Partial Hospitalization
    Settings **113**
    Katherine A. Halmi, M.D.
    Inpatient Hospitalization for Anorexia Nervosa:
        Inclusion Criteria. 114
    Inpatient Treatment of Anorexia Nervosa. 116
    Partial Hospitalization for Anorexia Nervosa 122
    References. 124

5   **Management of Anorexia Nervosa in an**
    Ambulatory Setting **127**
    Allan S. Kaplan, M.Sc., M.D., FRCPC, and
    Sarah Noble, M.D.
    Clinical Vignette 127
    Treatment Goals 129
    Psychosocial Approaches to the Outpatient
        Treatment of Anorexia Nervosa. 132
    Pharmacological Approaches to the
        Outpatient Treatment of Anorexia Nervosa. 138
    Long-Term Monitoring and Follow-Up: Indications
        for Hospitalization and Management of the
        Chronic Patient. 143
    References. 145

6   **Family Treatment of Eating Disorders** **149**
    James D. Lock, M.D., Ph.D., and Daniel le Grange, Ph.D.
    Why Families Have Been Targeted for Treatment 150
    Family Treatment for Adolescent Anorexia Nervosa . .152
    Family Treatment for Adults With Anorexia Nervosa. .161
    Family Therapy for Bulimia Nervosa and
        Eating Disorder Not Otherwise Specified. 162

Empirical Support for Family Therapy for Eating
    Disorders. 163
Future Directions in Family Therapy for Eating
    Disorders. 166
References. 167

7   **Management of Bulimia Nervosa. 171**
    *James E. Mitchell, M.D., Kristine J. Steffen, Pharm.D., and
    James L. Roerig, Pharm.D.*
    Clinical Vignette 172
    Target Symptoms and Treatment Goals. 173
    Nutritional Issues 173
    Psychosocial Approaches. 173
    Medication and Other Somatic Treatments. 174
    Combination CBT and Pharmacotherapy Trials. 184
    Sequential Treatment Studies 187
    Maintenance Studies 187
    Monitoring and Follow-Up. 188
    References. 188

8   **Management of Eating Disorders
    Not Otherwise Specified 195**
    *Michael J. Devlin, M.D., Kelly C. Allison, Ph.D.,
    Juli A. Goldfein, Ph.D., and Alexia Spanos*
    Binge-Eating Disorder. 197
    Night Eating and Nocturnal Eating Syndromes 207
    Other EDNOS Syndromes 218
    References. 219

9   **Psychiatric Aspects of
    Bariatric Surgery. 225**
    *James E. Mitchell, M.D., Lorraine Swan-Kremeier, Ph.D.,
    and Tricia Myers, Ph.D.*
    Overview of Bariatric Surgery Procedures 226
    Psychiatric Issues in Bariatric Surgery Candidates
        and Patients 235

Psychosocial Outcomes of Bariatric Surgery 238
Psychological Assessment for Bariatric Surgery 241
Psychological Management .246
References 250

10 Medication-Related Weight Changes:
Impact on Treatment of Eating Disorder
Patients 255
Pauline S. Powers, M.D., and Nancy L. Cloak, M.D.
Physiology of Weight Regulation 256
Medications That Affect Weight 259
Weight-Altering Medications and
Eating Disorders 269
Clinical Recommendations .276
References 278

11 Cognitive-Behavioral Therapy for
Eating Disorders 287
Joel Yager, M.D.
Distorted Cognitions and Maladaptive Behaviors
in Eating Disorders 288
Patient Selection for CBT 291
Applying CBT in Treating Patients
With Eating Disorders 292
When CBT Is Insufficient or Does Not Work 299
References 303

12 Psychodynamic Management of
Eating Disorders 307
Kathryn J. Zerbe, M.D.
Key Aspects of Psychodynamic Therapy 309
Additional Psychodynamic Considerations 318
Evolving Psychodynamic Research:
Implications for Therapeutic Change 326
Conclusion 328
References 330

13 Eating Disorders in Special Populations: Medical Comorbidities and Complicating or Unusual Conditions **335**
Stephanie L. Berg, M.D., and Arnold E. Andersen, M.D.
Diabetes Mellitus .... .336
Pregnancy .... .340
Nontraditional-Age Population .... .346
Males With Eating Disorders .... .349
Beyond the Narrow Diagnostic Boundaries in
  Anorexia Nervosa .... .353
References................................... .354

14 Athletes and Eating Disorders **357**
Pauline S. Powers, M.D., and Ron A. Thompson, Ph.D.
Role of the Athletic Environment in Predisposing
  Athletes to Eating Disorders .... .358
Identification and Assessment of Eating Disorders
  in Athletes.................................. .361
Sport Participation for Symptomatic Patients:
  Evaluation Criteria .... .366
Treatment for Athletes With Eating Disorders ...... .371
Prevention of Eating Disorders in Athletes......... .376
Conclusion................................... .370
References................................... .378
Appendix: Student Athletes and Eating Disorders:
  A Parents' Guide............................ .383

15 Cultural Considerations in Eating Disorders **387**
Tracy M. Anthony, M.D., and Joel Yager, M.D.
Epidemiology of Eating Disorders in
  Non-Caucasian Populations .... .389
Body Image and Eating and Dieting Behaviors in
  Non-Caucasian Women....................... .389
Eating Disorders in Non-Caucasian Men .... .397

International Trends in Eating and Dieting
  Behavior 397
Culturally Sensitive Assessment of Eating
  Disorders...................................398
Treatment of Eating Disorders in Non-Caucasian
  Patients 401
Conclusion...................................402
References...................................403

16 **Management of Patients With Chronic,
    Intractable Eating Disorders............407**
Joel Yager, M.D.
Chronicity of Illness 408
Treatment Nonresponse and Treatment
  Reluctance..................................412
Therapeutic Goals............................415
Psychiatric Management 418
Family Assessment and Treatment..............422
Choice of a Treatment Site 422
Medications and Other Somatic Treatments.......424
Legal, Ethical, and Humanistic Considerations 428
Countertransference Issues and Their
  Management.................................431
Compassionate Clinical Decision Making for
  Intractable Patients.........................432
References...................................436

Index 441

Contributors

Kelly C. Allison, Ph.D.
Research Assistant Professor and Co-Director of Education, Weight and Eating Disorders Program, University of Pennsylvania School of Medicine, Philadelphia, Pennsylvania

Arnold E. Andersen, M.D.
Professor, Department of Psychiatry, University of Iowa College of Medicine, Iowa City, Iowa

Tracy M. Anthony, M.D.
Staff Psychiatrist, The Oaks Treatment Center, Austin, Texas

Stephanie L. Berg, M.D.
Assistant Clinical Professor of Psychiatry, Department of Psychiatry, University of Iowa College of Medicine, Iowa City, Iowa

Nancy L. Cloak, M.D.
Staff Psychiatrist, MDSI Physicians, Inc., Portland, Oregon

Michael J. Devlin, M.D.
Associate Director, Eating Disorders Research Unit, New York State Psychiatric Institute, New York, New York

Kamryn T. Eddy, M.A.
Doctoral Candidate in Clinical Psychology, Center for Anxiety and Related Disorders, Boston University, Boston, Massachusetts

Juli A. Goldfein, Ph.D.
Research Scientist IV, Eating Disorders Research Unit, New York State Psychiatric Institute, New York, New York

Katherine A. Halmi, M.D.
Professor of Psychiatry, Weill Cornell Medical College; Director, Eating Disorder Program, New York Presbyterian Hospital–Westchester Division, White Plains, New York

David B. Herzog, M.D.
Director, Eating Disorders Unit, Child Psychiatry Service, Massachusetts General Hospital; Professor of Psychiatry (Pediatrics), Harvard Medical School, Boston, Massachusetts

Allan S. Kaplan, M.Sc., M.D., FRCPC
Loretta Anne Rogers Chair in Eating Disorders, Toronto General Hospital; Vice Chair for Research and Professor of Psychiatry, University of Toronto, Toronto, Ontario, Canada

Daniel le Grange, Ph.D.
Associate Professor, Department of Psychiatry, University of Chicago, Chicago, Illinois

James D. Lock, M.D., Ph.D.
Professor, Department of Psychiatry and Behavioral Sciences, Stanford University, Stanford, California

James E. Mitchell, M.D.
Chester Fritz Professor and Chair, Department of Clinical Neuroscience, University of North Dakota School of Medicine and Health Sciences; President and Scientific Director, Neuropsychiatric Research Institute, Fargo, North Dakota

Tricia Myers, Ph.D.
Assistant Professor, Department of Clinical Neuroscience, University of North Dakota School of Medicine and Health Sciences; Research Scientist, Neuropsychiatric Research Institute, Fargo, North Dakota

Sarah Noble, M.D.
Resident in Psychiatry, University of Toronto, Toronto, Ontario, Canada

Pauline S. Powers, M.D.
Professor of Psychiatry and Behavioral Medicine, College of Medicine, Health Sciences Center, University of South Florida, Tampa, Florida

James L. Roerig, Pharm.D.
Associate Professor, Department of Clinical Neuroscience, University of North Dakota School of Medicine and Health Sciences; Research Scientist, Neuropsychiatric Research Institute, Fargo, North Dakota

Lori A. Sansone, M.D.
Staff Physician (Family Medicine), Wright-Patterson Air Force Base, Dayton, Ohio

Randy A. Sansone, M.D.
Professor, Departments of Psychiatry and Internal Medicine, Wright State University School of Medicine, Dayton, Ohio; Director of Psychiatry Education, Kettering Medical Center, Kettering, Ohio

Alexia Spanos
Research Assistant, Eating Disorders Research Unit, New York State Psychiatric Institute, New York, New York

Kristine J. Steffen, Pharm.D.
Assistant Professor, Department of Clinical Neuroscience, University of North Dakota School of Medicine and Health Sciences; Research Scientist, Neuropsychiatric Research Institute, Fargo, North Dakota

Lorraine Swan-Kremeier, Ph.D.
Assistant Professor, Department of Clinical Neuroscience, University of North Dakota School of Medicine and Health Sciences; Research Scientist, Neuropsychiatric Research Institute, Fargo, North Dakota

Ron A. Thompson, Ph.D.
Psychiatrist, Private Practice, Bloomington Center for Counseling and Human Development, Bloomington, Indiana

Joel Yager, M.D.
Professor and Vice-Chair for Education and Academic Affairs, University of New Mexico School of Medicine, Albuquerque, New Mexico; Professor Emeritus, Department of Psychiatry and Biobehavioral Sciences, David Geffen School of Medicine, University of California at Los Angeles

Kathryn J. Zerbe, M.D.
Professor of Psychiatry and Obstetrics and Gynecology; Vice Chair for Psychotherapy and Director of Outpatient Services, Department of Psychiatry, Oregon Health Sciences University; Training and Supervising Analyst, Oregon Psychoanalytic Institute, Portland, Oregon

Disclosure of Competing Interests

The following authors have competing interests to declare:

Kelly C. Allison, Ph.D.—Receives royalties from a book (*Overcoming Night Eating Syndrome: A Step-by-Step Guide to Breaking the Cycle,* by Allison, Stunkard, and Thier) cited in her chapter.
Nancy L. Cloak, M.D.—*Stock:* Pfizer.
James D. Lock, M.D., Ph.D.—Receives royalties from a book (*Treatment Manual for Anorexia Nervosa: A Family-Based Approach,* by Lock, le Grange, Agras, et al.) cited in his chapter.
James E. Mitchell, M.D.—*Grant support:* Eli Lilly, Pfizer.
Pauline S. Powers, M.D.—*Grant support:* Astra-Zeneca (author is investigator on grant involving a double-blind, placebo-controlled study of quetiapine in anorexia nervosa).
James L. Roerig, Pharm.D.—*Grant support:* Eli Lilly, Corcept Therapeutics; *Speaker's bureau:* Bristol-Myers Squibb.

The following authors have no competing interests to report:

Arnold E. Andersen, M.D.
Tracy M. Anthony, M.D.

Stephanie L. Berg, M.D.
Michael J. Devlin, M.D.
Kamryn T. Eddy, M.A.
Juli A. Goldfein, Ph.D.
Katherine A. Halmi, M.D.
David B. Herzog, M.D.
Allan S. Kaplan, M.Sc., M.D., FRCPC
Daniel le Grange, Ph.D.
Tricia Myers, Ph.D.
Sarah Noble, M.D.
Lori A. Sansone, M.D.
Randy A. Sansone, M.D.
Alexia Spanos
Kristine J. Steffen, Pharm.D.
Lorraine Swan-Kremeier, Ph.D.
Ron A. Thompson, Ph.D.
Joel Yager, M.D.
Kathryn J. Zerbe, M.D.

Preface

This clinical manual evolved as an elaboration of the third edition of the American Psychiatric Association's "Practice Guideline for the Treatment of Patients With Eating Disorders," published in June 2006. A number of readers suggested that more detailed discussions of the various components of assessment and treatment would be helpful for clinicians grappling with treating patients with these disorders. To tackle this welcome task, we enlisted the members of the work group that authored the practice guideline, together with several other experts, to provide discussions to help clinicians better understand how to care for patients and families seeking help. Accordingly, most of this volume addresses the diagnosis, assessment, and treatment of patients with anorexia nervosa, bulimia nervosa, and eating disorder not otherwise specified, in particular binge-eating disorder.

In addition to building on sections addressed in the practice guideline, chapters in this volume also examine related topics that were not covered in the guideline: specifically, night-eating and related syndromes, obesity and weight management in relation to psychiatric medications, psychiatric aspects of bariatric surgery, and management of patients with chronic, intractable eating disorders.

Contributors were asked to use the practice guideline as a starting point for their presentations. Where suitable, we asked that clinical vignettes be presented as ways to anchor discussions in the concrete decision making required in clinical care. In this regard, the reader will find clinical examples sprinkled throughout several chapters in this volume. We asked that specific techniques and strategies be spelled out, although we realized that full and detailed presentations of how to conduct elaborate therapies were beyond the scope of this concise volume.

We trust that readers will find the material and discussions in this volume helpful, and we welcome feedback so that we can ensure that future publications addressing these issues are as user-friendly as possible.

Joel Yager, M.D.
Pauline S. Powers, M.D.

1

Diagnosis, Epidemiology, and Clinical Course of Eating Disorders

David B. Herzog, M.D.

Kamryn T. Eddy, M.A.

Eating disorders are significant problems most commonly occurring among late adolescent and young adult women. These conditions may be chronic and relapsing and are often associated with psychiatric comorbidity and medical sequelae. Among the eating disorders, anorexia nervosa and bulimia nervosa have received the most research attention over the past several decades, but other clinically significant eating disturbances, including binge-eating disorder (BED), have also been recognized. Although there are features common across eating disorders, including preoccupation with food, weight, and shape, notable differences exist in clinical presentation by eating disorder type. For example, both anorexia nervosa and bulimia nervosa are characterized by a desire for thinness; however, anorexia nervosa is marked by extreme weight loss, body image disturbance, and an intense fear of weight gain, while the hallmarks of bulimia nervosa are binge eating and compensatory behaviors within the normal weight range. The medical community has recognized anorexia nervosa as a diagnosis since the turn of the nineteenth century. By contrast, bulimia nervosa was not formally deemed a clinical diagnosis until Russell's description in 1979. Further, BED is currently identified in the *Diagnostic and Statistical Manual of Mental Disorders,* Fourth Edition, Text Revision (DSM-IV-TR; American Psychiatric Association 2000), as a provisional category in need of continued research.

In this chapter, we describe the diagnostic criteria, clinical features, epidemiology, and longitudinal outcome of eating disorders.

Anorexia Nervosa

Diagnosis

Diagnostic Criteria

Anorexia nervosa typically begins in adolescence but often persists into adulthood. Patients with anorexia nervosa lose weight by restricting their food intake and excessively exercising, and a subgroup also induces vomiting after meals and abuses laxatives, diuretics, or diet pills. Table 1–1 shows the DSM-IV-TR criteria for the disorder.

DSM-IV-TR distinguishes between two subtypes of anorexia nervosa—restricting and binge-eating/purging—based on the presence or absence of bulimic symptoms. Individuals with the binge-eating/purging type may be more likely than those with the restricting type to have comorbid impulsivity, including substance use disorders, cluster B personality disorders, mood lability, and suicidality (American Psychiatric Association 2000). Additionally, they may develop more severe medical complications as binge/purge behaviors compound their low weight.

Several questions concern the validity of the diagnostic criteria for anorexia nervosa. For example: Do patients who present with symptoms of anorexia nervosa that narrowly miss the full set of diagnostic criteria warrant a different diagnosis or treatment approach? The necessity of the amenorrhea criterion has been particularly controversial, since a subset of low-weight patients continue to menstruate, and the course and outcome in this subset differ little from the

Table 1–1. DSM-IV-TR diagnostic criteria for anorexia nervosa

A. Refusal to maintain body weight at or above a minimally normal weight for age and height (e.g., weight loss leading to maintenance of body weight less than 85% of that expected; or failure to make expected weight gain during period of growth, leading to body weight less than 85% of that expected).

B. Intense fear of gaining weight or becoming fat, even though underweight.

C. Disturbance in the way in which one's body weight or shape is experienced, undue influence of body weight or shape on self-evaluation, or denial of the seriousness of the current low body weight.

D. In postmenarcheal females, amenorrhea, i.e., the absence of at least three consecutive menstrual cycles. (A woman is considered to have amenorrhea if her periods occur only following hormone, e.g., estrogen, administration.)

Specify type:

Restricting type: during the current episode of anorexia nervosa, the person has not regularly engaged in binge-eating or purging behavior (i.e., self-induced vomiting or the misuse of laxatives, diuretics, or enemas)

Binge-eating/purging type: during the current episode of anorexia nervosa, the person has regularly engaged in binge-eating or purging behavior (i.e., self-induced vomiting or the misuse of laxatives, diuretics, or enemas)

Source.   Reprinted from American Psychiatric Association: *Diagnostic and Statistical Manual of Mental Disorders,* 4th Edition, Text Revision. Washington, DC, American Psychiatric Association, 2000. Used with permission.

course and outcome in patients with amenorrhea. General consensus suggests that patients with most of the key categorical criteria of anorexia nervosa deserve to be diagnosed with this disorder and treated accordingly.

Research on the clinical utility of distinguishing between individuals with anorexia nervosa and those with subthreshold variants of the disorder is crucial. Additionally, investigators and clinicians alike have noted that clinically significant eating disturbances can be present in children and adolescents even in the absence of established diagnostic criteria (Golden et al. 2003). Therefore, some have suggested lowering the threshold for intervention in children and adolescents, especially given that the physical consequences of the eating disorder may be particularly damaging or irreversible during periods of adolescent development (Golden et al. 2003). Further, bulimic symptoms are common among patients with anorexia nervosa, and the uncertainty about how to classify those patients who cross over between anorexia nervosa and bulimia nervosa poses another challenge for future research.

Clinical Features

Physical presentation.   Adolescent patients often appear physically younger than their chronological age, whereas those with chronic anorexia nervosa may look considerably older than their years. Cachexia and breast atrophy are apparent. Often skin is dry and yellow-tinged due to carotenemia. Physical signs commonly include bradycardia, hypotension, lanugo, alopecia, and edema. Patients who self-induce vomiting exhibit dental erosion and dorsal-surface hand lesions.

Individuals with anorexia nervosa may complain of cold intolerance, dizziness, constipation, and abdominal discomfort. Despite malnutrition, these patients are often hyperactive; lethargy may indicate fluid and electrolyte imbalance, dehydration, cardiovascular compromise, or severe depression.

Medical complications.   Anorexia nervosa is associated with numerous significant medical complications secondary to starvation. In patients with the binge-eating/purging type, these complications may also arise secondarily to bulimic symptoms (see Table 1–2).

Electrocardiographic abnormalities (e.g., low voltage, bradycardia, T-wave inversions, ST segment depression, and arrhythmias) are common and often normalize with refeeding. Other cardiac problems, including prolonged QT intervals, myocardial damage, and arrhythmias secondary to electrolyte imbalances, may be fatal. Endocrine sequelae include amenorrhea secondary to starvation-induced hypogonadism; hypothyroidism; a reduction in levels of growth hormones (insulin-like growth factor); and decreased serum levels of leptin (see, e.g., Misra Miller et al. 2004). Hormone levels generally improve with weight restoration. Related to the endocrine complications are skeletal problems; reductions in bone mineral density occur at several skeletal sites in most women with anorexia nervosa, leading to osteopenia and osteoporosis (Grinspoon et al. 2000). Although bone mineral density improves with weight gain, osteopenia often persists. Further, individuals with anorexia nervosa may experience infertility, premature births, and other perinatal complications (Wolfe 2005).

Laboratory findings may include electrolyte abnormalities, in particular hypokalemia. Gastrointestinal complications such as constipation, decreased gastric motility, and delayed gastric emptying are common. Patients may also report pancreatitis. High levels of blood urea nitrogen may reflect renal ab-

Table 1–2. Medical complications of anorexia nervosa

Cardiac	Low voltage, bradycardia, T-wave inversions, ST segment depression, arrhythmias Prolonged QT intervals, myocardial damage, arrhythmias
Endocrine	Amenorrhea, hypothyroidism Reduced growth hormone–binding protein, insulin-like growth factor, and serum leptin levels
Skeletal	Low bone mineral density, resulting in osteopenia or osteoporosis
Reproductive	Infertility, premature births, perinatal complications
Gastrointestinal	Decreased gastric motility, delayed gastric emptying, constipation
Renal	Elevated blood urea nitrogen, polyuria, peripheral edema (during refeeding)
Neurological	Decreased gray matter volume, increased sulcal cerebrospinal fluid volumes
Hematological	Anemia, leukopenia, thrombocytopenia

normalities resulting from dehydration. Polyuria related to an abnormality in vasopressin secretion may also develop. Approximately 20% of patients experience peripheral edema, usually during refeeding. Mild anemia, leukopenia, and thrombocytopenia are often observed but typically reverse with refeeding. Neurological abnormalities may include reduced gray matter volumes and increased sulcal cerebrospinal fluid volumes that persist postrecovery.

Psychological presentation.   Patients with anorexia nervosa prototypically present with severe body distortion, interoceptive disturbances, and dysthymia. Affect is restricted, and patients demonstrate minimal capacity for insight, often secondary to starvation-induced preoccupation with food, weight, and shape. Axis I comorbidity is common and most often includes major depression and anxiety disorders, although substance use disorders are also prevalent. With regard to personality, patients may be obsessional, interpersonally insecure, perfectionistic, intolerant of negative affect, rigidly controlling of impulses, unsure of their identity, competitive, and experiencing an increased sense of personal responsibility and guilt (Strober 2004; Westen and Harnden-Fischer 2001). A subset of patients, particularly those with binge/purge symptoms, may also demonstrate impulsivity and self-injurious behaviors. Often patients with anorexia nervosa experience conflict around tasks of emotional and sexual maturation, separation and individuation, and fears of being controlled. Comorbid conditions and their implications for treatment are more fully discussed in Chapter 3 ("Eating Disorders and Psychiatric Comorbidity: Prevalence and Treatment Modifications") in this volume.

Differential Diagnosis

Physical disorders, including diabetes mellitus, colitis, thyroid disease, inflammatory bowel disease, acid peptic diseases, Addison's disease, intestinal motility disorders such as achalasia, and brain tumors, all may display clinical symptoms common to those of anorexia nervosa and thus should be evaluated and ruled out. Further, conversion disorders, schizophrenia, and mood disorders are among the psychiatric disorders that may manifest weight loss and bingeing or purging.

Epidemiology

Epidemiological research in eating disorders is limited, particularly with respect to prevalence among adolescents, in whom onset of the disorder is most typically seen. According to large-scale population and archival surveys, lifetime prevalence of anorexia nervosa is estimated at 1% (for review, see Hoek 2002). Data from two recent, large population-based studies, one in the United States and one in Scandinavia, found lifetime prevalence rates of 0.9% and 1.20%, respectively, for women and 0.3% and 0.29%, respectively, for men (Bulik et al. 2006; Hudson et al. 2007). Research suggests that prevalence of anorexia nervosa has increased in recent years (Keel and Klump 2003). Approximately 90%–95% of patients with anorexia are female. Although males are less likely to develop anorexia nervosa, their symptom presentation is similar to that of females. Age at onset for anorexia nervosa ranges from preteen to adult, with bimodal peaks at ages 13–14 and 17–18 years. Prepubertal anorexia nervosa may be associated with a more severe profile, and adolescent onset is associated with a better prognosis than are prepubertal and adult onset.

While anorexia nervosa is most prevalent in industrialized societies where food is abundant and a thin body ideal is held, systematic research on the cross-cultural prevalence of anorexia nervosa is lacking. Some evidence suggests that women emigrating to more industrialized countries from countries in which the prevalence of anorexia nervosa is low may be at greater risk as they assimilate thin body ideals. Also, some data suggest that symptom presentation may differ cross-culturally: for example, cognitive criteria (e.g., fat phobia) do not seem to be present in certain Asian countries (Hsu and Lee 1993). Cross-cultural and ethnic issues in eating disorders are more fully described in Chapter 15 ("Cultural Considerations in Eating Disorders") in this volume.

In the United States, anorexia nervosa is prevalent across ethnicity and socioeconomic status, although younger, higher-weight, well-educated minority women who are more closely aligned with "white, middle-class values" may be at increased risk compared with other minorities (Crago et al. 1996). Although the research findings are conflicting, anorexia nervosa generally tends to be less common among African Americans than among Caucasian, Hispanic, and Asian American women.

Etiology

Multiple perspectives on the pathogenesis of anorexia nervosa exist, with the most comprehensive picture implicating a combination of biological, psychological, and sociocultural factors in the onset of the disorder.

Biological Factors

Population-based twin studies as well as clinical samples suggest significant genetic and nonshared environmental influences on anorexic symptomatology. Family studies suggest that anorexia nervosa is significantly more common in biological relatives of index patients with eating disorders than in the general population, with one study indicating a relative risk for the disorder in female relatives of 11.3 (Strober et al. 2000; for review, see Strober and Bulik 2002). Further, a recent multisite genetic study has provided initial evidence for the presence of a susceptibility locus on chromosome 1p (Grice et al. 2002).

Neurochemically, starvation itself produces changes in hypothalamic and metabolic functioning, and anorexia nervosa is further associated with changes in the noradrenergic, serotonergic, dopaminergic, and opioid neurotransmitter systems and with alterations in neuromodulators such as corticotropin-releasing hormone. Under certain circumstances, hypothalamic epinephrine and serotonin may induce loss of appetite, whereas norepinephrine increases food intake. Dysregulated serotonin levels in women with anorexia nervosa that persist postrecovery suggest this neurotransmitter may contribute to the development of the disorder (e.g., Frank et al. 2004).

Prevalence and demographics of anorexia nervosa

Lifetime prevalence of 1%.

90%–95% of individuals with anorexia nervosa are female.

Bimodal peaks for age at onset at 13–14 years and 17–18 years.

Most prevalent in industrialized nations where food is abundant and thin body ideals are held.

Prevalent across socioeconomic status and ethnicity; slightly less common among African Americans compared with Caucasian, Hispanic, and Asian Americans.

Cross-cultural symptom presentation may differ.

Further, individuals with anorexia nervosa exhibit abnormal taste profiles and sensory responses to high-calorie foods that may continue after weight recovery.

Psychological Factors

Personality characteristics, including emotional constraint, perfectionism, and rigidity, may represent risk factors for the development of anorexia nervosa (e.g., Fairburn et al. 1999; Westen and Harnden-Fischer 2001). During periods of stress and transition, individuals with these personality tendencies, who are temperamentally averse to sudden changes, may retreat into structure and rigidity (across multiple domains, including eating) that may provide a familiar sense of security. Adolescence, marked by physical and social change, may represent one of these periods of heightened risk. While providing relief from the physical and emotional changes and demands associated with adolescence, anorexia nervosa simultaneously causes physical and emotional debilitation; this dilemma renders the disorder all the more difficult for the patient to relinquish (Strober 2004).

From a psychodynamic perspective, anorexia nervosa results in a patient's attempts to solve intrapsychic conflicts, in which eating symptoms are conceptualized as a behavioral manifestation of emotional conflict. These conflicts often relate to issues of separation-individuation and control. Families of individuals with anorexia nervosa have been described as high in enmeshment and overprotection and lacking in intimacy and appropriate conflict resolution (Minuchin et al. 1978). Family systems theory posits that internal conflicts may be related to family dynamics, which for individuals with anorexia nervosa may be characterized by lack of intimacy, enmeshment, overprotection, rigidity, and lack of conflict resolution. In these formulations, the role of the patient with anorexia nervosa is to divert attention from impending family conflict; the symptoms serve as a stabilizing force for the family. As the patient continues to lose weight, she becomes increasingly dependent on and inseparable from the family. According to Minuchin, in these families excessive nurturance seemed to undermine the child's efforts at separation; the child's attempts at genuine self-expression were neglected.

Sociocultural Factors

Anorexia nervosa is far more prevalent in females than in males and tends to arise at times of sexual maturation, around menarche and puberty. Researchers have attributed this distribution to the greater cultural pressures on women toward thinness, which is commonly portrayed in Western culture as a prerequisite to success and beauty, and to the differences in socialization between girls and boys. Whereas girls are brought up to espouse "feminine" values, including service to others, attention to relationships, and interdependence, boys are trained to be autonomous, self-directed, and rule-oriented in their relationships. As modern culture transforms traditional models of female role definition by encouraging girls to be more autonomous, self-directed, and rule-oriented, girls are caught in severe role conflicts. For some, anorexia nervosa may be a response to these complex pressures of socialization.

High-Risk Populations

Individuals who participate in activities that require highly focused attention on weight and appearance, including ballet, long-distance running, gymnastics, ice-skating, and modeling, may be at increased risk for anorexia nervosa. Other susceptible groups include chronically ill women with diseases such as cystic fibrosis, diabetes, and spina bifida, and mood disorders, particularly depression; women with professions that require high standards of achievement; and homosexual men.

Course and Outcome

Recovery and Relapse

Anorexia nervosa typically first manifests in adolescence; midlife onset is rare (American Psychiatric Association 2000). Although the course of the disorder is variable, it is often marked by chronicity and relapse. Considerable longitudinal research has examined the course and outcome of anorexia nervosa. A comprehensive meta-analysis of 119 studies including 5,590 patients with anorexia indicated that over long-term follow-up (up to 29 years; mode = 5–10 years), less than one-half of surviving patients achieved full recovery, one-third improved but experienced lingering eating disorder symptoms, and one-fifth remained chronically ill (Steinhausen 2002). Even among those who achieve full recovery, up to one-third are likely to experience relapse.

Yet within this research, outlying findings suggest a more hopeful outcome. In one 10- to 15-year prospective study of adolescents receiving inpatient treatment for anorexia nervosa, three-fourths of patients met the criteria for full recovery, although the median time to recovery was approximately 5 years posttreatment (Strober et al. 1997). This and other research may suggest that early treatment of adolescent anorexia nervosa predicts a favorable outcome. General predictors of recovery include higher body weight at intake, shorter duration of intake episode, and atypical features (e.g., lack of cognitive symptoms, including fear of weight gain and body distortion) (see, e.g., Herzog et al. 1999).

Diagnostic Migration

The majority of individuals with anorexia nervosa engage in bingeing and purging behaviors during the course of the disorder; thus, diagnostic migration from the restricting type of anorexia nervosa to the binge/purge type or to bulimia nervosa is common, particularly within the first 5 years of illness (Eddy et al. 2002; Tozzi et al. 2005).

Mortality

Anorexia nervosa appears to have the highest mortality rate among psychiatric disorders. In spite of diagnostic and treatment advances, the prognosis of anorexia nervosa does not seem to have improved during the twentieth century (Steinhausen 2002). The mortality rate for women with anorexia nervosa, 0.56% per year, is more than 12 times higher than that for age-matched women in the general population (Sullivan 1995). The rate of suicide is also elevated, with one study demonstrating a 57-fold increase in death by suicide among individuals with anorexia nervosa (Keel et al. 2003). An 11-year follow-up study of women with eating disorders reported a mortality rate of 7.4% for the women with anorexia nervosa, with 4 of the 10 deaths due to suicide (Franko et al. 2004; Keel et al. 2003). In a survey of 14 outcome studies, Herzog et al. (1988) found that 24% of the deaths reported were due to suicide. Factors noted to predict death in women with anorexia nervosa include abnormally low serum albumin levels and low weight at intake, poor social functioning, longer duration of illness, bingeing and purging, comorbid substance abuse, and comorbid affective disorders (Keel et al. 2003). Although death is commonly due to suicide, it is also frequently ascribed to inanition and cardiac failure. However, the exact cause of death is often unclear.

Bulimia Nervosa

Diagnosis

Diagnostic Criteria

Bulimia nervosa typically has an onset in late adolescence or early adulthood in individuals who are of normal weight or slight overweight, and may have its onset following a period of dieting. Bulimia nervosa is characterized by recurrent binge eating (i.e., objective overeating marked by the subjective experience of loss of control over eating), compensatory behaviors, and related cognitions. Compensatory behaviors are used to counteract the effects of a binge and may include self-induced vomiting; misuse of laxatives, diuretics, and enemas; fasting; and excessive exercise. The DSM-IV-TR criteria for bulimia are shown in Table 1–3.

DSM-IV-TR distinguishes between two subtypes of bulimia nervosa—purging and nonpurging—based on the type of compensatory behaviors employed. The majority of patients with bulimia present with the purging type (i.e., compensatory behaviors, including vomiting and use of diuretics or laxatives). While individuals with bulimia often use more than one type of compensatory behavior, 80%–90% engage in self-induced vomiting (American Psychiatric Association 2000). Patients with purging-type bulimia tend to have more psychiatric and medical comorbidity than those with the nonpurging type.

Several issues have emerged with regard to the validity of the diagnostic criteria for bulimia nervosa. Some researchers have argued that the frequency criterion for "regular" binge eating and compensatory behaviors is arbitrary

Course and outcome of anorexia nervosa

<50% achieve full recovery, 33% improve, and 20% remain chronically ill, as suggested by longitudinal research.

33% of those who recover will experience relapse.

Prognosis may be better for individuals treated in adolescence.

Predictors of recovery include higher body weight at intake, shorter duration of illness, and atypical features.

Approximately 50% of individuals with anorexia nervosa will develop bulimic symptoms.

Mortality rate is 0.56% per year, and standardized mortality ratio is 12.

Common causes of death include suicide and cardiac failure.

and that a distinction between individuals who engage in binge/purge behaviors two or more times weekly and those who engage in the behaviors once weekly is not useful. Further, although binge eating has always been recognized as a defining feature of bulimia nervosa, recent studies have suggested that individuals who engage in purging without objective binge eating exhibit psychopathology that closely aligns them with individuals with bulimia nervosa. Research on these nosological issues is ongoing and will likely inform the next iteration of the *Diagnostic and Statistical Manual of Mental Disorders*.

Clinical Features

Physical presentation.   Patients with bulimia nervosa are typically within the healthy weight range, although a subset of patients are overweight or obese. Patients may complain of peripheral edema, bloating, weakness, fatigue, and dental problems. Facial swelling and peliosis and calluses or abrasions on the dorsal area of the hand may develop secondary to self-induced vomiting.

Medical complications.   Bulimia nervosa is associated with a number of medical complications. These complications are most often secondary to purging but may also be related to malnutrition and binge eating (see Table 1–4).

Purging through vomiting and misuse of laxatives or diuretics results in electrolyte and acid–base complications, including hypokalemia, arrhythmias, muscle weakness, tetany, and metabolic alkalosis (Lasater and Mehler 2001). Use of ipecac to induce vomiting can lead to skeletal muscle myopathy or even fatal cardiomyopathy. Rates of mitral valve prolapse are elevated in patients

Table 1–3.   DSM-IV-TR diagnostic criteria for bulimia nervosa

A.   Recurrent episodes of binge eating. An episode of binge eating is characterized by both of the following:

    (1)   eating, in a discrete period of time (e.g., within any 2-hour period), an amount of food that is definitely larger than most people would eat during a similar period of time and under similar circumstances

    (2)   a sense of lack of control over eating during the episode (e.g., a feeling that one cannot stop eating or control what or how much one is eating)

B.   Recurrent inappropriate compensatory behavior in order to prevent weight gain, such as self-induced vomiting; misuse of laxatives, diuretics, enemas, or other medications; fasting; or excessive exercise.

C.   The binge eating and inappropriate compensatory behaviors both occur, on average, at least twice a week for 3 months.

D.   Self-evaluation is unduly influenced by body shape and weight.

E.   The disturbance does not occur exclusively during episodes of anorexia nervosa.

Specify type:

    Purging type: during the current episode of bulimia nervosa, the person has regularly engaged in self-induced vomiting or the misuse of laxatives, diuretics, or enemas

    Nonpurging type: during the current episode of bulimia nervosa, the person has used other inappropriate compensatory behaviors, such as fasting or excessive exercise, but has not regularly engaged in self-induced vomiting or the misuse of laxatives, diuretics, or enemas

Source.   Reprinted from American Psychiatric Association: *Diagnostic and Statistical Manual of Mental Disorders,* 4th Edition, Text Revision. Washington, DC, American Psychiatric Association, 2000. Used with permission.

with bulimia nervosa. Gastrointestinal problems secondary to purging are also common. Self-induced vomiting may give rise to esophageal disorders, including esophagitis, chest pain, dyspepsia, gastroesophageal reflux disease, esophageal rupture, hiatal hernias, and Barrett's esophagus; patients who abuse laxatives may develop irritable bowel syndrome, melanosis coli, and atonic or cathartic colon. Although constipation often occurs when laxatives are discontinued, it usually remits within 3 weeks and responds well to exercise, fluid intake, and fiber increase. Oral complications secondary to chronic regurgitation of acidic gastric contents typically include enamel erosion and gum recession. Parotid gland swelling, due to salivary gland hypertrophy (sialadenosis), and el-

Table 1–4.   Medical complications of bulimia nervosa

Cardiac	Hypokalemia, arrhythmias, muscle weakness, tetany, and metabolic alkalosis (secondary to purging by vomiting/laxatives) Skeletal muscle myopathy and cardiomyopathy (secondary to ipecac use)
Gastrointestinal	Esophagitis, chest pain, dyspepsia, gastroesophageal reflux disease, esophageal rupture, hiatal hernias, and Barrett's esophagus (secondary to vomiting) Irritable bowel syndrome, melanosis coli, and atonic or cathartic colon (secondary to laxative abuse)
Oral/Dental	Enamel erosion, gum recession Swelling of the parotid gland, salivary gland hypertrophy, elevated serum amylase levels
Reproductive	Infertility Risk of spontaneous abortion, cesarean section, low birth weight, and postpartum depression

evated serum amylase levels are often present, and both remit when purging abates. Additionally, although a history of bulimia nervosa does not seem to impact women's ability to become pregnant, active bulimia nervosa may confer elevated risk for spontaneous abortion, cesarean section, low birth weight, and postpartum depression (e.g., Franko et al. 2001).

Psychological presentation.   Individuals with bulimia nervosa are preoccupied with eating, weight, and shape and tend to have marked body dissatisfaction and low mood. Patients with bulimia nervosa are generally less constricted and more aware of their feelings than patients with anorexia nervosa. They may demonstrate insight and articulate feelings and triggers associated with the binge-purge cycle, and often evince shame regarding bulimic behaviors. Axis I comorbidity is common and often includes mood, anxiety, and substance use disorders. Approximately half of patients with bulimia nervosa report a lifetime history of a mood or anxiety disorder, with depression, social phobia, and obsessive-compulsive disorder being particularly common. A substantial minority of patients with bulimia nervosa also report a lifetime history of substance use disorders, with alcohol abuse being the most common. In terms of personality, patients with bulimia nervosa manifest a range of traits, including perfectionism, identity confusion, impulse dysregulation, low self-esteem, guilt, and shame. A subset of patients with bulimia nervosa can be characterized as multi-impulsive or as exhibiting dysregulation across multiple domains, including eating, affect, interpersonal functioning, and sexuality, for example. Those with dysregulated personality styles are more likely to present with comorbid substance use disorders, Cluster B Axis II disorders, self-destructive and self-injurious behaviors, and kleptomania (Herzog et al. 1999). A full consideration of these comorbid conditions and their treatment implications can be found in Chapter 3 in this volume.

Differential Diagnosis

In performing a medical and psychiatric assessment, it is important to understand that a range of conditions may produce features similar to symptoms of bulimia nervosa. Neurological disorders that impact appetite regulation and eating behaviors, including brain tumors (e.g., pituitary or hypothalamic), and syndromes such as Kleine-Levin or Klüver-Bucy need to be ruled out, as do gastrointestinal disorders (e.g., malabsorption, ulcers, enteritis) and hormonal conditions relating to malnutrition and hypometabolism (e.g., adrenal disease, diabetes mellitus, pituitary dysfunction, hyperparathyroidism). Psychiatric illnesses, including major depressive disorder and borderline personality disorder, may be characterized by appetite dysregulation and binge eating or may be comorbid with bulimia nervosa. When binge eating and/or purging exists only in the context of anorexia nervosa, the bulimia nervosa diagnosis is not assigned.

Epidemiology

Epidemiological work in bulimia nervosa is limited. Population surveys indicate a lifetime prevalence rate for bulimia nervosa of 1%–4.2% (American Psychiatric Association 2000), although estimates are higher within certain population subsets, including college women. Research suggests that bulimia nervosa has decreased in prevalence in recent years (e.g., Keel et al. 2006). Data from the recent National Comorbidity Survey Replication study suggest a lifetime prevalence of 1.5% for women and 0.5% for men (Hudson et al. 2007).

As with anorexia nervosa, approximately 90%–95% of patients with bulimia nervosa are female (Hoek 2002). Onset tends to be somewhat later than in anorexia nervosa, occurring in late adolescence and early adulthood, and may coincide with an important transition (e.g., high school to college) or psychosocial stress. Bulimic attitudes and behaviors are widespread across ethnic and racial groups, but bulimia nervosa appears to be equally common among Caucasian and Hispanic American women and less common among African American women (Crago et al. 1996; Striegel-Moore et al. 2003).

Etiology

The pathogenesis of bulimia nervosa, like that of anorexia nervosa, is conceptualized as multifactorial, implicating biological, psychological, and sociocultural factors.

Biological Factors

The role of biology and genetic factors in the development of bulimia nervosa has received considerable attention in the last decade. The higher concordance of monozygotic twins compared with dizygotic twins for bulimia nervosa supports the biological model. Heritability estimates for bulimia nervosa from twin studies range from 31% to 83% (see Strober and Bulik 2002 for review). Further, first-degree relatives of patients with bulimia nervosa have higher rates of eating disorders than do control subjects. Although it is unlikely that research will identify a single gene to predict bulimia nervosa, preliminary findings suggest there are significant links between presence of bulimia nervosa and chromosome 10p (Bulik et al. 2003a, 2003b).

Further support for biological factors includes the dietary restraint model of bulimia nervosa, which suggests that patient-induced dietary restraint leads to binge eating. Neurotransmitters, including serotonin, play a role in appetite, satiation, food selection, and eating patterns, all of which may be disrupted in patients with bulimia nervosa. Additional findings point to elevations in the appetite-inducing neuropeptide Y and peptide YY in patients with bulimia nervosa. Levels of cholecystokinin, a hormone associated with the experience of satiety and discontinuation of eating behavior, have tended to be low in some patients with bulimia nervosa. The disruption of these neuronal systems may be implicated in bulimia nervosa (for review, see Bailer and Kaye 2003).

Psychological Factors

Individuals with bulimia nervosa exhibit perfectionism, affect dysregulation, impulsivity, self-destructiveness, pervasive low self-esteem, conflict aversion,

Prevalence and demographics of bulimia nervosa

Lifetime prevalence of 1%–4.2%.

90%–95% individuals with bulimia nervosa are female.

Onset typically in late adolescence or early adulthood.

Less common among African American women compared with Caucasian and Hispanic American women.

and fear of abandonment—all of which represent vulnerability factors predictive of the bulimic symptoms that emerge. Perfectionism is often characterized by dichotomous thinking, in which something or someone is either all-good or all-bad. This type of thinking may relate to the bulimia patient's alternation between strict dieting and binge eating; the individual on a strict diet may have difficulty maintaining her limited intake and, believing she has already failed, overeat (Polivy and Herman 1993). At the same time, failure to adhere to her diet and engagement in binge eating leave the patient feeling out of control and lower her self-esteem and efficacy. In order to regain that sense of control, and to improve her self-esteem, she resumes the cycle of dieting.

Another hypothesis is that binge eating and purging serve as regulation strategies for coping with negative affect (Polivy and Herman 1993). In this regard, both overeating and purging are acts of self-destruction, which may reflect the patient's internalized emotionality (e.g., anger) that she is averse to expressing outwardly. As in anorexia nervosa, the symptoms of bulimia are ultimately ineffective coping strategies consonant with the patient's personality style and simultaneously result in physical deterioration.

Families of individuals with bulimia nervosa are often marked by conflict, achievement orientation, dependence, and lack of cohesion. Disturbances in family functioning, particularly in the mother–child dyadic relationship, are common, leading to attachment disruptions and associated personality patterns. The findings from one large community-based study indicated that parental problems, including low child–parent contact and high parental expectations, as well as parent difficulties with alcohol, may be risk factors for bulimia nervosa (Fairburn et al. 1997). Yet the nature of the relationship between family dysfunction variables and bulimic symptoms is often unclear with regard to directionality. History of sexual abuse may also be an additional risk factor.

Sociocultural Factors

The increased prevalence of bulimia nervosa in industrialized nations supports the role of sociocultural factors in the pathogenesis of the disorder. Media images of ideal beauty inundate Western society and yet are unrealistically thin for most women; women with a childhood history of overweight and obesity may be at particular risk (e.g., Fairburn et al. 1997). Over time, the presentation of these unrealistic images leads to internalization of a thin body ideal and associated body dissatisfaction, both of which predict dieting and bulimic symptoms (for review, see Stice 2002). Further, cross-cultural research discerns that exposure to Western beauty ideals influences the development of eating disorder pathology. It is likely that the confluence of multiple psychological, biological, and sociocultural factors predicts the development of bulimia nervosa. These issues are further discussed in Chapter 15 in this volume.

High-Risk Populations

Given the etiological framework described above, a subgroup of individuals may be at increased risk for the development of bulimia nervosa. These at-risk groups may include individuals involved in activities in which weight and appearance are central (e.g., ballet, long-distance running, wrestling); individuals with certain physical conditions such as insulin-dependent diabetes mellitus; and homosexual males.

Course and Outcome

Recovery and Relapse

The longitudinal course of bulimia nervosa is variable, but, as with anorexia nervosa, the course of bulimia nervosa may be chronic and relapsing (for review, see Keel and Mitchell 1997). Longitudinal research suggests that approximately one-half of patients with bulimia nervosa will achieve full recovery from the eating disorder at 5- to 12-year follow-up, although approximately one-third of these will go on to experience relapse (e.g., Herzog et al. 1999). A subset of individuals with bulimia nervosa will receive cognitive-behavioral therapy, which has demonstrated clinical efficacy, with approximately one-half of individuals achieving full recovery and most of the remaining achieving symptomatic improvement. A small minority of patients present with chronic bulimia nervosa. It appears that a longer duration of illness, a history of unsuccessful treatment attempts, comorbid substance abuse, and Cluster B personality disorders are predictive of a worse outcome for patients with bulimia nervosa.

Diagnostic Migration

As noted previously, up to 50% of patients with anorexia nervosa will develop bulimic symptomatology; crossover from bulimia nervosa to anorexia nervosa is less likely (e.g., Tozzi et al. 2005).

Mortality

In contrast to the high mortality rates in patients with anorexia nervosa, mortality does not appear to be elevated in patients with bulimia nervosa (Nielsen et al. 1998). One review of 88 studies demonstrated a crude mortality rate of 0.3% at longitudinal follow-up, although the authors cautioned that this finding may be an underestimate due to variable lengths of follow-up (6 months to 10 years) and low ascertainment across follow-up (Keel and Mitchell 1997).

Eating Disorder Not Otherwise Specified

Diagnostic Features

Eating disorder not otherwise specified (EDNOS) is the diagnostic category used to describe individuals with clinically significant eating disturbances that do not fit into the narrowly defined categories of anorexia nervosa and bulimia nervosa. It is a comparatively large and heterogeneous diagnostic group; approximately half of individuals presenting for eating disorder treatment in the community meet the EDNOS criteria (Fairburn and Bohn 2005), and EDNOS appears to be particularly common among adolescents. A subset of those with EDNOS consists of individuals whose symptom presentation closely aligns with anorexia or bulimia nervosa but falls outside these classifications on the basis of one criterion (e.g., amenorrhea, binge/purge frequency). Other examples of patients with an EDNOS symptom cluster are those who engage in chewing and spitting and those who regularly engage in nighttime eating. Examples of EDNOS are provided in the DSM-IV-TR diagnostic criteria (Table 1–5).

In spite of the prevalence of EDNOS—particularly in comparison with the prevalence of anorexia nervosa and bulimia nervosa—there is a paucity of research on the epidemiology, course, and outcome of this heterogeneous diagnostic group. Within the category of EDNOS, the one symptom cluster presentation that has received comparative attention is BED.

Course and outcome of bulimia nervosa

50% of patients will achieve full recovery, while a small minority remain chronically ill, as suggested by longitudinal research.

33% of those who recover will experience relapse.

Cognitive-behavioral treatment is associated with symptom improvement and recovery.

Predictors of poor outcome include longer duration of illness, a history of unsuccessful treatment attempts, comorbid substance abuse, and Cluster B personality disorders.

Diagnostic migration from bulimia nervosa to anorexia nervosa is uncommon.

Binge-Eating Disorder

Diagnostic Criteria

Although descriptions of the clinical phenomenon of binge eating in the absence of compensatory behaviors date back a half century, BED was not formally recognized until 1994. DSM-IV (American Psychiatric Association 1994) introduced BED as a specific example within the heterogeneous category of EDNOS. As a provisional diagnosis, BED has received significant research and clinical attention during the last decade, and DSM-IV-TR offers research criteria for making the diagnosis (see Table 1–6).

BED is characterized by recurrent binge eating (i.e., objective overeating accompanied by the subjective experience of loss of control over eating) and marked distress in the absence of the regular compensatory behaviors that characterize bulimia nervosa. The binge episodes may be associated with a cluster of symptoms, including eating more rapidly than normal, eating until feeling uncomfortably full, eating large amounts in the absence of physical hunger, eating in secret due to embarrassment around overeating, and feeling disgusted, depressed, or guilty after eating. The phenomenon of binge eating in patients with BED is similar to bulimic behaviors in individuals with bulimia nervosa; yet there are differences. Whereas in bulimia nervosa, episodes of binge eating represent lapses in overcontrol in the context of overall dietary restraint, in BED, binge eating tends to occur in the context of generally chaotic food patterns and overeating (Wilfley et al. 2000).

Table 1–5.   DSM-IV-TR diagnostic criteria for eating disorder not otherwise specified

The eating disorder not otherwise specified category is for disorders of eating that do not meet the criteria for any specific eating disorder. Examples include

1. For females, all of the criteria for anorexia nervosa are met except that the individual has regular menses.

2. All of the criteria for anorexia nervosa are met except that, despite significant weight loss, the individual's current weight is in the normal range.

3. All of the criteria for bulimia nervosa are met except that the binge eating and inappropriate compensatory mechanisms occur at a frequency of less than twice a week or for a duration of less than 3 months.

4. The regular use of inappropriate compensatory behavior by an individual of normal body weight after eating small amounts of food (e.g., self-induced vomiting after the consumption of two cookies).

5. Repeatedly chewing and spitting out, but not swallowing, large amounts of food.

6. Binge-eating disorder: recurrent episodes of binge eating in the absence of the regular use of inappropriate compensatory behaviors characteristic of bulimia nervosa [see Table 1–6 for suggested research criteria].

Source.   Reprinted from American Psychiatric Association: *Diagnostic and Statistical Manual of Mental Disorders,* 4th Edition, Text Revision. Washington, DC, American Psychiatric Association, 2000. Used with permission.

Clinical Features

Physical presentation.   Patients with BED are often overweight or obese; although the disorder may be present in normal-weight individuals, overweight/ obesity is more commonly observed. Individuals presenting in clinical settings often have a history of marked weight fluctuations and repeated failed efforts at weight control.

Medical complications.   BED is associated with overweight and obesity, both of which are related to a number of health-related problems as well as increased mortality. Medical complications of overweight and obesity include hypertension, dyslipidemia, type 2 diabetes, coronary heart disease, stroke, gallbladder disease, osteoarthritis, sleep apnea, respiratory problems, and cancer (i.e., endometrial, breast, colon). Further, BED has been associated with increased health risk independent of body mass index (e.g., Bulik et al. 2003a). In one large population-based twin study, obese individuals with BED tended to

Table 1–6.   DSM-IV-TR research diagnostic criteria for binge-eating disorder

A.   Recurrent episodes of binge eating. An episode of binge eating is characterized by both of the following:

(1)   eating, in a discrete period of time (e.g., within any 2-hour period), an amount of food that is definitely larger than most people would eat in a similar period of time under similar circumstances

(2)   a sense of lack of control over eating during the episode (e.g., a feeling that one cannot stop eating or control what or how much one is eating)

B.   The binge-eating episodes are associated with three (or more) of the following:

(1)   eating much more rapidly than normal

(2)   eating until feeling uncomfortably full

(3)   eating large amounts of food when not feeling physically hungry

(4)   eating alone because of being embarrassed by how much one is eating

(5)   feeling disgusted with oneself, depressed, or very guilty after overeating

C.   Marked distress regarding binge eating is present.

D.   The binge eating occurs, on average, at least 2 days a week for 6 months.

Note: The method of determining frequency differs from that used for bulimia nervosa; future research should address whether the preferred method of setting a frequency threshold is counting the number of days on which binges occur or counting the number of episodes of binge eating.

E.   The binge eating is not associated with the regular use of inappropriate compensatory behaviors (e.g., purging, fasting, excessive exercise) and does not occur exclusively during the course of anorexia nervosa or bulimia nervosa.

Source.   Reprinted from American Psychiatric Association: *Diagnostic and Statistical Manual of Mental Disorders,* 4th Edition, Text Revision. Washington, DC, American Psychiatric Association, 2000. Used with permission.

have an increase in health problems and were significantly more likely to demonstrate dissatisfaction with their health (Bulik et al. 2003b).

Psychological presentation.   Like individuals with anorexia nervosa and bulimia nervosa, those with BED are preoccupied with weight and shape concerns and overvalue the importance of weight and shape in self-worth. Patients with BED often present with self-loathing, disgust with body weight and shape, frustration at their inability to control eating, dysphoric affect, somatic concerns, and interpersonal sensitivity (American Psychiatric Association 2000).

Both psychosocial and physical quality of life are compromised in individuals with BED; however, the extent to which quality of life is impaired because of the BED above and beyond the overweight associated with BED is unclear. For some patients, binge eating may be triggered by dysphoric mood and may be tension-relieving; others describe an experience of dissociation and "numbing out" while binge eating. Axis I comorbidity commonly includes depressive disorders and anxiety disorders. Personality patterns have not been carefully delineated, but there is some suggestion that patients with BED exhibit impulsive traits and elevated Cluster B and Cluster C Axis II disorders (e.g., Marcus et al. 1996).

Although the presentation in eating disturbance is similar for men and women, men may be more likely to have Axis I disorders (and in particular a lifetime history of substance dependence) when compared with women, and women may be more likely than men to binge eat in response to emotional triggers (Tanofsky et al. 1997).

Differential Diagnosis

In making a differential diagnosis of BED, clinicians should consider other medical and psychiatric disorders. Neurological disorders that impact appetite regulation and eating behaviors, and syndromes associated with hyperphagia such as Kleine-Levin or Prader-Willi, need to be ruled out, as do psychiatric disorders such as bulimia nervosa and major depressive disorder. In BED—in contrast to bulimia nervosa—the binge eating occurs in the *absence* of recurrent compensatory behaviors (e.g., purging, excessive exercise, fasting). Although patients with BED may occasionally make use of compensatory behaviors, these behaviors do not occur "regularly," which is typically defined as an average of twice weekly. Additionally, episodes of overeating are commonly associated with major depressive disorder; however, such episodes are not typically characterized by a sense of loss of control over eating.

Epidemiology

Epidemiological research on BED began only a decade ago and is still considered preliminary (for review, see Striegel-Moore and Franko 2003). One limitation of this initial research is that the majority of community-based prevalence studies of BED have used samples of convenience, rather than representative samples; another drawback is that assessment of BED has largely been by self-report questionnaire rather than interview.

In spite of these limitations, the research indicates that BED is significantly more prevalent than either anorexia or bulimia nervosa. Prevalence rates based on community samples are estimated to be between 0.7% and 4%. Data from the recent large National Comorbidity Survey Replication study suggest that the lifetime community prevalence of BED is 3.5% in women and 2.0% in men (Hudson et al. 2007). Within specific populations, particularly among those seeking weight-loss treatment, prevalence rates are considerably higher, estimated at between 20% and 30% (e.g., Spitzer et al. 1992, 1993).

With regard to demographic features, unlike anorexia and bulimia nervosa, BED appears to affect a more diverse population. The ratio of females to males with BED has been estimated to be 3:2 (Spitzer et al. 1992, 1993). There does not seem to be a significant difference in prevalence of BED by ethnicity. Research yields conflicting reports on the prevalence of BED across the life span, with some studies indicating comparable prevalence rates in young adult and older adult populations and others suggesting that the prevalence decreases after the age of 25. Additional demographic variables, including socioeconomic status, and cross-cultural research have not yet been examined.

Notably, a small minority of individuals with BED will have a history of anorexia nervosa or bulimia nervosa.

Etiology

Research on the etiology of BED is limited. Preliminary study suggests that overweight and obesity are risk factors for the development of binge eating and BED. One population-based longitudinal twin study demonstrated unique and shared genetic risk factors for developing obesity and binge eating; the investigators found substantial heritability for obesity and a moderate heritability for binge eating, with a modest genetic correlation between the traits (Bulik et al. 2003a). These study findings argue against the notion that obesity causes binge eating or vice versa.

Psychosocial variables, including a history of teasing or bullying, physical or sexual abuse, and discrimination, are increased in individuals who develop BED. Additionally, a childhood history of overweight, family overeating/binge eating, family discord, and high parental demands may be risk factors (Striegel-Moore et al. 2005).

Dieting does not appear to play an etiological role in the development of BED. The majority of individuals with BED report the onset of binge eating

Prevalence and demographics of binge-eating disorder

Limited existing research given provisional diagnostic status.

0.7%–4% prevalence based on community samples.

20%–30% prevalence among individuals seeking weight-loss treatment.

3:2 ratio of females to males.

Prevalent across ethnicity.

prior to the onset of dieting, and only a minority report dieting first—an order of onset that contrasts with the pathway from dieting to binge eating in bulimia nervosa.

BED appears to be more prevalent among certain clinical populations, including individuals with type 2 diabetes.

Course and Outcome

Recovery and relapse.   Research on the longitudinal course and outcome of BED is currently limited but suggests that the diagnosis is unstable. The findings from one prospective study of women in the community with BED suggested that by 5-year follow-up, less than one-fifth of the sample still had clinically significant eating disorder symptoms (Fairburn et al. 2000). Notably, the rate of concomitant obesity in the sample increased by follow-up (from 21% to 39%); thus, concomitant obesity may be an important health outcome to assess in addition to the BED. Further, a 6-month prospective study of BED in the community demonstrated that by 6 months of follow-up, approximately half of those remaining in the study still met the criteria for BED; however, one-third of the initial sample dropped out, and external validity was therefore limited (Cachelin et al. 1999). Taken together, these findings suggest that BED may not be a stable diagnosis.

Research on individuals with BED who have received treatment has also demonstrated that good outcomes are achieved in the majority of cases and that relapse is less likely than in anorexia and bulimia nervosa.

Diagnostic migration.   Diagnostic migration from BED to bulimia nervosa or anorexia nervosa appears, on the basis of the limited existing prospective research in this area, to be rare (Cachelin et al. 1999; Fairburn et al. 1999, 2000).

Course and outcome of binge-eating disorder (BED)

Findings on course and outcome (based on limited research) are mixed. Some suggestion that BED may not be a stable diagnosis.

Conclusion

Eating disorders are life-threatening conditions that have come to the forefront of public attention in the last several decades. Successful collaboration of clinical researchers from all disciplines is necessary to further the understanding of the diagnosis, pathogenesis, and treatment of these disorders.

References

American Psychiatric Association: Diagnostic and Statistical Manual of Mental Disorders, 4th Edition. Washington, DC, American Psychiatric Association, 1994

American Psychiatric Association: Diagnostic and Statistical Manual of Mental Disorders, 4th Edition, Text Revision. Washington, DC, American Psychiatric Association, 2000

Bailer UF, Kaye WH: A review of neuropeptide and neuroendocrine dysregulation in anorexia and bulimia nervosa. Curr Drug Targets CNS Neurol Disord 2:53–59, 2003

Bulik CM, Sullivan PF, Kendler KS: Genetic and environmental contributions to obesity and binge eating. Int J Eat Disord 33:293–298, 2003a

Bulik CM, Sullivan PF, Wade TD, et al: Twin studies of eating disorders: a review. Int J Eat Disord 27:1–20, 2003b

Bulik CM, Sullivan PF, Tozzi F, et al: Prevalence, heritability and prospective risk factors for anorexia nervosa. Arch Gen Psychiatry 63:305–312, 2006

Cachelin FM, Striegel-Moore RH, Elder KA, et al: Natural course of a community sample of women with binge eating disorder. Int J Eat Disord 25:45–54, 1999

Crago M, Shisslak CM, Estes LS: Eating disturbances among American minority groups: a review. Int J Eat Disord 19:239–248, 1996

Eddy KT, Keel PK, Dorer DJ, et al: A longitudinal comparison of anorexia nervosa subtypes. Int J Eat Disord 31:191–201, 2002

Fairburn CG, Bohn K: Eating disorder NOS (EDNOS): an example of the troublesome "not otherwise specified" (NOS) category in DSM-IV. Behav Res Ther 43:691–701, 2005

Fairburn CG, Welch SL, Doll HA, et al: Risk factors for bulimia nervosa: a community-based case-control study. Arch Gen Psychiatry 54:509–517, 1997

Fairburn CG, Cooper Z, Doll HA, et al: Risk factors for anorexia nervosa: three integrated case-control comparisons. Arch Gen Psychiatry 56:468–476, 1999

Fairburn CG, Cooper Z, Doll HA, et al: The natural course of bulimia nervosa and binge eating disorder in young women. Arch Gen Psychiatry 57:659–665, 2000

Frank GK, Bailer UF, Henry S, et al: Neuroimaging studies in eating disorders. CNS Spectr 9:539–548, 2004

Franko DL, Blais MA, Becker AE, et al: Pregnancy complications and neonatal outcomes in women with eating disorders. Am J Psychiatry 158:1461–1466, 2001

Franko DL, Keel PK, Dorer DJ, et al: What predicts suicide attempts in women with eating disorders? Psychol Med 34:843–853, 2004

Golden NH, Katzman DK, Kreipe RE, et al: Eating disorders in adolescents. Position paper of the Society for Adolescent Medicine. J Adolesc Health 33:496–503, 2003

Grice DE, Halmi KA, Fichter MM, et al: Evidence for a susceptibility gene for anorexia nervosa on chromosome 1. Am J Hum Genet 70:787–792, 2002

Grinspoon S, Thomas E, Pitts S, et al: Prevalence and predictive factors for regional osteopenia in women with anorexia nervosa. Ann Intern Med 133:790–794, 2000

Herzog DB, Keller MB, Lavori PW: Outcome in anorexia nervosa and bulimia nervosa: a review of the literature. J Nerv Ment Dis 176:131–143, 1988

Herzog DB, Dorer DJ, Keel PK, et al: Recovery and relapse in anorexia and bulimia nervosa: a 7.5 year follow-up study. J Am Acad Child Adolesc Psychiatry 38:829–837, 1999

Hoek HW: Distribution of eating disorders, in Eating Disorders and Obesity: A Comprehensive Handbook. Edited by Fairburn CG, Brownell KD. New York, Guilford, 2002, pp 233–237

Hsu LK, Lee S: Is weight phobia always necessary for a diagnosis of anorexia nervosa? Am J Psychiatry 150:1466–1471, 1993

Hudson JI, Hiripi E, Pope HG Jr, et al: The prevalence and correlates of eating disorders in the National Comorbidity Survey Replication. Biol Psychiatry 61:348–358, 2007

Keel PK, Klump KL: Are eating disorders culture-bound syndromes? Implications for conceptualizing their etiology. Psychol Bull 129:747–769, 2003

Keel PK, Mitchell JE: Outcome in bulimia nervosa. Am J Psychiatry 154:313–321, 1997

Keel PK, Dorer DJ, Eddy KT, et al: Predictors of mortality in eating disorders. Arch Gen Psychiatry 60:179–183, 2003

Keel PK, Heatherton TF, Dorer DJ, et al: Point prevalence of bulimia nervosa in 1982, 1992, and 2002. Psychol Med 3:119–127, 2006

Lasater LM, Mehler PS: Medical complications of bulimia nervosa. Eat Behav 2:279–292, 2001

Marcus MD, Wing RR, Ewing L, et al: Psychiatric disorders among obese binge eaters. Int J Eat Disord 9:69–77, 1996

Minuchin S, Rosman BL, Baker L: Psychosomatic Families: Anorexia Nervosa in Context. Cambridge, MA, Harvard University Press, 1978

Misra Miller KK, Almazan C, et al: Hormonal and body composition predictors of soluble leptin receptor, leptin, and free leptin index in adolescent girls with anorexia nervosa and controls and relation to insulin sensitivity. J Clin Endocrinol Metab 89:3486–3495, 2004

Nielsen S, Moller-Madsen S, Isager T, et al: Standardized mortality in eating disorders— a quantitative summary of previously published and new evidence. J Psychosom Res 44:413–434, 1998

Polivy J, Herman CP: Etiology of binge eating: psychological mechanisms, in Binge Eating. Edited by Fairburn CG, Wilson GT. New York, Guilford, 1993, pp 173–205

Russell G: Bulimia nervosa: an ominous variant of anorexia nervosa. Psychol Med 9:429–448, 1979

Spitzer RL, Devlin MJ, Walsh BT, et al: Binge eating disorder: a multisite field trial of the diagnostic criteria. Int J Eat Disord 11:191–203, 1992

Spitzer RL, Yanovski SZ, Wadden T, et al: Binge eating disorder: its further validation in a multisite study. Int J Eat Disord 13:137–153, 1993

Steinhausen HC: The outcome of anorexia nervosa in the 20th century. Am J Psychiatry 159:1284–1293, 2002

Stice E: Risk and maintenance factors for eating pathology: a meta-analytic review. Psychol Bull 128:825–848, 2002

Striegel-Moore RH, Franko DL: Epidemiology of binge eating disorder. Int J Eat Disord 34(suppl):S19–S29, 2003

Striegel-Moore RH, Dohm FA, Kraemer HC, et al: Eating disorders in white and black women. Am J Psychiatry 160:1326–1331, 2003

Striegel-Moore RH, Fairburn CG, Wilfley DE, et al: Toward an understanding of risk factors for binge-eating disorder in black and white women: a community-based case-control study. Psychol Med 35:907–917, 2005

Strober M: Managing the chronic, treatment-resistant patient with anorexia nervosa. Int J Eat Disord 36:245–255, 2004

Strober M, Bulik CM: Genetic epidemiology of eating disorders, in Eating Disorders and Obesity: A Comprehensive Handbook. Edited by Fairburn CG, Brownell KD. New York, Guilford, 2002, pp 238–242

Strober M, Freeman R, Morrell W: The long-term course of severe anorexia nervosa in adolescents: survival analysis of recovery, relapse, and outcome predictors over 10–15 years in a prospective study. Int J Eat Disord 22:339–360, 1997

Strober M, Freeman R, Lampert C, et al: Controlled family study of anorexia nervosa and bulimia nervosa: evidence of shared liability and transmission of partial phenotypes. Am J Psychiatry 157:393–401, 2000

Sullivan PF: Mortality in anorexia nervosa. Am J Psychiatry 152:1073–1074, 1995

Tanofsky MB, Wilfley DE, Spurrell EB, et al: Comparison of men and women with binge eating disorder. Int J Eat Disord 21:49–54, 1997

Tozzi F, Thornton LM, Klump KL, et al: Symptom fluctuation in eating disorders: correlates of diagnostic crossover. Am J Psychiatry 162:732–740, 2005

Westen D, Harnden-Fischer J: Personality profiles in eating disorders: rethinking the distinction between Axis I and Axis II. Am J Psychiatry 158:547–562, 2001

Wilfley DE, Schwartz MB, Spurrell EB, et al: Using the Eating Disorder Examination to identify the specific psychopathology of binge eating disorder. Int J Eat Disord 27:259–269, 2000

Wolfe BE: Reproductive health in women with eating disorders. J Obstet Gynecol Neonatal Nurs 34:255–263, 2005

2

Assessment and Determination of Initial Treatment Approaches for Patients With Eating Disorders

Joel Yager, M.D.

This chapter reviews the initial assessment and decision-making processes regarding treatment planning for patients with eating disorders. The diagnostic criteria for the eating disorders described in Chapter 1 ("Diagnosis, Epidemiology, and Clinical Course of Eating Disorders") of this volume should by now be familiar to the clinician. However, comprehensive assessment of the patient goes far beyond simply establishing the presence of diagnostic criteria according to the latest edition of the *Diagnostic and Statistical Manual of Mental Disorders* (DSM). Furthermore, many patients who fail to meet the strictly stated DSM criteria for anorexia nervosa or bulimia nervosa, and whose conditions fall into the large category of eating disorder not otherwise specified (EDNOS), still suffer from considerable degrees of impairment and often have an outcome not very different from those of patients carrying these strictly defined entities (Garfinkel et al. 1996; Woodside et al. 2001).

Assessing the Patient

At the outset, it should be clear that for younger patients who are still living at home and for many others who are still heavily involved with their families, comprehensive assessment requires the participation of family members and sometimes other collateral informants (Lock 2002). Second, the comprehensive assessment of patients is most frequently a team effort, involving, along with a psychiatrist, a pediatrician, adolescent physician, family physician, internist, or other primary care health professional; often a registered dietician; and sometimes other health care professionals trained in psychology, social work, and/or nursing, depending on circumstances, professional availability, and individual skill sets. Third, comprehensive assessment of patients with eating disorders often requires more than a single hour, certainly if the patient is a child or adolescent and the family is to be seen as well. Often, the clinical picture is complex, with multiple medical and psychiatric comorbid conditions, ambivalent motivational states, and involved family and social situations. Eliciting the history and all associated phenomena typically requires not only several visits but also a certain amount of time and trust before all important features emerge and can be verified and placed in context.

When a patient with an eating disorder is referred by other health professionals, the psychiatrist should obtain as much information about the patient and her circumstances as possible in advance of the initial consultation.

When psychiatrists are the first health care professionals to see the patient, they should appraise how much of the comprehensive assessment and workup they are personally qualified and prepared to undertake, and make certain to refer the patient and her family to others who will fill in the gaps.

Increasingly, where possible, and when appointments are scheduled sufficiently far in advance, busy practitioners are asking patients and their families to complete assessment instruments in advance and to bring the completed questionnaires along with them to the initial visit. Many clinicians have found, among the available symptom checklists and life history questionnaires, the Eating Disorders Questionnaire (currently EDQ 9.0 of James Mitchell, M.D., and colleagues) to be very useful for these purposes. (The EDQ 9.0 is presented as an appendix to this chapter.) Patients who complete this instrument usually have the positive sense that regardless of other aspects of psychiatric history and symptomatology to be covered, the clinician is quickly focusing in on highly specific and relevant eating disorder issues of the kind that unprepared mental health clinicians may never get around to assessing in depth.

Psychiatrists and their associates should carefully assess the patient's recent history—the "history of the present episode"—along the four primary dimensions that will need to be addressed in treatment planning: physical and nutritional status; eating behaviors and eating disorder–related behaviors; core beliefs and attitudes associated with the eating disorder; and comorbid psychiatric symptomatology. As with all good history taking, the specific signs and symptoms should be framed in terms of time (initial onset and course) and examined for the following:

- Intensity and duration of the signs and symptoms, with quantitative appraisals whenever possible
- Sequencing, clustering, or cascading of the signs and symptoms
- Correlation of the initial appearance and course with the appearance of external precipitants, stressors, or inciting events
- Points and manner in which these symptoms produced subjective impairment or impairment in the minds of significant others
- Efforts at compensation and self-correction, if any
- Outcomes
- Specific circumstances prompting the clinical visit at which the patient is first encountered

For patients with eating disorders, these initial questions often begin with discussions of earlier developmental issues: temperament; childhood signs and symptoms of anxiety or mood dysregulation; perfectionism; obsessive and/or compulsive traits; unusual attitudes, overvalued ideas, and behavioral patterns regarding food and exercise; and preoccupations with appearance. Specific aspects of perfectionism that have been associated with vulnerability to eating disorders include exhibiting unusual degrees of orderliness and neatness and being rule-bound (Anderluh et al. 2003). Initially observed events, sometimes grasped by patients and their families only in retrospect, may include such seemingly innocuous shifts as becoming vegetarian or otherwise becoming more restrictive in eating patterns than family and peers; spending increasing amounts of time preening and mirror-gazing; and developing what might sometimes be an encouraged intense desire to diet and lose weight. A variety of normative and non-normative, developmentally expected or undesirable and unexpected life events, physiological stresses, and peer pressures have been associated with the onset of eating disorders, with very little specificity demonstrated. On balance, however, the higher the number and intensity of stressors, the higher the likelihood of some form of individual breakdown. Depending on individual temperamental vulnerabilities, the timing, intensity, and chronicity of various life factors such as intra- and extrafamilial pressures, conflicts, shaming, neglect, abuse, teasing, losses, disappointments, peer pressures, and so forth will inflict variable degrees of distress, adaptive and/or maladaptive coping responses, and, ultimately, cognitive-emotional and behavioral expressions of maladaptive coping and psychopathology.

Addressing the patient's safety must be the first order of consideration, and particular attention needs to be given to suicidal ideation, plans, intentions, and attempts, as well as impulsive and compulsive self-harm behaviors. Assessment for suicidality is of particular importance in patients with comorbid alcohol and/or substance use disorders. Furthermore, even among patients who are not frankly or overtly suicidal, the eating disorder patient's sense of being attached to life may be less than that of patients without eating disorders (Bachar et al. 2002).

Physical Status

It is important to determine the point at which the patient as a youth started to deviate from a previous growth curve—when, why, and under what circumstances did the patient fail to continue to gain appropriate weight? The use of a growth chart of standardized values for pediatric populations may permit identification of patients who have failed to gain weight and who have growth retardation (Golden 2003a); such charts are readily available at a Centers for Disease Control and Prevention (CDC) Web site (http://www. cdc.gov/growth-charts/).

Along with obtaining a careful history, a treatment team member must measure weight and height and, during the course of treatment, must continue to measure weight in a consistent manner, under similar conditions—for example, at the same time of day, postvoiding, and with the patient in similar garb. In addition to determination of the patient's weight and height, calculation of body mass index (BMI) has gained increasing attention in both research and clinical settings. BMI is calculated using the formula weight (in kg)/height (in meters)^2 and is particularly useful for adults. Adults with a BMI < 18.5 are considered to be underweight. In children and adolescents, age-adjusted BMI is used (see http://www.cdc.gov/nccdphp/dnpa/growthcharts/bmi_tools.htm). Children and adolescents with a BMI below the fifth percentile for age are considered to be underweight. It is important to remember that BMI is a calculation based only on height and weight and does not provide any further measure of body composition. Except at extremes, it is often not useful in estimating an individual's nutritional status. Abnormal muscularity, body frame status, constipation, fluid loading, and other factors influence the relevance of BMI (Chanoine et al. 2002; Lear et al. 2003). Furthermore, considerable debate in the scientific community exists about appropriate BMI ranges for various ethnic groups. Among Caucasian women, for example, the range of healthy BMIs may be higher than for some groups of Asian women (see Yates et al. 2004).

For patients who are extremely resistant to knowing their weight, being weighed without being told the weight may be acceptable initially, but as quickly as possible patients need to know what they actually weigh, for purposes of reality checks and so that education about their own healthy weights may be incorporated into early discussions. The initial assessment of weight is a good time to inquire about the highest weight the patient has ever attained, the lowest weight (at the current height), the weight trajectory over the past few years, the patient's desired weight (both from an "emotional" perspective and from the perspective of "logic and health"), and the weight the patient would settle for to achieve good health.

The clinician must inquire about the onset and pattern of menses. If menses ceased, when did that occur, and what were the patient's weight and eating pattern at the time of the cessation of menses? Is the patient taking birth control pills or other agents that might distort an appraisal of normal menstruation?

Eliciting associated physical signs and symptoms requires appreciation of the myriad forms they may take, with particular attention to systemic features of poor health such as weakness, fatigue, increasing cold intolerance, and other nonspecific complaints. For all of these features, family members are often keener observers than patients themselves about a declining course from previous states of well-being. Most commonly, few symptoms are reported in office practice, and there may be few obvious physical signs as well. However, occult abnormalities (e.g., for bone, heart, and brain) may be significant despite lack of symptoms, signs, and abnormalities in routine laboratory test results.

Table 2–1 lists appropriate initial laboratory assessments that the primary care physician or psychiatrist should obtain and monitor. Attention to the simplest and most basic features is often the most important clinical action: vital signs, heart rate and rhythm, orthostatic pulse and blood pressure changes, general physical appearance (including evidence of malnutrition and dehydration), skin appearance and turgor, obvious signs of poor dentition, and physical signs of self-harming behaviors. These features are easily observed and assessed and are most telling. Clinicians must be vigilant regarding shifts in weight, blood pressure, pulse, other cardiovascular parameters, and behaviors likely to provoke physiological decline and collapse. They should be quick to act in these situations to avert medically dangerous situations and to prevent chronicity. Referral for a dental examination should also be given when indicated by history.

Findings of objective abnormalities on standard laboratory tests are important not only for medical appraisal and treatment planning but often as motivators for ambivalent patients as well. In particular, findings of borderline cardiac abnormalities found on the electrocardiogram or echocardiogram (Ramacciotti et al. 2003) and deficiencies in bone density pointing to osteopenia or osteoporosis assessed via bone dual-energy X-ray absorptiometry (DEXA) scans (Golden 2003b) may serve several clinical functions.

Eating Disorder Behaviors

Assessment of eating disorder behaviors should include evaluation of the following:

- Restrictive, avoidant, and changed eating patterns (quality and quantity)
- Exercise patterns
- Compensatory behaviors such as binge eating
- Purging by self-induced vomiting, laxatives, enemas, or diuretics
- Patterns of spitting and chewing food without swallowing
- Use of prescribed, over-the counter, complementary–alternative medicine
- Use of illicit diet pills or illicit drugs

Other behaviors, particularly of a compulsive or impulsive nature, that seem to have increased over the course of the eating disorder should be identified. Having a meal together with the patient or observing a meal (sometimes with her family as well) may provide useful information, permitting the clinician to observe difficulties the patient may have in eating particular foods, anxieties that erupt in the course of a meal, and rituals concerning food (e.g., cutting, separating, or mashing) that she may feel compelled to perform.

With regard to eating patterns, a highly specific description and recording of what the patient has eaten that day, on several prior days, and over the past few weeks is essential and may be illuminating. Obtaining a detailed report of a single day or using a calendar as a prompt may help elicit specific information, particularly regarding perceived intake. For example, if a patient with highly restrictive patterns of eating decided to become a "strict vegan" or to stop eating protein in the past few weeks, rapid nutritional deficiencies, including deterioration of muscles and brain, may emerge. The development of highly restrictive and avoidant patterns of eating is usually accompanied by marked changes in social behaviors. Avoiding family meals or no longer eating with friends is often cause of others' concerns, as they notice increasing social isolation.

Increasing exercise to unhealthy degrees may start insidiously and may progress to hours per day of compulsive exercise. In some studies, exercise compulsion seems to be the first symptom to appear and is often the last to remit as patients recover (Kron et al. 1978). The compulsion to exercise may be associated with unrelenting pacing and fidgeting, and even an inability to sit down. Dog owners may sometimes walk their dogs to the point that the dogs show inanition.

Binge eating is relatively easy for most patients to quantitate in terms of frequency, intensity, duration, triggers, settings, and consequences. If binge eating has occurred, at what point did it start? Did the patient previously become chubby or obese? Did the eating binges seem to occur de novo without evident overweight, in settings of frustration, or premenstrually, or in association with starting a birth control pill or psychiatric medication?

Like binge eating, purging behaviors are usually relatively easy to characterize and quantitate. If purging occurs, what have been the circumstances? In some patients with anorexia nervosa, purging occurs in the absence of binge eating, as a ritual of purification or of emptying the gastrointestinal tract of

Table 2-1.   Suggested laboratory assessments for patients with eating disorders

Assessment	Patient indication
Basic analyses	For all patients with eating disorders
Blood chemistry studies	
Serum electrolytes	
Blood urea nitrogen (BUN)	
Serum creatinine (interpretations must incorporate assessments of weight)	
Thyroid-stimulating hormone (TSH); if indicated free T_4, T_3	
Complete blood cell count (CBC), including differential and erythrocyte sedimentation rate	
Aspartate aminotransferase (AST), alanine aminotranferease (ALT), alkaline phosphatase	
Urinalysis	
Additional analyses	
Complement component C3[a]	For malnourished and severely symptomatic patients. Serum magnesium should be obtained prior to beginning certain medications if QTc is prolonged. *Note:* During hospital refeeding, serum potassium, magnesium, and phosphorus should be followed daily for 5 days and thereafter at least three times a week for 3 weeks.
Blood chemistry studies	
Serum calcium	
Serum magnesium	
Serum phosphorus	
Serum ferritin	
Electrocardiogram	
24-hour urine for creatinine clearance[b]	
Osteopenia and osteoporosis assessments	For patients with amenorrhea of more than 6 months' duration
Dual-energy X-ray absorptiometry (DEXA)	
Serum estradiol in females	
Serum testosterone in males	

Table 2–1.   Suggested laboratory assessments for patients with eating disorders *(continued)*

Assessment	Patient indication
Nonroutine assessments	
Drug screen	For patients with suspected substance abuse, particularly patients with anorexia nervosa, binge/purge subtype, or bulimia nervosa
Serum amylase (fractionated for salivary gland isoenzyme if available, to rule out pancreatic involvement)	
Serum luteinizing hormone (LH), follicle-stimulating hormone (FSH); beta-human chorionic gonadotropin (bHCG) and prolactin	For patients with persistent amenorrhea at normal weight
Brain magnetic resonance imaging (MRI) and computed tomography (CT)	For patients with significant cognitive deficits, other neurological soft signs, unremitting course, or other atypical features
Stool for guaiac	For patients with suspected gastrointestinal bleeding
Stool or urine for bisacodyl, emodin, aloe-emodin, rhein	For patients with suspected laxative abuse

Note. T_3 = triiodothyronine; T_4 = thyroxine.
[a]Some experts recommend the routine use of complement component C3 as a sensitive marker that may indicate nutritional deficiencies even when other laboratory test results are apparently normal (Nova et al. 2004; Wyatt et al. 1982).
[b]Boag et al. 1985. *Note:* Creatinine clearance should be calculated using equations that involve body surface based on assessments of height and weight.
Source.   Adapted with permission from "Practice Guideline for the Treatment of Patients With Eating Disorders, Third Edition." American Psychiatric Association. *American Journal of Psychiatry* 163 (7, suppl):4–54, 2006. Copyright 2006, American Psychiatric Association.

any contents, or after the smallest amounts of nonpermitted foods have been ingested. Does the purging require the patient to vigorously self-induce vomiting by forced gagging, or is she capable of "automatic purging" via a relatively easily induced eructation? Does the patient consume large quantities of fluid and induce repeated multiple episodes of vomiting each time to ensure complete emptying?

Asking patients about other forms of compensatory behaviors to control weight and mood, in addition to those mentioned above and the use of various substances, may uncover other behavioral adaptations, such as chewing and spitting large quantities of food, by means of which the patient may experience the taste of food while reducing the caloric intake.

Assessment of eating disorder behaviors is best conducted together with an appraisal of initiating triggers (e.g., environmental and social circumstances most likely to elicit negative self-feelings or eating binges) and the consequences or aftermath of these behaviors.

Core Beliefs and Attitudes Associated With Eating Disorders

The cognitive underpinnings of eating disorders, anchored in tightly bound cognitive emotion structures, are central to our current understanding of eating disorders and their treatment. From the cognitive perspective, these ideas need to be characterized by when and how they initially appeared and in terms of the internal, family, peer, and media sources, pervasiveness, emotional strength, and the degree of unswerving allegiance with which they are held. To what extent can the individual step back and examine them objectively and consider that they may be false or untrustworthy? How much power to do they hold over the individual? It is also helpful to assess the ongoing reinforcing factors that sustain or challenge these beliefs. Cognitive disturbances form the basis for several psychotherapeutic approaches, including cognitive-behavioral therapy, motivational interviewing, and psychodynamic therapy. In assessing cognitions, clinicians should assess not only the cognitions themselves but also the meta-cognitions (the patient's beliefs about her beliefs), such as why they came about, where they came from, how believable they are, and the extent to which they fit and dovetail with broader, deeper primary beliefs in personal and social values, spirituality and religion, and existential attitudes. A sizable percentage of eating disorder patients recall specific, often minor and otherwise innocuous events that served as "tipping points" to trigger an avalanche of eating disorder–related thoughts and behaviors. These events were often well-intentioned remarks made by family members, teachers, or friends regarding appearance, to which the patient reacted with feelings of shame, humiliation, and determined resolve to diet. Examples of seemingly innocuous statements include "You don't really want that ice cream—you'll wind up fat like me and your mother"; "You'd really look better in that tank top if you took a little off that midriff"; and "I think you'd be a better swimmer if you lost a few pounds."

Core beliefs in eating disorders focus on shape, weight, and the self. Appraisal of the self is equated with how one perceives one's success or failure in the contest with impossible-to-achieve, perfectionistic goals related to shape and weight. These goals are often based on overvalued ideals regarding purity, perfection, or attractiveness, and on incorrect assumptions about physiology and health (e.g., "You can never be too thin"; "Any fat at all is bad"; "Having anything in your stomach or intestine is bad"). Failure to meet self-imposed perfectionistic standards often results in self-derogatory assessments (e.g., "I'm too fat"; "I'm ugly"; "If I'm too heavy I'm worthless, unattractive, a failure"; "If I eat a bite I'll gain a pound"; "Anything I eat immediately turns into fat that everyone else can see"; "If I'm able to pinch any skin, anywhere on my body, that's evidence of excessive fat").

Although the content of these beliefs can be understood in terms of culture, family attitudes, and peer pressure, their structural features are better understood as forms of strongly held, core beliefs, and inflexible thought processes, which range from overvalued ideas and religious zeal to frank delusions. The capacity for these unswerving, maladaptive patterns of thought may have temperamental roots and may be reinforced by individual biological circumstances, some of which may be exacerbated by the physiological effects of undernutrition, semistarvation, and excessive exercise, in a vicious positive-feedback cycle.

To some patients, these overvalued ideas and the resulting compulsive behaviors regarding eating and exercise have an alien, ego-dystonic quality—they feel imposed from the outside, as if a possessing external force is taking over the mind and body. These patients retain the capacity to reflect on what is occurring to them and may retain sufficient objectivity to realize they must fight against these destructive tendencies. They may be able to acknowledge that there is something wrong with their assessment and beliefs about their own weight and shape.

In contrast, some patients feel from the outset—or may bring themselves to feel via self-deception and the various attempts at internal alignment of attitude and behavior driven by cognitive dissonance—that they themselves strongly hold to these values and desire to behave as they do. These patients have distorted self-images with respect to their weight and shape, but they fully believe that their perceptions and appraisals are accurate. They strongly identify with their beliefs and behaviors—and, indeed, draw their core sense of self and identity from these beliefs and behaviors, even if these perverse manners of eating, exercise, and purging will inevitably impair or even kill them. Such individuals may entirely lack reflective capacity and may fight attempts to get them to change their thoughts about themselves or their behaviors.

These differences have important clinical implications. Those individuals who strongly identify with their disorders, whose "selves" are rooted in these attitudes and behaviors, who fight off suggestions that they have problems or that they ought to change, constitute the so-called typical patients. Their beliefs assume an almost delusional quality. From the motivational analysis perspective, they appear in most cases to be in the "precontemplative" stage or in "denial." Such individuals are much less likely to seek treatment on their own or engage in treatment easily, and are more likely to require external reinforcement and structured interventions, sometimes to save their lives.

Those individuals who can appreciate the fact that they have a problem— that their attitudes and behaviors may be problematic and indicative of psychopathology—are the so-called atypical patients (Strober et al. 1999). From a motivational analysis perspective, they are often in the "contemplative" stage and are more ready to undertake personal actions to combat their eating disorders. They may be more likely to seek and stay with treatment and to have the capacity to perceive and reflect on their unreasonable and distorted cognitions and compulsive urges with greater objectivity. The prognosis tends to be somewhat better for these patients than for "typical" patients.

Co-occurring Psychiatric and Medical Conditions

The most common co-occurring psychiatric and medical conditions are detailed elsewhere in Chapter 3 ("Eating Disorders and Psychiatric Comorbidity: Prevalence and Treatment Modifications") and Chapter 13 ("Eating Disorders in Special Populations: Medical Comorbidities and Complicating or Unusual Conditions") in this volume and thus will not be covered in depth here. Suffice it to say that the presence of comorbid psychiatric conditions on both Axis I and Axis II is the rule rather than the exception for patients with eating disorders and that initial treatment decisions often derive from the presence, nature, intensity and severity of these comorbidities in addition to the eating disorders themselves. The most prominent Axis I conditions are mood disorders (most notably major depressive disorders, dysthymic disorders, and bipolar I and II disorders), generalized anxiety disorder, panic disorder, obsessive-compulsive disorder, posttraumatic stress disorder, and alcohol- and drug-related disorders. Axis II disorders most prominently include Cluster C (avoidant and obsessive-compulsive) and Cluster B (narcissistic, histrionic, and borderline) personality disorders (Halmi et al. 1991). Most prominent medical conditions are seen only in the wake of severe and chronic semistarvation and malnutrition (Herzog et al. 1997; Mehler and Krantz 2003). Assessment should include inquiries about the signs and symptoms of co-occurring conditions (e.g., when they began, their temporal association with the onset and course of the eating disorders) and treatment histories for the conditions, including medications, that may have helped or exacerbated the course of the eating disorder.

Assessing the Family

Family assessment is needed across several dimensions: the family history of eating and other psychiatric disorders (e.g., for information on genetic vulnerability and familial transmission that may be used to inform treatment); a developmental and dynamic family history to reveal parenting patterns and the family environment; and an assessment of current family resources, intentions, interaction styles, loyalties, and commitments that may allow the clinician to gauge whether the family can be recruited in the service of treatment or whether treatment or return to the family setting will be more difficult.

The clinician should first assess families for evidence of eating disorders and other psychiatric disorders, alcoholism, substance use disorders, and obesity in first-degree relatives and extended family, including important nonbiological relatives who might have served as role models.

Family dynamic history assessment includes appraisal of parenting patterns, including evidence of neglect; psychological-emotional, physical, or sexual abuse; family communication styles; structural family patterns; intergenerational influences; helpful and deleterious factors stemming from extended family influences beyond the boundaries of the nuclear family; and family attitudes toward eating, exercise, and appearance. In this assessment, it is essential not to articulate theories that imply blame or permit family members to blame one another or themselves. No evidence exists to prove that families *cause* eating disorders. Furthermore, blaming families harms their psychological well-being and often impairs their desire, willingness, and capacity to be helpful to patients and to participate actively and constructively in treatment and recovery.

Finally, it is important to identify family stressors whose amelioration may facilitate recovery (Lock 2002) and particular interactions with the patient around eating disorder issues. It is helpful to assess the extent to which the family's attitude toward the patient is loyal, devoted, and encouraging; blaming, resentful, and critical; or frankly indicative of burnout. This information will help the clinician determine the extent to which the initial and longer-term treatment plan may count on the family's involvement and participation in actually helping the patient to deal with eating and other behaviors and providing a safe haven for recovery and additional practical and emotional support (Yager 1982).

In assessing young patients, it is useful to involve not only parents but also, whenever appropriate, school personnel, athletic coaches, and others who routinely work with the child or adolescent.

Choosing Initial Treatment Approaches and the Initial Site of Treatment

Initial Approach to Psychiatric Management

Initial psychiatric management includes a broad range of actions that the psychiatrist performs or ensures for all patients with eating disorders in combination with other specific treatment modalities. Such management begins with the establishment of a therapeutic alliance, which is enhanced by empathic comments and behaviors, positive regard, reassurance, and support (McIntosh et al. 2005). It is helpful to provide educational materials, including self-help workbooks, information on community and Internet resources (Myers et al. 2004), and direct advice to the patient and to families when they are involved. Selected resources for patients and families are presented in Table 2–2.

Table 2–2.   Self-help books and Internet resources on eating disorders

Cognitive-behavioral therapy–oriented workbooks

Agras WS, Apple RF: *Overcoming Eating Disorders: A Cognitive-Behavioral Treatment for Bulimia Nervosa.* New York, Oxford University Press, 1997 (both client and therapist workbooks available)

Cash TF: *The Body Image Workbook: An 8-Step Program for Learning to Like Your Looks.* Oakland, CA, New Harbinger Publications, 1997

Fairburn C: *Overcoming Binge Eating.* New York, Guilford, 1995

Goodman LJ, Villapiano M: *Eating Disorders: The Journey to Recovery Workbook.* Oxford, UK, Brunner-Routledge, 2001 (client workbook)

Schmidt U, Treasure J: *Getting Better Bit(e) by Bit(e): A Survival Kit for Sufferers of Bulimia Nervosa and Binge Eating Disorder.* Hillsdale, NJ, Lawrence Erlbaum, 1993

Villapiano M, Goodman LJ: *Eating Disorders: Time for Change: Plans, Strategies, and Worksheets.* Oxford, UK, Brunner-Routledge, 2001 (therapist workbook)

Other books reported to be helpful by patients and families

Bulik CM, Taylor N: *Runaway Eating: The 8-Point Plan to Conquer Adult Food and Weight Obsessions.* Emmaus, PA, Rodale Books, 2005

Ellis A, Abrams M, Dengelegi L: *The Art and Science of Rational Eating.* Fort Lee, NJ, Barricade Books, 1992

Hall L: *Full Lives: Women Who Have Freed Themselves From Food and Weight Obsessions.* Carlsbad, CA, Gurze Books, 1993

Lock J, Le Grange D: *Help Your Teenager Beat an Eating Disorder.* New York, Guilford, 2005

Michel DM, Willard SG: *When Dieting Becomes Dangerous.* New Haven, CT, Yale University Press, 2003

Walsh BT, Cameron VL: *If Your Child Has an Eating Disorder: An Essential Resource for Parents.* New York, Guilford, 2005

Zerbe K: *The Body Betrayed: A Deeper Understanding of Women, Eating Disorders and Treatment.* Carlsbad, CA, Gurze Books, 1995

Books reported to be helpful for males

Andersen AE, Cohn L, Holbrook T: *Making Weight: Men's Conflicts With Food, Weight, Shape and Appearance.* Carlsbad, CA, Gurze Books, 2000

Table 2–2.   Self-help books and Internet resources on
eating disorders *(continued)*

Internet resources for health care professionals

Academy for Eating Disorders (http://www.aedweb.org)

Internet resources for patients, families, and professionals

National Eating Disorders Association (http://www.nationaleatingdisorders.org)

National Association of Anorexia Nervosa and Associated Disorders
(http://www.anad.org)

http://www.edreferral.com

http://www.Something-fishy.org (a well-monitored advocacy site)

Source.   Adapted with permission from "Practice Guideline for the Treatment of Patients With
Eating Disorders, Third Edition." American Psychiatric Association. *American Journal of Psychiatry* 163 (7, suppl):4–54, 2006. Copyright 2006, American Psychiatric Association.

Depending on variations in individual professional qualifications and training and comfort level, the availability of other health professionals with experience and qualifications in treating patients with eating disorders, and the structure of local eating disorder programs, the psychiatrist may assume a leadership role as part of an informal team or structured program or work collaboratively on a team led by other health professionals, including other physicians or psychologists. Professionals from several disciplines often collaborate in the patient's care. For example, registered dietitians with specialized training in eating disorders often provide nutritional counseling; therapists from a variety of professional fields may provide family, individual, or group psychotherapy, including cognitive-behavioral therapy; and other physician specialists and dentists should be consulted for management of acute and ongoing medical and dental complications.

Although a variety of different management models are used for adult patients with eating disorders, no data exist on their comparative effectiveness. Psychiatrists who choose to manage both general medical and psychiatric issues should have appropriate training and experience as well as appropriate levels of medical backup to treat the medical complications associated with eating disorders. Some eating disorder programs routinely arrange for interdisciplinary team management models of treatment (often referred to as *split management*), in which a psychiatrist handles administrative and general medical requirements, prescribes medications as necessary, and recommends specific interventions targeted at disturbed cognitions, eating patterns, and maladaptive weight-reducing behaviors. In these models, other clinicians provide individual and/or group psychotherapies (e.g., cognitive-behavioral psychotherapy, psychodynamic psychotherapy, family therapy). For this approach to work effectively, all health professionals must maintain frequent and open communication and mutual respect in order to minimize the possibility that patients play staff off one another (i.e., to "split" the staff) (Garcia de Amusquibar 2000; Joy et al. 2003).

For children and adolescents, the *team approach* is the recommended treatment (Golden et al. 2003). This interdisciplinary approach is based on management of general medical issues, such as nutrition, weight gain, exercise, and eating patterns, by general medical care professionals (e.g., specialists in internal medicine, pediatrics, adolescent medicine, and nutrition) and management of psychiatric issues by psychiatrists (Golden 2003b; Kreipe and Yussman 2003). In unusual circumstances, psychiatrists may be qualified to act as the primary provider of comprehensive medical care.

When a patient is managed by an interdisciplinary team in an outpatient setting, communication among the professionals is essential so that each one is clear on what is expected of him or her and what the others are doing. For example, in team management of outpatients with anorexia nervosa, one professional must be designated to consistently monitor weights so that this essential function is not inadvertently omitted from care.

Choosing the Initial Site of Treatment

Details on how to provide treatment in different settings are provided elsewhere in this book. Here we present considerations regarding how clinicians go about choosing the most appropriate site of treatment for a given patient. Available services for treating patients with eating disorders range from varying levels of outpatient care (in which the patient can receive psychiatric care; general medical care; nutritional counseling; individual, group, and/or family-based education; and counseling and/or psychotherapy supplied by a formal or informal network of health care professionals) through intensive outpatient programs, to residential and partial hospital programs, to intensive inpatient settings (in which subspecialty general medical consultation is readily available). Because specialized programs are not available in all geographic areas, and since financial considerations are often significant, it may be difficult to access care, and the psychiatrist and others may be required to administratively intervene with insurance companies on behalf of patients and families.

In determining an initial level of care or a change to a different level of care, it is important to consider the overall physical condition, psychology, behavior, and social circumstances of the patient rather than simply to rely on one or more physical parameters such as weight. Weight (in relation to estimated individually healthy weight and rate of weight loss), cardiac function, and metabolic status are the most important *physical* parameters for determining choice of setting, but psychosocial parameters are also important. Admission to or continuation at an intensive level of care (e.g., hospitalization) may be necessary when access to a less intensive level of care (e.g., partial hospitalization) is absent because of lack of resources or geography.

Generally, adult patients who weigh less than approximately 85% of their individually estimated healthy weights have considerable difficulty gaining weight outside of a highly structured program. It is important to underscore that these are *individually estimated healthy weights,* not weights that are simply read off a standard insurance table. Rather, healthy weight estimates for a given individual must be determined by that person's physicians on the basis of historical considerations, often including that person's growth chart (Golden 2003a) and, for women, weights at which healthy menstruation and ovulation resume (which may be higher than weights at which menstruation and ovulation became impaired).

Highly structured programs, including inpatient care, may be medically and psychiatrically necessary for some patients who are above 85% of their individually estimated healthy weight. Factors that suggest hospitalization may appropriately include the following:

- Rapid or persistent decline in oral intake
- Decline in weight despite maximally intensive available outpatient or partial hospitalization interventions
- Knowledge of weight at which instability previously occurred

- Presence of additional stressors that may additionally interfere with the patient's ability to eat
- Degree to which the patient is in denial and resists participating in her own care in less supervised settings
- Notable comorbid psychiatric problems that would ordinarily merit hospitalization on their own

Once weight loss is severe enough to cause the indications for immediate medical hospitalization, treatment may be less effective, refeeding may entail greater risks, and prognosis may be more problematic than when intervention is provided earlier. Since cortical gray matter deficits result from malnutrition and persist following refeeding earlier rather than later (Lambe et al. 1997), interventions may be important in minimizing the persistent effects of these physiological impairments. Therefore, hospitalization should occur *before* the onset of medical instability as manifested by abnormalities in vital signs (e.g., marked orthostatic hypotension with an increase in pulse of 20 bpm or a drop in blood pressure of 20 mm Hg standing, or bradycardia below 40 bpm, tachycardia over 110 bpm, or inability to sustain core body temperature), physical findings, or laboratory tests.

Many children and adolescents whose weight loss, while rapid, may not have been as severe as in adult patients nonetheless require inpatient treatment, because physiological abnormalities may be more likely to develop in the child or adolescent. Earlier inpatient treatment may be needed to avert potentially irreversible effects on physical growth and development. Children may become dehydrated quickly because they may refuse both water and food, believing that either could cause them to become fat. Also, a child's small size may mean that relatively smaller weight losses result in greater physiological danger.

Although most patients with uncomplicated bulimia nervosa do not require hospitalization, indications for hospitalization for bulimia nervosa include severe disabling symptoms that have not responded to adequate trials of outpatient treatment, serious concurrent general medical problems (e.g., metabolic abnormalities, hematemesis, vital sign changes, uncontrolled vomiting), suicidality, psychiatric disturbances that would warrant the patient's hospitalization independently of the eating disorder diagnosis, and severe concurrent alcohol or drug dependence or abuse.

Legal interventions, including involuntary hospitalization and legal guard-
ianship, may be necessary to address the safety of patients who are reluctant
to seek treatment but whose general medical conditions are life threatening
(Appelbaum and Rumpf 1998; Russell 2001; Watson et al. 2000).

Decisions to hospitalize on a psychiatric versus general medical or adoles-
cent/pediatric unit depend on the patient's general medical and psychiatric status, the skills and abilities of local psychiatric and general medical staffs, and the
availability of suitable programs to care for the patient's general medical and psychiatric problems.

Some evidence suggests that patients treated on inpatient units that specialize in eating disorders have better outcomes than patients treated in general
inpatient settings whose staff lack expertise and experience in treating patients
with eating disorders (Palmer and Treasure 1999). Outcomes from partial hospital programs that specialize in eating disorders are highly correlated with treatment intensity. The more successful programs involve patients at least 5 days per
week for 8 hours per day, and partial hospital programs should be structured
to provide at least that level of care (Olmsted et al. 2003).

Patients who are considerably below healthy body weight and have high
motivation to comply with treatment, cooperative families, and brief symptom
duration may benefit from treatment in outpatient settings, but only if they
are carefully monitored and if they and their families understand that a more
restrictive setting may be necessary if persistent progress is not evident in a few
weeks. Careful monitoring includes weighing the patient at least once a week
(and often two to three times a week) directly after the patient voids and while
the patient is wearing the same class of garment (e.g., hospital gown, standard
exercise clothing). In purging patients, serum electrolytes should be routinely
monitored. Urine-specific gravity, orthostatic vital signs, and oral tempera-
tures may also need to be monitored on a regular basis.

Suggested guidelines for the selection of initial treatment settings are provided in Table 2–3.

Although patients treated in the outpatient setting can remain with their
families and continue to attend school or work, these concerns should not by
themselves take priority over safe and adequate treatment of a rapidly progressing or otherwise unresponsive disorder for which hospital care might be
necessary. Choice of the specific outpatient team, outpatient therapy approaches, whether or not to medicate, and various elements of the overall out-

Table 2–3. Level-of-care guidelines for patients with eating disorders

Characteristic	Level of care[a]				
	Level 1: Outpatient	Level 2: Intensive outpatient	Level 3: Partial hospitalization (full-day outpatient care)[b]	Level 4: Residential treatment center	Level 5: Inpatient hospitalization
Medical status	Medically stable to the extent that more extensive medical monitoring, as defined in levels 4 and 5, is not required.			Medically stable to the extent that intravenous fluids, nasogastric tube feedings, and multiple daily laboratory tests are not needed.	*For adults*: heart rate <40 bpm; blood pressure <90/60 mm Hg; glucose <60 mg/dL; potassium <3 mEq/L; electrolyte imbalance; temperature <97.0°F; dehydration; or hepatic, renal, or cardiovascular organ compromise requiring acute treatment. Poorly controlled diabetes mellitus.

Table 2–3.   Level-of-care guidelines for patients with eating disorders *(continued)*

	Level of care[a]				
Characteristic	Level 1: Outpatient	Level 2: Intensive outpatient	Level 3: Partial hospitalization (full-day outpatient care)[b]	Level 4: Residential treatment center	Level 5: Inpatient hospitalization
Medical status *(continued)*					*For children and adolescents:* heart rate in the 40s; orthostatic blood pressure changes (>20-bpm increase in heart rate or >10- to 20-mm Hg drop); blood pressure below 80/50 mm Hg; hypokalemia,[c] hypophosphatemia, or hypomagnesemia.
Suicidality[d]	If suicidality is present, level of risk may require inpatient monitoring and treatment.				Specific plan with high lethality or intent; admission may also be indicated in patients with suicidal ideas or after a suicide attempt or aborted attempt, depending on the presence or absence of other factors modulating suicide risk.

Table 2–3.   Level-of-care guidelines for patients with eating disorders (continued)

Characteristic	Level of care[a]				
	Level 1: Outpatient	Level 2: Intensive outpatient	Level 3: Partial hospitalization (full-day outpatient care)[b]	Level 4: Residential treatment center	Level 5: Inpatient hospitalization
Weight as percentage of healthy body weight (for children, an additional determining factor is rate of weight loss)[c]	Generally >85%. See text for discussion regarding weight.	Generally >80%. See text for discussion regarding weight.	Generally >80%. See text for discussion regarding weight.	Generally <85%. See text for discussion regarding weight.	Generally <85%. See text for discussion regarding weight. Acute weight decline with food refusal even if not <85% below healthy body weight.[f]
Motivation to recover, including cooperativeness, insight, and ability to control obsessive thoughts	Fair to good.	Fair.	Partial; preoccupied with intrusive repetitive thoughts[g] more than 3 hours a day; cooperative.	Poor to fair; preoccupied with intrusive repetitive thoughts[g] 4–6 hours a day; cooperative with highly structured treatment.	Very poor to poor; preoccupied with intrusive repetitive thoughts[g]; uncooperative with treatment or cooperative only in highly structured environment.

Table 2–3.   Level-of-care guidelines for patients with eating disorders *(continued)*

			Level of care[a]		
Characteristic	Level 1: Outpatient	Level 2: Intensive outpatient	Level 3: Partial hospitalization (full-day outpatient care)[b]	Level 4: Residential treatment center	Level 5: Inpatient hospitalization
Comorbid disorders (substance abuse, depression, anxiety)	Presence of comorbid condition may influence choice of level of care.				Any existing psychiatric disorder that would require hospitalization.
Structure needed for eating/ gaining weight	Self-sufficient.	Self-sufficient.	Needs some structure to gain weight.	Needs supervision at all meals or will restrict eating.	Needs supervision during and after all meals or nasogastric/special feeding.
Ability to control compulsive exercise	Able to control; manages compulsive exercising via self-control.	Rarely a sole indication for increased levels of care. Some degree of external structure beyond self-control required to prevent patient from compulsive exercising.			

Table 2–3. Level-of-care guidelines for patients with eating disorders *(continued)*

Characteristic	Level of care[a]				
	Level 1: Outpatient	Level 2: Intensive outpatient	Level 3: Partial hospitalization (full-day outpatient care)[b]	Level 4: Residential treatment center	Level 5: Inpatient hospitalization
Purging behavior (laxatives and diuretics)	Can greatly reduce purging in nonstructured settings; no significant medical complications such as electrocardiographic or other abnormalities suggesting the need for hospitalization.			Can ask for and use support from others or use cognitive and behavioral skills to inhibit purging.	Needs supervision during and after all meals and in bathrooms. Inability to control multiple daily episodes of purging behavior that are severe, persistent, and disabling, despite appropriate trials of outpatient care, even if routine laboratory test results reveal no obvious metabolic abnormalities.
Environmental stress	Others able to provide adequate emotional and practical support and structure.		Others able to provide at least limited support and structure.	Severe family conflict, problems, or absence, so unable to have structured treatment at home, or lives alone without adequate support system.	
Treatment availability/ living situation	Lives near treatment setting.		Lives near treatment setting.	Too distant to live at home.	

Table 2–3.　Level-of-care guidelines for patients with eating disorders (continued)

	Level of care[a]				
Characteristic	Level 1: Outpatient	Level 2: Intensive outpatient	Level 3: Partial hospitalization (full-day outpatient care)[b]	Level 4: Residential treatment center	Level 5: Inpatient hospitalization

[a]In general, a given level of care should be considered for patients who meet one or more criteria under that particular level. These guidelines are not absolutes, however, and their application requires physician judgment.

[b]This level of care is most effective if administered for at least 8 hours per day, 5 days per week. Dropping below 5 days per week, 8 hours per day is demonstrably less effective.

[c]Total body potassium may be low even if the serum potassium value is normal, if the patient is dehydrated. Thus, determination of concurrent urine specific gravity can be used to help assess for dehydration.

[d]Determination of suicide risk is a complex clinical judgment, as is determination of the most appropriate treatment setting for care of patients at suicide risk. Factors such as concurrent medical conditions, psychosis, substance use, and other psychiatric symptoms or syndromes; psychosocial supports; past suicidal behaviors; treatment adherence; and the quality of existing physician–patient relationships may all be relevant and are described in greater detail in the American Psychiatric Association's "Practice Guideline for the Assessment and Treatment of Patients With Suicidal Behaviors" (2003).

[e]Although this table lists percentages of expected healthy body weight in relation to suggested levels of care, these percentages are only approximations and do not correspond to percentages based on standardized values for the population as a whole. For any given individual, differences in body build, body composition, and other physiological variables may result in considerable differences as to what constitutes a healthy body weight in relation to "norms." For some, a healthy body weight may be 110% of standardized value for the population, whereas for other individuals it may be 98%. Each individual's physiological differences must be assessed and appreciated.

[f]Weight level per se should never be used as the sole criterion for discharge from inpatient care. Many patients require inpatient admission at higher weights and should not be automatically discharged just because they have achieved a certain weight level unless all other factors are appropriately considered. See text for details.

[g]Individuals may experience these thoughts as consistent with their own deeply held beliefs (in which case they seem to be ego-syntonic and "overvalued") or as unwanted and ego-alien repetitive thoughts, consistent with classic obsessive-compulsive disorder phenomenology.

Source. Adapted and modified from Lavia et al. 1998. Adapted with permission from "Practice Guideline for the Treatment of Patients With Eating Disorders, Third Edition." American Psychiatric Association. *American Journal of Psychiatry* 163 (7, suppl):4–54, 2006. Copyright 2006, American Psychiatric Association.

patient treatment plan are addressed elsewhere in this book (see Chapter 5, "Management of Anorexia Nervosa in an Ambulatory Setting," Chapter 6, "Family Treatment of Eating Disorders," and Chapter 11, "Cognitive-Behavioral Therapy for Eating Disorders").

References

Anderluh MB, Tchanturia K, Rabe-Hesketh S, et al: Childhood obsessive-compulsive personality traits in adult women with eating disorders: defining a broader eating disorder phenotype. Am J Psychiatry 160:242–247, 2003

Appelbaum PS, Rumpf T: Civil commitment of the anorexic patient. Gen Hosp Psychiatry 20:225–230, 1998

Bachar E, Latzer Y, Canetti L, et al: Rejection of life in anorexic and bulimic patients. Int J Eat Disord 31:43–48, 2002

Boag F, Weerakoon J, Ginsburg J, et al: Diminished creatinine clearance in anorexia nervosa: reversal with weight gain. J Clin Pathol 38:60–63, 1985

Chanoine JP, Yeung LP, Wong AC, et al: Immunoreactive ghrelin in human cord blood: relation to anthropometry, leptin, and growth hormone. J Pediatr Gastroenterol Nutr 35:282–286, 2002

Garcia de Amusquibar AM: Interdisciplinary team for the treatment of eating disorders. Eat Weight Disord 5:223–227, 2000

Garfinkel PE, Lin E, Goering P, et al: Should amenorrhoea be necessary for the diagnosis of anorexia nervosa? Evidence from a Canadian community sample. Br J Psychiatry 168:500–506, 1996

Golden NH: Eating disorders in adolescence and their sequelae. Best Pract Res Clin Obstet Gynaecol 17:57–73, 2003a

Golden NH: Osteopenia and osteoporosis in anorexia nervosa. Adolesc Med 14:97–108, 2003b

Golden NH, Katzman DK, Kreipe RE, et al: Eating disorders in adolescents: position paper of the Society for Adolescent Medicine. J Adolesc Health 33:496–503, 2003

Halmi KA, Eckert E, Marchi P, et al: Comorbidity of psychiatric diagnoses in anorexia nervosa. Arch Gen Psychiatry 48:712–718, 1991

Herzog W, Deter HC, Fiehn W, et al: Medical findings and predictors of long-term physical outcome in anorexia nervosa: a prospective, 12-year follow-up study. Psychol Med 27:269–279, 1997

Joy EA, Wilson C, Varechok S: The multidisciplinary team approach to the outpatient treatment of disordered eating. Curr Sports Med Rep 2:331–336, 2003

Kreipe RE, Yussman SM: The role of the primary care practitioner in the treatment of eating disorders. Adolesc Med 14:133–147, 2003

Kron L, Katz JL, Gorzynski G, et al: Hyperactivity in anorexia nervosa: a fundamental clinical feature. Compr Psychiatry 19:433–440, 1978

Lambe EK, Katzman DK, Mikulis DJ, et al: Cerebral gray matter volume deficits after weight recovery from anorexia nervosa. Arch Gen Psychiatry 54:537–542, 1997

Lear SA, Toma M, Birmingham CL, et al: Modification of the relationship between simple anthropometric indices and risk factors by ethnic background. Metabolism 52:1295–1301, 2003

Lock J: Treating adolescents with eating disorders in the family context: empirical and theoretical considerations. Child Adolesc Psychiatr Clin N Am 11:331–342, 2002

McIntosh VV, Jordan J, Carter FA, et al: Three psychotherapies for anorexia nervosa: a randomized controlled trial. Am J Psychiatry 16:741–747, 2005

Mehler PS, Krantz M: Anorexia nervosa medical issues. J Womens Health (Larchmt) 12:331–340, 2003

Myers TC, Swan-Kremeier L, Wonderlich S, et al: The use of alternative delivery systems and new technologies in the treatment of patients with eating disorders. Int J Eat Disord 36:123–143, 2004

Nova E, Lopez-Vidriero I, Varela O, et al: Indicators of nutritional status in restricting-type anorexia nervosa patients: a 1-year follow-up study. Clin Nutr 23:1353–1359, 2004

Olmsted MP, Kaplan AS, Rockert W: Relative efficacy of a 4-day versus a 5-day day hospital program. Int J Eat Disord 34:441–449, 2003

Palmer RL, Treasure J: Providing specialised services for anorexia nervosa. Br J Psychiatry 175:306–309, 1999

Practice guideline for the assessment and treatment of patients with suicidal behaviors. Am J Psychiatry 160 (11, suppl):1–60, 2003

Practice guideline for the treatment of patients with eating disorders, third edition. American Psychiatric Association. Am J Psychiatry 163 (7, suppl):4–54, 2006

Ramacciotti CE, Coli E, Biadi O, et al: Silent pericardial effusion in a sample of anorexic patients. Eat Weight Disord 8:68–71, 2003

Russell GF: Involuntary treatment in anorexia nervosa. Psychiatr Clin North Am 24:337–349, 2001

Strober M, Freeman R, Morrell W: Atypical anorexia nervosa: separation from typical cases in course and outcome in a long-term prospective study. Int J Eat Disord 25:135–142, 1999

Watson TL, Bowers WA, Andersen AE: Involuntary treatment of eating disorders. Am J Psychiatry 157:1806–1810, 2000

Woodside DB, Garfinkel PE, Lin E, et al: Comparisons of men with full or partial eating disorders, men without eating disorders, and women with eating disorders in the community. Am J Psychiatry 158:570–574, 2001

Wyatt RJ, Farrell M, Berry PL, et al: Reduced alternative complement pathway control protein levels in anorexia nervosa: response to parenteral alimentation. Am J Clin Nutr 35:973–980, 1982

Yager J: Family issues in the pathogenesis of anorexia nervosa. Psychosom Med 44:43–60, 1982

Yates A, Edman J, Aruguete M: Ethnic differences in BMI and body/self-dissatisfaction among Whites, Asian subgroups, Pacific Islanders, and African-Americans. J Adolesc Health 34:300–307, 2004

Appendix: Eating Disorders Questionnaire (EDQ), Version 9.0

INSTRUCTIONS: Please fill in the circle that best describes you for each item.

A. DEMOGRAPHIC INFORMATION

1. Sex: O Female   O Male

2. Current Age: _____ years

   Date of Birth:

   ☐☐ / ☐☐ / ☐☐☐☐

3. Race (fill in only one):
   O White
   O African American
   O Native American
   O Hispanic
   O Asian
   O Other (please specify) _____

4. Marital Status (fill in only one):
   O Never married
   O Married (first marriage)
   O Divorced or widowed and presently remarried
   O Monogamous relationship, living with partner (but not married)
   O Monogamous relationship, not living with partner
   O Divorced and not presently married
   O Widowed and not presently remarried

5. What is your primary role? (fill in only one)
   O Wage earner, full-time
   O Wage earner, part-time
   O Student, full-time
   O Student, part-time
   O Homemaker
   O Unemployed
   O Other (specify) _____

B. WEIGHT HISTORY

1. Current Weight:

   ☐☐☐ lbs.

2. Current Height:

   ☐ ft. ☐☐ in.

3. I would like to weigh:

   ☐☐☐ lbs.

4. **Highest Weight** (non-pregnancy) since age 18:

   Weight   Age
   ☐☐☐ lbs. at   ☐☐ yrs.

5. **Lowest Weight** since age 18:

   Weight   Age
   ☐☐☐ lbs. at   ☐☐ yrs.

6. **Highest Weight between ages 12 and 18:**

   Weight   Height
   ☐☐☐ lbs. at   ☐ ft. ☐☐ in.   at age

   O 12
   O 13
   O 14
   O 15
   O 16
   O 17

7. **Lowest Weight between ages 12 and 18:**

   Weight   Height
   ☐☐☐ lbs. at   ☐ ft. ☐☐ in.   at age

   O 12
   O 13
   O 14
   O 15
   O 16
   O 17

8. At your current weight, do you feel that you are:
   O Extremely thin   O Slightly overweight
   O Moderately thin   O Moderately overweight
   O Slightly thin   O Extremely overweight
   O Normal weight

9. How much do you fear <u>gaining</u> weight?
   O Not at all
   O Slightly
   O Moderately
   O Very much
   O Extremely

Continue on Next Page

EDQ - continued, pg. 2

10. How <u>dissatisfied</u> are you with the way your body is proportioned?

○ Not at all dissatisfied
○ Slightly dissatisfied
○ Moderately dissatisfied
○ Very dissatisfied
○ Extremely dissatisfied

11. How important are your weight & shape in affecting how you feel about yourself as a person?

○ Not at all important
○ Slightly important
○ Moderately important
○ Very important
○ Extremely important

12. How fat do you currently feel?

○ Not at all fat
○ Slightly fat
○ Fat
○ Very fat
○ Extremely fat

13. **Please indicate on the scales below how you feel about different areas of your body.**
(Fill in the circle of best response for each body part.)

	(a) Face	(b) Arms	(c) Shoulders	(d) Breasts	(e) Stomach	(f) Waist	(g) Hips	(h) Buttocks	(i) Thighs
Extremely positive	○	○	○	○	○	○	○	○	○
Moderately positive	○	○	○	○	○	○	○	○	○
Slightly positive	○	○	○	○	○	○	○	○	○
Neutral	○	○	○	○	○	○	○	○	○
Slightly negative	○	○	○	○	○	○	○	○	○
Moderately negative	○	○	○	○	○	○	○	○	○
Extremely negative	○	○	○	○	○	○	○	○	○

14. On the average, how often do you weigh yourself?

○ Never
○ Less than monthly
○ Monthly
○ Several times/month
○ Weekly
○ Several times/week
○ Daily
○ 2 or 3 times/day
○ 4 or 5 times/day
○ More than 5 times/day

C. DIETING BEHAVIOR

1. On the average, how many main meals do you eat each day?

2. On the average, how many snacks do you eat each day?

3. On the average, how many days a week do you eat the following meals?

<u>Breakfast:</u> ___ days a week   <u>Lunch:</u> ___ days a week   <u>Dinner:</u> ___ days a week

4. Do you try to avoid certain foods in order to influence your shape or weight?
○ Yes (If Yes, what?) _____
○ No

5. Have you ever been on a diet, restricted your food intake, and/or reduced the amounts or types of food eaten to control your weight?
○ Yes
○ No (If No, go to section D, "BINGE EATING BEHAVIOR.")

6. At what age did you first begin to diet, restrict your food intake, and/or reduce the amount or types of food eaten to <u>control</u> your weight?

___ years old

7. At what age did you first begin to diet, restrict your food intake, and/or reduce the amount or types of food eaten to <u>lose</u> weight?

___ years old

Continue on Next Page

EDQ - continued, pg. 3

8. Over the last year, how often have you begun a diet that lasted for more than 3 days?

[ ][ ][ ] times

9. Over the last year, how often have you begun a diet that lasted for 3 days or less?

[ ][ ][ ] times

10. Indicate your preferred ways of dieting (fill in all that apply).

   O Skip meals
   O Completely fast for 24 hours or more
   O Restrict carbohydrates
   O Restrict sweets/sugar
   O Reduce fats

   O Reduce portion size
   O Exercise more
   O Reduce calories
   O Other: _____

11. In which of the following treatments or types of treatment for eating or weight problems have you participated?

(a) Supervised Diets:	Yes	No	If Yes, ages used	Weight at Start	Weight at End
Weight Watchers ®	O	O			
Jenny Craig ®	O	O			
NutriSystem ®	O	O			
Optifast ®	O	O			
Procal ®	O	O			
Nutramed ®	O	O			
Liquid protein diet	O	O			
Others: _____	O	O			

(b) Medication for Obesity:	Yes	No	If Yes, ages used	Weight at Start	Weight at End
Phentermine	O	O			
Fenfluramine	O	O			
Xenical (Orlistat ®)	O	O			
Sibutramine (Meridia ®)	O	O			
Topiramate (Topamax ®)	O	O			
Wellbutrin (Bupropion ®)	O	O			
Over-the-counter diet pills (specify): _____	O	O			
Other medication treatment (specify): _____	O	O			
Human chorionic gonadotropin (HCG)	O	O			
Others: _____	O	O			

(c) Psychotherapy for Eating Problems, Weight Loss, or Weight Gain:	Yes	No	If Yes, ages used	Weight at Start	Weight at End
Behavior Modification	O	O			
Individual Psychotherapy	O	O			
Group Psychotherapy	O	O			
Hypnosis	O	O			
Others: _____	O	O			

(d) Psychotherapy for Eating Disorder:	Yes	No	If Yes, ages used	Weight at Start	Weight at End
Individual Cognitive Behavioral	O	O			
Group Cognitive Behavioral	O	O			
Interpersonal Psychotherapy	O	O			
Nutritional Counseling	O	O			
Others: _____	O	O			

Continue on Next Page

EDQ - continued, pg. 4

(e) Medication for Eating Problems/Weight Problems:	Yes	No	If Yes, ages used	If Yes, maximum dosage
Fluoxetine (Prozac ®)	O	O		
Desipramine (Norpramin ®)	O	O		
Paroxetine HCl (Paxil ®)	O	O		
Sertraline HCl (Zoloft ®)	O	O		
Citalopram (Celexa ®)	O	O		
Fluvoxamine (Luvox ®)	O	O		
Naltrexone (Trexan ®)	O	O		
Escitalopram (Lexapro ®)	O	O		
Quetiapine (Seroquel ®)	O	O		
Olanzapine (Zyprexa ®)	O	O		
Risperidone (Risperdal ®)	O	O		
Others: _____	O	O		

(f) Self-help groups:	Yes	No	If Yes, ages used
Bulimia Anonymous	O	O	
Overeaters Anonymous	O	O	
Anorexics Anonymous	O	O	
Others: _____	O	O	

(g) Surgical Procedures:	Yes	No	If Yes, at what age	Weight at Start	Weight at End
Liposuction	O	O			
Gastric bypass	O	O			
Gastric banding	O	O			
Other intestinal surgery (specify): _____	O	O			
Gastric balloon/"bubble"	O	O			
Others: _____	O	O			

12. Please record your major diets which resulted in a weight loss of 10 pounds or more.

	Age at time of diet	Weight at start of diet	# lbs. lost	Type of diet
(1)				
(2)				
(3)				
(4)				
(5)				
(6)				
(7)				
(8)				
(9)				
(10)				

13. Have you ever had any significant physical or emotional symptoms while attempting to lose weight or after losing weight?

O Yes   O No

If Yes, describe your symptoms, how long they lasted, if they made you stop your weight loss program, and if they made you seek professional help.

Problem	Year	Duration (weeks)	Stopped weight loss program? Yes No	Type of professional help, if any
			O O	
			O O	
			O O	
			O O	
			O O	

EDQ 9.0. Copyright © 2004, The Neuropsychiatric Research Institute. Used with permission.

Continue on Next Page

EDQ - continued, pg. 5

D. BINGE EATING BEHAVIOR

1. Have you ever had an episode of binge eating characterized by:

    (a) eating, in a discrete period of time (e.g., within any two hour period), an amount of food that is definitely larger than most people eat in a similar period of time?
    O Yes   O No

    (b) a sense of lack of control over eating during the episode (e.g., a feeling that one cannot stop eating or control what or how much one is eating)?
    O Yes   O No

    If No to either a) or b), go to section E, "WEIGHT CONTROL BEHAVIOR."

2. Please indicate on the scales below how <u>characteristic</u> the following symptoms are or were of your <u>binge eating</u>.

	Never	Rarely	Sometimes	Often	Always
(a) feeling that I can't stop eating or control what or how much I eat	O	O	O	O	O
(b) eating much more rapidly than usual	O	O	O	O	O
(c) eating until I feel uncomfortably full	O	O	O	O	O
(d) eating large amounts of food when not feeling physically hungry	O	O	O	O	O
(e) eating alone because I am embarrassed by how much I am eating	O	O	O	O	O
(f) feeling disgusted with myself, depressed, or very guilty after overeating	O	O	O	O	O
(g) feeling very distressed about binge eating	O	O	O	O	O

3. How old were you when you began binge eating?

    ☐☐ years old

4. When did binge eating start to occur on a regular basis, on average at least 2 times each week?

    ☐☐ years old

5. What were your height & weight at that time?

    Weight   **Height**
    ☐☐☐ lbs. at   ☐ ft. ☐☐ in.

6. What is the total duration of time you had a problem with binge eating (whether or not you are binge eating now)?

    Days   **Months**   **Years**
    ☐☐   ☐☐   ☐☐

E. WEIGHT CONTROL BEHAVIOR

1. Have you ever self-induced vomiting after eating in order to get rid of the food eaten?
    O Yes   O No (If No, go to question 8.)

2. How old were you when you induced vomiting for the first time?

    ☐☐ years old

3. How old were you when you first induced vomiting on a regular basis (on average at least two times each week)?

    ☐☐ years old

4. How long did you self-induce vomiting?

    Days   **Months**   **Years**
    ☐☐   ☐☐   ☐☐

Continue on Next Page

EDQ - continued, pg. 6

5. Have you ever taken syrup of ipecac to control your weight?

   ○ Yes   ○ No

6. How old were you when you took ipecac for the first time?

   ☐☐ years old

7. How long did you use ipecac to control your weight?

Days	Months	Years
☐☐	☐☐	☐☐

8. Have you ever used laxatives to control your weight or "get rid of food"?

   ○ Yes   ○ No (If No, go to question 13.)

9. How old were you when you first took laxatives for weight control?

   ☐☐ years old

10. How old were you when you first took laxatives for weight control (on a regular basis on average at least two times each week)?

    ☐☐ years old

11. How long did you use laxatives for weight control?

Days	Months	Years
☐☐	☐☐	☐☐

12. What type and amounts of laxatives have you used? (Indicate all types that apply and the maximum number used per day.)

			Maximum Number per Day							
	Yes	No	1	2	3	4	5	6-10	11-20	>20
Ex-Lax ®	○	○	○	○	○	○	○	○	○	○
Correctol ®	○	○	○	○	○	○	○	○	○	○
Metamucil ®	○	○	○	○	○	○	○	○	○	○
Colace ®	○	○	○	○	○	○	○	○	○	○
Dulcolax ®	○	○	○	○	○	○	○	○	○	○
Phillips' Milk of Magnesia ®	○	○	○	○	○	○	○	○	○	○
Senokot ®	○	○	○	○	○	○	○	○	○	○
Perdiem ®	○	○	○	○	○	○	○	○	○	○
Fleet ®	○	○	○	○	○	○	○	○	○	○
Other (specify).	○	○	○	○	○	○	○	○	○	○

13. Have you ever used diuretics (water pills) to control your weight?

    ○ Yes   ○ No (If No, go to question 18.)

14. How old were you when you first took diuretics for weight control?

    ☐☐ years old

15. How old were you when you first took diuretics for weight control (on a regular basis, on average at least two times each week)?

    ☐☐ years old

16. How long did you use diuretics for weight control?

Days	Months	Years
☐☐	☐☐	☐☐

17. What type and amount of diuretics have you used? (Indicate all that apply and the maximum number used per day.)

(a) Over-the-counter Diuretics:			Maximum Number per Day									
	Yes	No	1	2	3	4	5	6	7	8	9	10	>10
Aqua-Ban ®	○	○	○	○	○	○	○	○	○	○	○	○	○
Diurex ®	○	○	○	○	○	○	○	○	○	○	○	○	○
Midol ®	○	○	○	○	○	○	○	○	○	○	○	○	○
Pamprin ®	○	○	○	○	○	○	○	○	○	○	○	○	○
Others (specify):	○	○	○	○	○	○	○	○	○	○	○	○	○

Continue on Next Page

EDQ - continued, pg. 7

(b) Prescription Diuretics:	Yes	No		1	2	3	Maximum Number per Day 4	5	6	7	8	9	10	>10
	O	O		O	O	O	O	O	O	O	O	O	O	O
	O	O		O	O	O	O	O	O	O	O	O	O	O

18. Have you ever used diet pills to control your weight?
    O Yes   O No (If No, please go to question 22.)

19. How old were you when you first used diet pills for weight control?

    ☐☐ years old

20. How long did you use diet pills to control your weight?

    Days   Months   Years
    ☐☐   ☐☐   ☐☐

21. What types and amounts of diet pills have you used **within the last month**? (Indicate all that apply and the maximum number per day.)

(a) Over-the-counter:	Yes	No		1	2	3	Maximum Number per Day 4	5	6	7	8	9	10	>10
Dexatrim ®	O	O		O	O	O	O	O	O	O	O	O	O	O
Dietac ®	O	O		O	O	O	O	O	O	O	O	O	O	O
Acutrim ®	O	O		O	O	O	O	O	O	O	O	O	O	O
ProTrim ®	O	O		O	O	O	O	O	O	O	O	O	O	O
Ma huang	O	O		O	O	O	O	O	O	O	O	O	O	O
Ephedrine	O	O		O	O	O	O	O	O	O	O	O	O	O
Chromium	O	O		O	O	O	O	O	O	O	O	O	O	O
Guarana seed	O	O		O	O	O	O	O	O	O	O	O	O	O
Garcinia cambogia	O	O		O	O	O	O	O	O	O	O	O	O	O
Caffeine	O	O		O	O	O	O	O	O	O	O	O	O	O
Other (specify):	O	O		O	O	O	O	O	O	O	O	O	O	O

(b) Prescription:	Yes	No		1	2	3	Maximum Number per Day 4	5	6	7	8	9	10	>10
	O	O		O	O	O	O	O	O	O	O	O	O	O
	O	O		O	O	O	O	O	O	O	O	O	O	O

22. During the entire LAST MONTH, what is the average frequency that you have engaged in the following behaviors? (Please fill in one circle for each behavior.)

	Never	Once a Month or Less	Several Times a Month	Once a Week	Twice a Week	Three to Six Times a Week	Once a Day	More Than Once a Day
Binge eating (as defined on pg. 5, D.1.)	O	O	O	O	O	O	O	O
Vomiting	O	O	O	O	O	O	O	O
Laxative use to control weight	O	O	O	O	O	O	O	O
Use of diet pills	O	O	O	O	O	O	O	O
Use of diuretics	O	O	O	O	O	O	O	O
Use of enemas	O	O	O	O	O	O	O	O
Use of ipecac syrup	O	O	O	O	O	O	O	O
Exercise to control weight	O	O	O	O	O	O	O	O
Fasting (skipping meals for entire day)	O	O	O	O	O	O	O	O
Skipping meals	O	O	O	O	O	O	O	O
Eating very small meals	O	O	O	O	O	O	O	O
Eating meals low in calories and/or fat grams	O	O	O	O	O	O	O	O
Chewing and spitting out food	O	O	O	O	O	O	O	O
Rumination (vomit food into mouth, chew, and re-swallow	O	O	O	O	O	O	O	O
Saunas to control weight	O	O	O	O	O	O	O	O
Herbal products ("fat burners")	O	O	O	O	O	O	O	O

Continue on Next Page

EDQ - continued, pg. 8

23. During **any one-month period**, what is the HIGHEST frequency that you have engaged in the following behaviors?
(Please fill in one circle for each behavior.)

	Never	Once a Month or Less	Several Times a Month	Once a Week	Twice a Week	Three to Six Times a Week	Once a Day	More Than Once a Day
Binge eating (as defined on pg. 5, D.1.)	O	O	O	O	O	O	O	O
Vomiting	O	O	O	O	O	O	O	O
Laxative use to control weight	O	O	O	O	O	O	O	O
Use of diet pills	O	O	O	O	O	O	O	O
Use of diuretics	O	O	O	O	O	O	O	O
Use of enemas	O	O	O	O	O	O	O	O
Use of ipecac syrup	O	O	O	O	O	O	O	O
Exercise to control weight	O	O	O	O	O	O	O	O
Fasting (skipping meals for entire day)	O	O	O	O	O	O	O	O
Skipping meals	O	O	O	O	O	O	O	O
Eating very small meals	O	O	O	O	O	O	O	O
Eating meals low in calories and/or fat grams	O	O	O	O	O	O	O	O
Chewing and spitting out food	O	O	O	O	O	O	O	O
Rumination (vomit food into mouth, chew, and re-swallow)	O	O	O	O	O	O	O	O
Saunas to control weight	O	O	O	O	O	O	O	O
Herbal products ("fat burners")	O	O	O	O	O	O	O	O

F. EXERCISE

1. How frequently do you exercise?

O Not at all   O Several times per week
O Once per month or less O Once per day
O Several times per month O Several times a day
O Once per week

2. If you exercise, how long do you usually exercise each time?

O Less than 15 minutes
O 15 - 30 minutes
O 31 - 60 minutes
O 61 - 120 minutes
O More than 120 minutes

3. If you exercise, please indicate the types of exercise you do (fill in all that apply)

O Biking   O Walking
O Running   O In-line skating
O Swimming   O Stairmaster
O Weight training   O Treadmill
O Aerobics   O Stationary bike
O Calisthenics   O Other: _____

G. MENSTRUAL HISTORY

1. Age at onset of menses: ☐☐ years

2. Have you ever had periods of time when you stopped menstruating for three months or more (which were unrelated to pregnancy)?

   O Yes   O No   If Yes, number of times: ☐☐

3. Did weight loss ever cause irregularities of your cycle?

   O Yes   O No   If Yes, describe:
   _____
   _____

4. Have you menstruated during the last three months?

   O Yes   O No

Continue on Next Page

EDQ - continued, pg. 9

5. Are you on birth control pills?   O Yes   O No

6. Are you on hormone replacement?   O Yes   O No

7. Are you postmenopausal?   O Yes   O No

8. Please indicate when during your cycle you feel most vulnerable to binge eating. Please fill in the single best response.

O I do not binge eat during menstruation   O 1 - 2 days prior to menstruation
O 11 - 14 days prior to menstruation   O After menstruation onset
O 7 - 10 days prior to menstruation   O No particular time
O 3 - 6 days prior to menstruation

9. Do you crave particular foods (have a desire or urge to consume a specific food item or drink) for the <u>few days prior to</u> menstruation?

O Yes   O No   If Yes, what foods do you crave?
_____
_____

10. Do you crave particular foods (have a desire or urge to consume a specific food item or drink) <u>during</u> your menstruation?

O Yes   O No   If Yes, what foods do you crave?
_____
_____

11. Marriage and pregnancy:

	Yes	No	Does Not Apply
(a) Did problems with weight and/or binge eating begin before you were married?	O	O	O
(b) Did problems with weight and/or binge eating begin after you were married?	O	O	O
(c) Did problems with weight and/or binge eating begin before your first pregnancy?	O	O	O
(d) Did problems with weight and/or binge eating begin after your first pregnancy?	O	O	O

12. Do you have children?

O Yes   O No (If No, skip to section H, "HISTORY OF ABUSE.")

(a) For your FIRST child, what was your...
...weight at the start of your pregnancy?   ...weight at delivery?   ...lowest weight in the first year after delivery?

(b) For your SECOND child, what was your...
...weight at the start of your pregnancy?   ...weight at delivery?   ...lowest weight in the first year after delivery?

(c) For your THIRD child, what was your...
...weight at the start of your pregnancy?   ...weight at delivery?   ...lowest weight in the first year after delivery?

(d) For your FOURTH child, what was your...
...weight at the start of your pregnancy?   ...weight at delivery?   ...lowest weight in the first year after delivery?

Continue on Next Page

EDQ - continued, pg. 10

H. HISTORY OF ABUSE

1. <u>Before</u> you were 18, did any of the following happen to you?

Yes	No	
O	O	Someone constantly criticized you and blamed you for minor things.
O	O	Someone physically beat you (hit you, slapped you, threw something at you, pushed you).
O	O	Someone threatened to hurt or kill you, or do something sexual to you.
O	O	Someone threatened to abandon or leave you.
O	O	You watched one parent physically beat (hit, slap) the other parent.
O	O	Someone from your family forced you to have sexual relations (unwanted touching, fondling, sexual kissing, sexual intercourse).
O	O	Someone outside your family forced you to have sexual relations (unwanted touching, fondling, sexual kissing, sexual intercourse).

2. <u>After</u> you were 18, did any of the following happen to you?

Yes	No	
O	O	Someone constantly criticized you and blamed you for minor things.
O	O	Someone physically beat you (hit you, slapped you, threw something at you, pushed you).
O	O	Someone threatened to hurt or kill you, or do something sexual to you.
O	O	Someone threatened to abandon or leave you.
O	O	You watched one parent physically beat (hit, slap) the other parent.
O	O	Someone from your family forced you to have sexual relations (unwanted touching, fondling, sexual kissing, sexual intercourse).
O	O	Someone outside your family forced you to have sexual relations (unwanted touching, fondling, sexual kissing, sexual intercourse).

I. PSYCHIATRIC HISTORY

1. Have you ever been hospitalized for psychiatric problems?

   O Yes (If Yes, please complete the section below.)
   O No

HOSPITAL NAME & ADDRESS (CITY, STATE)	WHAT YEAR	DIAGNOSIS (IF KNOWN) OR PROBLEMS YOU WERE HAVING	RECEIVED	WAS THIS HELPFUL? Yes No
				O O
				O O
				O O
				O O
				O O

Continue on Next Page

EDQ - continued, pg. 11

2. Have you ever been treated out of the hospital for psychiatric problems?

○ Yes (If Yes, please complete the section below.)

○ No

YEAR(S) WHEN TREATED	DOCTOR OR THERAPIST'S NAME & ADDRESS (CITY, STATE)	DIAGNOSIS (IF KNOWN) OR PROBLEMS YOU WERE HAVING	TREATMENT YOU RECEIVED	WAS THIS HELPFUL? Yes No
				○ ○
				○ ○
				○ ○
				○ ○
				○ ○

3. Complete the following information for any of the following types of medications you are now taking or have ever taken:

		Took Previously	On Currently	Current Dosage	If taking currently, for what problem?
(a) ANTIDEPRESSANTS					
Prozac ®	(Fluoxetine)	○	○		
Zoloft ®	(Sertraline)	○	○		
Paxil ®	(Paroxetine)	○	○		
Luvox ®	(Fluvoxamine)	○	○		
Celexa ®	(Citalopram)	○	○		
Effexor ®	(Venlafaxine)	○	○		
Wellbutrin ®	(Bupropion)	○	○		
Elavil ®	(Amitriptyline)	○	○		
Tofranil ®	(Imipramine)	○	○		
Sinequan ®	(Doxepin)	○	○		
Norpramin ®	(Desipramine)	○	○		
Vivactil ®	(Protriptyline)	○	○		
Desyrel ®	(Trazodone)	○	○		
Parnate ®	(Tranylcypromine)	○	○		
Nardil ®	(Phenelzine)	○	○		
Anafranil ®	(Clomipramine)	○	○		
Remeron ®	(Mirtazapine)	○	○		
Serzone ®	(Nefazodone)	○	○		
St. John's wort		○	○		
Lexapro ®	(Escitalopram)	○	○		
(b) MAJOR TRANQUILIZERS					
Clozaril ®	(Clozapine)	○	○		
Zyprexa ®	(Olanzapine)	○	○		
Risperdal ®	(Risperidone)	○	○		
Haldol ®	(Haloperidol)	○	○		
Navane ®	(Thiothixene)	○	○		
Trilafon ®	(Perphenazine)	○	○		
Thorazine ®	(Chlorpromazine)	○	○		
Stelazine ®	(Trifluoperazine)	○	○		
Prolixin ®	(Fluphenazine)	○	○		
Orap ®	(Pimozide)	○	○		
Moban ®	(Molindone)	○	○		
Loxitane ®	(Loxapine)	○	○		
Seroquil ®	(Quetiapine)	○	○		
Mellaril ®	(Thioridazine)	○	○		
Geodon ®	(Ziprasidone)	○	○		
Abilify ®	(Aripiprazole)	○	○		

Continue on Next Page

EDQ - continued, pg. 12

		Took Previously	On Currently	Current Dosage	If taking currently, for what problem?
(c) MINOR TRANQUILIZERS					
Valium ®	(Diazepam)	O	O		
Librium ®	(Chlordiazepoxide)	O	O		
Serax ®	(Oxazepam)	O	O		
Halcion ®	(Triazolam)	O	O		
Tranxene ®	(Clorazepate)	O	O		
Ambien ®	(Zolpidem)	O	O		
Klonopin ®	(Clonazepam)	O	O		
Ativan ®	(Lorazepam)	O	O		
BuSpar ®	(Buspirone)	O	O		
Dalmane ®	(Flurazepam)	O	O		
Xanax ®	(Alprazolam)	O	O		
Sonata ®	(Zaleplon)	O	O		

		Took Previously	On Currently	Current Dosage	If taking currently, for what problem?
(d) MOOD STABILIZERS					
Lithobid ®	(Lithium)	O	O		
Depakote ®	(Sodium valproate)	O	O		
Tegretol ®	(Carbamazepine)	O	O		
Topamax ®	(Topiramate)	O	O		
Lamictal ®	(Lamotrigine)	O	O		
OTHER:		O	O		
OTHER:		O	O		
OTHER:		O	O		
OTHER:		O	O		

J. MEDICAL HISTORY

1. Please list all medical hospitalizations:

WHEN? YEAR(S)	WHERE? (Hospital Name & City)	PROBLEM	DIAGNOSIS	TREATMENT YOU RECEIVED

2. Please list all other medical treatment you've received. (Include any significant problem, but do not include flu, colds, routine exams.)

WHEN? YEAR(S)	WHERE? (Doctor's Name & Address)	PROBLEM	DIAGNOSIS	TREATMENT YOU RECEIVED

Continue on Next Page

EDQ - continued, pg. 13

K. CHEMICAL USE HISTORY

1. In the last six months, how often have you taken these drugs?

	Not At All	Less Than Monthly	About Once a Month	Several Times a Month	About Once a Week	Several Times a Week	Daily	Several Times a Day
ALCOHOL	O	O	O	O	O	O	O	O
STIMULANTS (Amphetamines, Uppers, Crank, Speed)	O	O	O	O	O	O	O	O
DIET PILLS	O	O	O	O	O	O	O	O
SEDATIVES (Barbiturates, Sleeping pills, Valium ®, Librium ®, Downers)	O	O	O	O	O	O	O	O
MARIJUANA/HASHISH	O	O	O	O	O	O	O	O
HALLUCINOGENS (LSD, Mescaline, Mushrooms, Ectasy)	O	O	O	O	O	O	O	O
OPIATES (Heroin, Morphine, Opium)	O	O	O	O	O	O	O	O
COCAINE/CRACK	O	O	O	O	O	O	O	O
PCP (Angel dust, Phencyclidine)	O	O	O	O	O	O	O	O
INHALANTS (Glue, Gasoline, etc.)	O	O	O	O	O	O	O	O
CAFFEINE PILLS (NoDoz ®, Vivarin ®, etc.)	O	O	O	O	O	O	O	O
OTHER: _____	O	O	O	O	O	O	O	O
_____	O	O	O	O	O	O	O	O

2. What is the most you have used any of these drugs during a one-month period (month of heaviest use)?

(Example: If you used sleeping pills about once a month many years ago, but not at all now, you would fill in the circle under "About Once a Month" on the line "Sedatives - Barbiturates...")

	Not At All	Less Than Monthly	About Once a Month	Several Times a Month	About Once a Week	Several Times a Week	Daily	Several Times a Day
ALCOHOL	O	O	O	O	O	O	O	O
STIMULANTS (Amphetamines, Uppers, Crank, Speed)	O	O	O	O	O	O	O	O
DIET PILLS	O	O	O	O	O	O	O	O
SEDATIVES (Barbiturates, Sleeping pills, Valium ®, Librium ®, Downers)	O	O	O	O	O	O	O	O
MARIJUANA/HASHISH	O	O	O	O	O	O	O	O
HALLUCINOGENS (LSD, Mescaline, Mushrooms, Ectasy)	O	O	O	O	O	O	O	O
OPIATES (Heroin, Morphine, Opium)	O	O	O	O	O	O	O	O
COCAINE/CRACK	O	O	O	O	O	O	O	O
PCP (Angel dust, Phencyclidine)	O	O	O	O	O	O	O	O
INHALANTS (Glue, Gasoline, etc.)	O	O	O	O	O	O	O	O
CAFFEINE PILLS (NoDoz ®, Vivarin ®, etc.)	O	O	O	O	O	O	O	O
OTHER: _____	O	O	O	O	O	O	O	O
_____	O	O	O	O	O	O	O	O

3. Assuming all the drugs mentioned above were readily available, which would you prefer? _____

Continue on Next Page

EDQ 9.0. Copyright © 2004, The Neuropsychiatric Research Institute. Used with permission.

EDQ - continued, pg. 14

Have you ever had any of the following problems because of your alcohol or drug use? (If Yes, please specify.)

4. Drinking and driving when unsafe?
   - O Yes......When?
   - O No
   - O More than 6 months ago
   - O During the past 6 months
   - O Both

5. Medical problems?
   - O Yes......When?
   - O No
   - O More than 6 months ago
   - O During the past 6 months
   - O Both

6. Problems at work or school?
   - O Yes......When?
   - O No
   - O More than 6 months ago
   - O During the past 6 months
   - O Both

7. An arrest?
   - O Yes......When?
   - O No
   - O More than 6 months ago
   - O During the past 6 months
   - O Both

8. Family trouble?
   - O Yes......When?
   - O No
   - O More than 6 months ago
   - O During the past 6 months
   - O Both

---

9. Have you ever smoked cigarettes?

O Yes
O No (If No, go to question 10.)

What was the most you ever smoked?

O Only occasionally
O Less than one pack per day
O About one pack per day
O One to two packs per day
O About two packs per day
O More than two packs per day

If you are smoking now, how much do you smoke?

O Only occasionally
O Less than one pack per day
O About one pack per day
O One to two packs per day
O About two packs per day
O More than two packs per day

---

10. Do you drink coffee?

O Yes
O No (If No, go to question 11.)

On the average, how many cups of caffeinated coffee do you drink per day?

O Less than 1   O 4 cups
O 1 cup per day   O 5 cups
O 2 cups   O 6 - 10 cups
O 3 cups   O More than 10 cups

On the average, how many cups of decaffeinated coffee do you drink per day?

O Less than 1   O 4 cups
O 1 cup per day   O 5 cups
O 2 cups   O 6 - 10 cups
O 3 cups   O More than 10 cups

---

11. Do you drink tea?

O Yes
O No (If No, go to question 12.)

On the average, how many cups of caffeinated tea do you drink per day?

O Less than 1   O 4 cups
O 1 cup per day   O 5 cups
O 2 cups   O 6 - 10 cups
O 3 cups   O More than 10 cups

On the average, how many cups of decaffeinated tea do you drink per day?

O Less than 1   O 4 cups
O 1 cup per day   O 5 cups
O 2 cups   O 6 - 10 cups
O 3 cups   O More than 10 cups

---

12. Do you drink cola or soft drinks?

O Yes
O No (If No, go to next section.)

On the average, how many cans/glasses of caffeinated cola or soft drinks do you drink per day?

O Less than 1   O 4 cans
O 1 can per day   O 5 cans
O 2 cans   O 6 - 10 cans
O 3 cans   O More than 10 cans

On the average, how many cans/glasses of decaffeinated cola or soft drinks do you drink per day?

O Less than 1   O 4 cans
O 1 can per day   O 5 cans
O 2 cans   O 6 - 10 cans
O 3 cans   O More than 10 cans

Continue on Next Page

EDQ - continued, pg. 15

L. FAMILY MEMBERS

1.

	NAME	AGE IF LIVING	CAUSE OF DEATH	AGE AT DEATH
FATHER				
MOTHER				
BROTHERS & SISTERS				
SPOUSE				
CHILD 1				
CHILD 2				
CHILD 3				
CHILD 4				

2. Are you a twin?   ○ Yes   ○ No

(If Yes, is your twin identical?   ____Yes   ____No)

3. Were you adopted?   ○ Yes   ○ No

(If Yes, at what age were you adopted? _____)

M. FAMILY MEDICAL AND PSYCHIATRIC HISTORY

1. Fill in the circle in the column of any of your *blood relatives* who has, or has had, the following conditions or problems:

   * Include half brothers/half sisters

Columns: MOTHER | FATHER | *BROTHERS | *SISTERS | UNCLES | AUNTS | GRANDPARENTS | CHILDREN

CONDITIONS

CONDITIONS	M	F	B	S	U	A	G	C
Alcoholism or Drug Abuse	○	○	○	○	○	○	○	○
Anorexia Nervosa	○	○	○	○	○	○	○	○
Anxiety	○	○	○	○	○	○	○	○
Arthritis/Rheumatism	○	○	○	○	○	○	○	○
Asthma, Hay Fever, or Allergies	○	○	○	○	○	○	○	○
Binge Eating	○	○	○	○	○	○	○	○
Birth Defects	○	○	○	○	○	○	○	○
Bleeding Problems	○	○	○	○	○	○	○	○
Bulimia Nervosa	○	○	○	○	○	○	○	○
Cataracts	○	○	○	○	○	○	○	○
Cancer or Leukemia	○	○	○	○	○	○	○	○
Colitis	○	○	○	○	○	○	○	○
Deafness	○	○	○	○	○	○	○	○
Depression	○	○	○	○	○	○	○	○
Diabetes	○	○	○	○	○	○	○	○
Drug Abuse	○	○	○	○	○	○	○	○
Epilepsy (seizures, fits)	○	○	○	○	○	○	○	○
Eczema	○	○	○	○	○	○	○	○
Gall Bladder Malfunction	○	○	○	○	○	○	○	○
Gambling	○	○	○	○	○	○	○	○
Glaucoma	○	○	○	○	○	○	○	○
Gout	○	○	○	○	○	○	○	○
Heart Attack	○	○	○	○	○	○	○	○
Heart Disease	○	○	○	○	○	○	○	○
Hyperlipidemia (excessive fat in blood)	○	○	○	○	○	○	○	○

CONDITIONS

CONDITIONS	M	F	B	S	U	A	G	C
Hypertension (high blood pressure)	○	○	○	○	○	○	○	○
Jail or Prison	○	○	○	○	○	○	○	○
Kidney Disease	○	○	○	○	○	○	○	○
Liver Cirrhosis	○	○	○	○	○	○	○	○
Manic Depression (Bipolar)	○	○	○	○	○	○	○	○
Mental Retardation	○	○	○	○	○	○	○	○
Migraine or Sick Headaches	○	○	○	○	○	○	○	○
Nerve Diseases (Parkinson's, MS, etc.)	○	○	○	○	○	○	○	○
Obesity (overweight)	○	○	○	○	○	○	○	○
Psychiatric Hospitalization	○	○	○	○	○	○	○	○
Thyroid Disease/Goiter	○	○	○	○	○	○	○	○
Pernicious Anemia	○	○	○	○	○	○	○	○
Psychosis	○	○	○	○	○	○	○	○
Rheumatic Fever	○	○	○	○	○	○	○	○
Schizophrenia	○	○	○	○	○	○	○	○
Sickle Cell Disease	○	○	○	○	○	○	○	○
Stroke	○	○	○	○	○	○	○	○
Suicide Attempt	○	○	○	○	○	○	○	○
Suicide (completed)	○	○	○	○	○	○	○	○
Syphilis	○	○	○	○	○	○	○	○
Tuberculosis (TB)	○	○	○	○	○	○	○	○
Other Glandular Diseases	○	○	○	○	○	○	○	○
Ulcers	○	○	○	○	○	○	○	○
Yellow Jaundice	○	○	○	○	○	○	○	○
Other: _____	○	○	○	○	○	○	○	○

EDQ 9.0. Copyright © 2004, The Neuropsychiatric Research Institute. Used with permission.

Continue on Next Page

EDQ - continued, pg. 16

2. If any of your *blood relatives* have not had ANY of the above conditions or problems, please indicate here:

O Mother   O Brothers   O Uncles   O Grandparents
O Father   O Sisters   O Aunts   O Children

N. MEDICATION HISTORY

1. What medications are you now taking?

MEDICATION NAME	DOSAGE	HOW LONG HAVE YOU BEEN TAKING THIS MEDICATION?

2. What drugs, medications, or shots are you allergic to?

MEDICATION/DRUG/SHOT NAME	REACTION

O. SOCIAL HISTORY

1. Highest level achieved in school (choose one):

O 8th grade or less   O College graduate
O Some high school   O Graduate study
O High school graduate   O Graduate degree
O Trade or technical school   O Post-graduate degree
O Some college

Specify highest degree attained:

O M.D./D.O.
O Ph.D./Psy.D./Ed.D.
O Pharm.D.
O M.A. or M.S.
O B.A. or B.S.
O B.S.N.
O Other: _____

2. Are you now employed?   O Yes O No   If No, when were you last employed? _____

3. Current occupation or last work if now unemployed: _____

4. Were you ever in the armed services?   O Yes O No

Years of service (from when to when?) _____   Highest rank achieved _____

5. Have you ever been arrested? O Yes O No

Age(s) when arrested: Reason(s) for arrest: Did you spend time in jail?

_____   _____   _____

_____   _____   _____

Continue on Next Page

EDQ - continued, pg. 17

P. MEDICAL CHECKLIST

Fill in the circle of any of the following that you have experienced during the last four weeks. You should indicate items which are very noticeable to you and not those things which, even if present, are minor.

GENERAL:
- O Severe loss of appetite
- O Severe weakness
- O Fever
- O Chills
- O Heavy sweats
- O Heavy night sweats - bed linens wet
- O Fatigue
- O Sudden change in sleep

SKIN:
- O Itching
- O Easy bruising that represents a change in the way you normally bruise
- O Sores
- O Marked dryness
- O Hair fragile - comes out in comb
- O Hair has become fine and silky
- O Hair has become coarse and brittle

HEAD:
- O Struck on head - knocked out
- O Frequent dizziness that makes you stop your normal activity and lasts at least 5 minutes
- O Headaches that are different from those you normally have
- O Headaches that awaken you
- O Headaches with vomiting

EYES:
- O Pain in your eyes
- O Need new glasses
- O Seeing double
- O Loss of part of your vision
- O Seeing flashing lights or forms
- O Seeing halos around lights

EARS:
- O Pain in your ears
- O Ringing in your ears
- O Change in hearing
- O Room spins around you

NOSE:
- O Bleeding
- O Pain
- O Cannot breathe well
- O Unusual smells

MOUTH:
- O Toothache
  Soreness or bleeding of:
  - O Lips
  - O Tongue
  - O Gums
- O Unusual tastes
- O Hoarseness

NECK:
- O Pain
- O Cannot move well
- O Lumps
- O Difficulty swallowing
- O Pain on swallowing

NODES:
- O Swollen or tender lymph nodes (Kernals)

BREASTS:
- O Pain
- O New lumps
- O Discharge from nipples

LUNGS:
- O Pain in chest
- O Pain when you take a deep breath
- O New cough
- O Coughing up blood
- O Green, white, or yellow phlegm
- O Wheezing
- O Short of breath (sudden)
- O Wake up at night - can't catch breath
- O Unable to climb stairs

HEART:
- O Pain behind breastbone
- O Pain behind left nipple
- O Pain on left side of neck or jaw
- O Heart racing
- O Heart thumps and misses beats
- O Short of breath when walking
- O Need 2 or more pillows to sleep
- O Legs and ankles swelling (not with menstrual period)
- O Blue lips/fingers/toes when indoors and warm

GASTRO-INTESTINAL:
- O Have lost all desire to eat
- O Food makes me ill
- O Cannot swallow normally
- O Pain on swallowing
- O Food comes halfway up again
- O Sudden persistent heartburn
- O Pain or discomfort after eating
- O Bloating
- O Sharp, stabbing pains in side or shoulder after eating

Continue on Next Page

EDQ - continued, pg. 18

GENITO-URINARY:
O Stabbing pain in back by lower ribs
O Urinating much more frequently
O Sudden awakening at night to urinate
O Passing much more urine
O Not making much urine
O Unable to start to urinate
O Must go to urinate quickly or afraid of losing
   urine
O Pain on urination
O Wetting yourself
O Blood in urine
O Pus in urine

NEUROLOGICAL:
O Fainting
O Fits
O Weakness in arms or legs
O Change in speech
O Loss of coordination
O Sudden periods or onset of confusion
O Sudden changes in personality (suddenly not the
   same person)
O Loss of ability to concentrate
O Seeing things
O Loss of touch
O Tingling in arms or legs
O Unable to chew properly
O Memory loss
O Tremulous or shaky

MALE:
O Pain in testicles
O Swelling of testicles
O Swelling of scrotum

FEMALE:
O Sudden change in periods
O Between-periods bleeding

LIST ANY OTHERS NOT MENTIONED ABOVE:
_____
_____
_____

3

Eating Disorders and Psychiatric Comorbidity

Prevalence and Treatment Modifications

Randy A. Sansone, M.D.

Lori A. Sansone, M.D.

Patients with eating disorders appear to have high rates, as well as wide ranges, of psychiatric comorbidity (Hudson et al. 2005, 2007). The most prevalent Axis I disorders seem to be mood and anxiety disorders, followed by alcohol and substance abuse and bipolar disorder. Axis II disorders are commonplace as well. In this chapter, we briefly review exemplary studies relating to the prevalence rates of comorbidity and then recommend eating disorder treatment modifications for several common comorbid psychiatric disorders. We believe that the effective management of comorbid psychiatric conditions will ultimately enhance the overall treatment response in these polysymptomatic patients.

Prevalence of Axis I and Axis II Disorders in Patients With Eating Disorders

To provide a sense of psychiatric comorbidity loadings among patients with eating disorders, we offer the following examples of prevalence studies, beginning with those relating to mood disorders.

Mood Disorders

Anorexia Nervosa

Mood disorders are fairly common among patients with anorexia nervosa. Milos and colleagues (2003) examined 77 women with anorexia nervosa and found that 53% had a comorbid affective disorder. In a review of the literature, Pearlstein (2002) found that the lifetime prevalence of major depression in patients with restricting anorexia nervosa and binge-eating/purging anorexia nervosa was 15%–50% and 46%–80%, respectively, and that the lifetime prevalence of dysthymia in patients with anorexia nervosa was 19%–93%.

Bulimia Nervosa

Brewerton and colleagues (1995) examined 59 adult female patients with bulimia nervosa and found that 75% had an affective disorder, with 63% having major depression. Milos and colleagues (2003) examined 137 women with bulimia nervosa and found that 52% had an affective disorder. In a review of the literature, Pearlstein (2002) found that the lifetime prevalence rates of major depression and dysthymia in bulimia nervosa were 50%–65% and 6%–95%, respectively.

Unspecified Diagnosis

Striegel-Moore and colleagues (1999) examined 161 female veterans with eating disorders and found that 60% had comorbid diagnoses of affective disorders.

Bipolar Disorder

As with other Axis I mood disorders, higher-than-expected rates of bipolar disorder have been reported among eating disorder patients (Kawa et al. 2005; Krishnan 2005; McElroy et al. 2005).

Anxiety Disorders

Any Anxiety Disorders

Anorexia nervosa.   Among study samples with restricting and binge-eating/purging anorexia nervosa, Iwasaki and colleagues (1999) found prevalence rates for *any* anxiety disorder to be 24% and 71%, respectively. Bulik and colleagues (1997) found similarly high rates of anxiety disorders among 68 individuals with anorexia (60%). In a 2002 literature review, Godart and colleagues analyzed the lifetime prevalence rates for anxiety disorders in restricting and binge-eating/purging anorexia nervosa and found rates of 33%–72% and 55%, respectively. Finally, Kaye and colleagues (2004) found rates for generalized anxiety disorder (GAD) and panic disorder of 13% and 9%, respectively, in patients with restricting anorexia nervosa and 10% and 11%, respectively, in patients with binge-eating/purging anorexia nervosa.

Bulimia nervosa.   Among a sample of patients with bulimia, Brewerton and colleagues (1995) found prevalence rates for *any* anxiety disorder, social phobia, GAD, and panic disorder to be 36%, 17%, 12%, and 10%, respectively. Iwasaki and colleagues (1999) found that the prevalence rate for *any* anxiety disorder was 58%. Bulik and colleagues (1997) found high rates of anxiety disorders among 116 bulimic patients (57%). In a 2002 literature review, Godart and colleagues found that lifetime prevalence rates for anxiety disorders in patients with bulimia nervosa ranged from 41% to 75%. Finally, Kaye and colleagues (2004) found prevalence rates of 8% and 11% for GAD and panic disorder, respectively, in patients with bulimia.

Unspecified diagnosis.   In their patient sample of veterans with eating disorders, Striegel-Moore and colleagues (1999) found the comorbid prevalence of *any* anxiety disorder to be 36%.

Obsessive-Compulsive Disorder

Investigators have also examined the prevalence of obsessive-compulsive disorder (OCD) among individuals with eating disorders.

Anorexia nervosa.   Kaye and colleagues (2004) found that 35% of their sample of individuals with restricting anorexia had OCD, compared with 44% of those with binge-eating/purging anorexia. Speranza and colleagues (2001) examined individuals with restricting anorexia and purging anorexia and found current and lifetime rates for OCD of 19% and 22%, and 29% and 43%, respectively. Milos and colleagues (2002) examined the prevalence of comorbid OCD among 84 anorexia patients and found a prevalence rate of 29%. In a literature review, Pearlstein (2002) found that 11%–69% of women with anorexia nervosa had either OCD or obsessional personality characteristics. Finally, in their literature review, Godart and colleagues (2002) found the lifetime prevalence rates for OCD among women with restricting anorexia nervosa and binge-eating/purging anorexia nervosa to be 10%–62% and 10%–66%, respectively.

Bulimia nervosa.   Kaye and colleagues (2004) found that 40% of their sample of bulimia patients had OCD. Speranza and colleagues (2001) determined current and lifetime rates of OCD among bulimic individuals to be 10% and 13%, respectively. Milos and colleagues (2002) examined the prevalence of comorbid OCD among 84 bulimia patients and found a rate of 30%. In a literature review, Pearlstein (2002) found that 3%–43% of women with bulimia nervosa had either OCD or obsessional personality characteristics. Finally, in their literature review, Godart and colleagues (2002) found the lifetime prevalence rate for OCD among women with bulimia nervosa to be between 0% and 43%.

Alcohol and Substance Abuse

While mood and anxiety disorders are associated with the highest rates of psychiatric comorbidity among eating disorder patients, other types of comorbidity, including alcohol and substance abuse/dependence, have been examined as well.

Anorexia Nervosa

Bulik and colleagues (2004) explored rates of alcohol abuse, dependence, and both abuse and dependence in a sample of 97 individuals with restricting anorexia and reported prevalence rates of 10%, 10%, and 17%, respectively; for individuals with binge-eating/purging anorexia, the corresponding rates were 15%, 28%, and 38%. Jordan and colleagues (2003) examined anorexic individuals for alcohol abuse or dependence and reported a rate of 28%.

Milos and colleagues (2003) reported the lifetime prevalence of any substance-related disorder in anorexia to be 22%. Jordan and colleagues (2003) examined anorexic individuals for cannabis abuse or dependence and any lifetime psychoactive substance use disorder and reported corresponding rates of 20% and 33%, respectively. Finally, in Pearlstein's (2002) review, lifetime prevalence rates of substance abuse in anorexia nervosa ranged from 12% to 18%.

Bulimia Nervosa

Bulik and colleagues (2004) examined bulimic individuals for alcohol abuse, dependence, and both abuse and dependence and reported corresponding rates of 25%, 26%, and 46%—rates that were considerably higher than the rates encountered in their samples of anorexic individuals.

With regard to substance abuse, Brewerton and colleagues (1995) reported a rate of 20% among individuals with bulimia nervosa. Milos and colleagues found the lifetime prevalence of any substance-related disorder in patients with bulimia to be 26%. Finally, in the review by Pearlstein (2002), lifetime prevalence rates of substance abuse in bulimia nervosa ranged from 30% to 70%.

Unspecified Diagnosis

Striegel-Moore and colleagues (1999) reported substance abuse rates of 33% in a sample of veterans with eating disorders.

Other Axis I Disorders

Among 164 eating disorder patients, Turnbull and colleagues (1997) found that 11% had posttraumatic stress disorder (PTSD). In a sample of 26 individuals with restricting anorexia, Lilenfeld and colleagues (1998) found that 8% of the sample had PTSD.

Limitations of Axis I Data Comparisons

We have not included all comorbidity studies in these various Axis I areas, because we quickly realized that methodological issues hampered any reasonable scientific comparison, which explains the wide ranges in findings. These methodological issues include sample variability (e.g., inpatient versus outpatient, primary- versus tertiary-care treatment settings), varying assessment tools for Axis I diagnoses, controlled and noncontrolled studies, recruitment variability, and various types of prevalence rates (e.g., point vs. lifetime). Therefore, we elected to highlight comorbidity *themes* rather than attempt to compare and analyze conglomerate data. However, our conclusion is that eating disorders are highly comorbid with other Axis I psychiatric disorders, particularly mood and anxiety disorders, although the *explicit* comorbidity rates remain empirically unknown.

Axis II Disorders

We recently reviewed the literature on the prevalence of Axis II disorders among individuals with eating disorders (Sansone et al. 2005); our findings are summarized in Figures 3–1 through 3–3.

Anorexia Nervosa

In restricting anorexia nervosa, the most frequent Axis II disorder is obsessive-compulsive personality disorder (22%), followed by avoidant personality disorder (19%). In the binge-eating/purging type of anorexia nervosa, the most common Axis II disorder is borderline personality disorder (BPD) (26%), followed by avoidant personality disorder (17%).

Bulimia Nervosa

In bulimia nervosa, the most common Axis II disorder is BPD (28%), followed by dependent (21%), histrionic (20%), and avoidant (19%) personality disorders. It appears that the eating disorders with impulsive eating pathology (i.e., binge eating, purging) tend to be associated with relatively high rates of BPD.

Treatment Modifications for Comorbid Psychiatric Disorders and Eating Disorders

In this section, we highlight the major treatment modifications in eating disorder patients with various types of Axis I and Axis II comorbidities. Because of space limitations, we cannot overview the general treatment for these individual comorbidities. However, for each comorbid condition, we describe up to three areas of modification in patients with eating disorders: 1) assessment; 2) psychotherapy intervention; and 3) psychotropic medications. We also provide general recommendations for hospitalization.

Comorbid Axis I Disorders and Eating Disorders

To illustrate the complexities often encountered in clinical practice, we offer the following case vignette, illustrating the co-occurrence of eating disorders and mood disorders and other Axis I conditions.

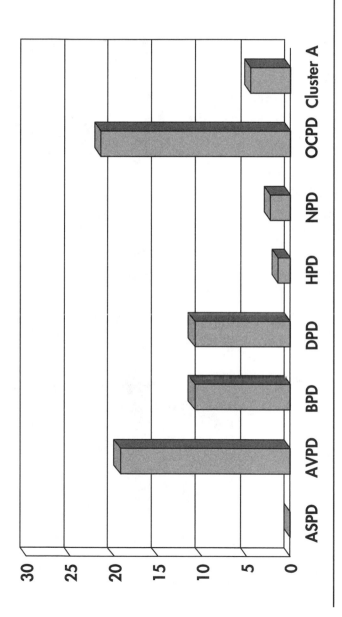

Figure 3–1. Prevalence (%) of personality disorders in anorexia nervosa, restricting type.

Note. ASPD = antisocial; AVPD = avoidant; BPD = borderline; DPD = dependent; HPD = histrionic; NPD = narcissistic; OCPD = obsessive-compulsive.

Source. Sansone et al. 2005.

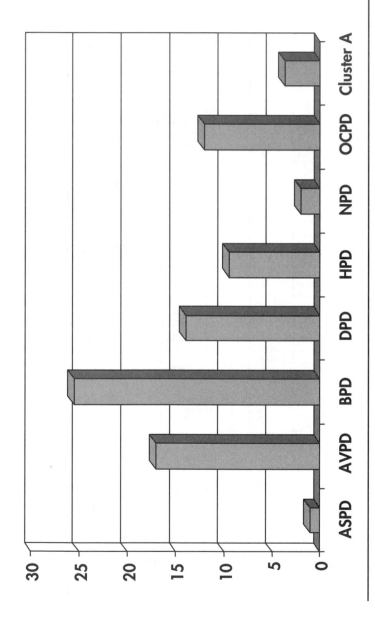

Figure 3–2. Prevalence (%) of personality disorders in anorexia nervosa, binge-eating/purging type.

Note. ASPD=antisocial; AVPD=avoidant; BPD=borderline; DPD=dependent; HPD=histrionic; NPD=narcissistic; OCPD = obsessive-compulsive.

Source. Sansone et al. 2005.

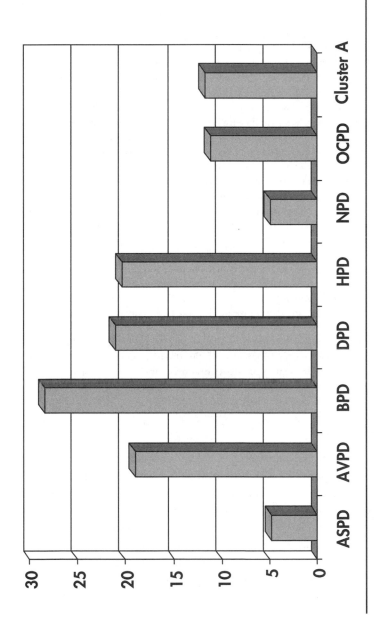

Figure 3–3.   Prevalence (%) of personality disorders in bulimia nervosa.

Note.   ASPD=antisocial; AVPD=avoidant; BPD=borderline; DPD=dependent; HPD=histrionic; NPD=narcissistic; OCPD = obsessive-compulsive.

Source.   Sansone et al. 2005.

Clinical Vignette

Carla, an 18-year-old high school senior, was diagnosed with bipolar I disorder at age 13 and anorexia nervosa, binge/purge type, at age 14, at which point her body mass index dropped from 21 to 16. Her family included several close relatives with severe mood and anxiety disorders. As a child, Carla was described as "hyper," "irritable," and "violently volatile" at times, and as extremely moody, shy, withdrawn, and fearful at other times. Her ability to concentrate in school was impaired. She was extremely concerned about social evaluation and had strong visceral reactions to the idea that peers might be gossiping about her. She had frequent frank panic attacks in school settings, sometimes in anticipation of public speaking. In addition to constant ruminations concerning body shape and weight, Carla also acknowledged preoccupations with other "body defects," particularly what she thought to be her fat ankles. She was highly phobic about insects and fearful of germs and contamination. In addition to her earlier diagnoses, she also merited diagnoses of GAD with panic, social phobia, OCD, and body dysmorphic disorder. Attention-deficit disorder was considered. Personality traits included features consistent with Cluster B and C conditions.

The treatment program included weekly individual psychotherapy (with elements drawn from cognitive-behavioral, interpersonal, and psychodynamic schools), weekly family therapy, dietary counseling, and a complex medication regimen that included, ultimately, valproic acid 1,000 mg/day, lamotrigine 100 mg/day, fluoxetine 80 mg/day, and mixed amphetamine salts sustained-release 20 mg/day for daytime fatigue and attention-concentration difficulties. This program empirically evolved over months of trial and error. With this regimen, Carla's mood and eating disorder symptoms, and symptoms of all of the aforementioned anxiety disorders, ameliorated substantially, and she was able to achieve A's and B's in advanced high school courses and to maintain a steady relationship with a suitable boyfriend.

Mood Disorders

Assessment of anorexia nervosa.   The nutritional effects of dieting and starvation can complicate the assessment of mood disorders in individuals with eating disorders characterized by dieting and weight loss. For example, dieting, alone, tends to produce mood lability, and experimental starvation has resulted in irritability, dysphoria, and a deterioration in social behavior (Keys et al. 1950). In minimizing these nutritional effects on mood assessment in anorexia nervosa, it is most clinically feasible, we believe, to assess underlying mood disorders when the patient's weight is within 10% of a normal weight for height.

Assessment of bulimia nervosa. Because of the concern about the nutritional effects of dieting and starvation on mood in patients with bulimia nervosa, we believe that it is most feasible to assess for mood disorders when reasonable nutritional stabilization occurs. However, in both anorexia nervosa and bulimia nervosa patients, these recommendations are not meant to exclude the meaningful diagnosis of mood disorders among individuals with active eating disorder symptoms when dramatic depressive symptoms are present.

Psychotherapy. With comorbid mood disorders, we generally recommend the addition of cognitive-behavioral therapy (CBT) for depression. CBT for depression has been effective in the treatment of both children and adolescents (Compton et al. 2004) as well as adults. This technique entails the systematic elicitation of faulty or pathology-promoting thought patterns, identification of these patterns with the patient, restructuring of the content of the thoughts, and ongoing self-monitoring. Most forms of CBT include education about the process itself. This type of intervention can be provided by the therapist or in book form (we provide a booklist to patients) and is also available as electronic products (e.g., CD-ROM). We do not promote a single book or training program, as the content of each varies. Some programs are in workbook format with high levels of interaction with the reader, whereas others are more focused, concentrated, and didactic. We suggest to patients that they peruse the available offerings and elect the approach that most suits their needs.

In addition to CBT, which can be used with most patients, interpersonal psychotherapy is effective in the treatment of depression (de Mello et al. 2005; Roelofs and Muris 2005) and has been empirically effective in adolescent populations (Mufson et al. 2004). Other approaches to psychotherapy may be used as well. For more psychologically developed or mature patients, psychodynamic approaches may be useful. Problem-solving approaches may be effective in specific patients, particularly for those in time-limited treatment or in patients who are uninterested in psychodynamic intervention. Supportive psychotherapy may be an adjunctive intervention to the aforementioned psychotherapy approaches or may be employed alone in treating lower-functioning or medically compromised patients. In clinical practice, we sense that most clinicians use a combination of approaches (i.e., an eclectic approach) that includes cognitive-behavioral, interpersonal, supportive, psychodynamic, and problem-solving elements, and titrate these approaches on the basis of their experience with the patient.

Medications. Although all antidepressants are effective in the treatment of mood disorders, we avoid those that may result in weight gain, such as paroxetine, mirtazapine, most tricyclic antidepressants (TCAs), and monoamine oxidase inhibitors (MAOIs). On an additional precautionary note, TCAs can accentuate any underlying cardiovascular symptoms because of their tendency to cause tachycardia and orthostatic hypotension. Although effective, MAOIs are not routinely advised in anorexic patients because of these patients' young age or in bulimic patients because of the inability to guarantee careful food scrutiny during binge-eating episodes.

In general, relatively weight-neutral selective serotonin reuptake inhibitors (SSRIs)—namely, sertraline, citalopram, and fluoxetine—are our antidepressants of first choice because of their efficacy in mood disorders and their antiobsessive effects. The next preferred medication is venlafaxine extended-release. When augmentation strategies are indicated (i.e., the addition of a second drug to enhance the efficacy of the antidepressant), we avoid those that cause weight gain, such as valproate, lithium, and olanzapine, and elect to use buspirone, low-dose gabapentin (e.g., 200–400 mg/day; little risk of weight gain at these dosages), and weight-neutral atypical antipsychotics such as aripiprazole, ziprasidone, and low-dose risperidone. In nutritionally depleted patients, we begin all medications at a low dose and increase the dose slowly. For example, with sertraline, we typically begin at 12.5 mg.

Hospitalization. While moderate to severe mood disorders, alone, are of concern, these may significantly impede the effectiveness of an attempt at outpatient treatment of eating disorder patients, particularly in medically stressed patients (i.e., those metabolically and/or nutritionally depleted). Therefore, we advise clinicians to continually monitor the overall outpatient progress of the patient as well as the cumulative effects of comorbidity. In our experience, comorbidity *always* necessitates addition of another treatment layer and generally tends to impede treatment efforts directed at the eating pathology.

Bipolar Disorder

Assessment. On the basis of self-report alone, bipolar disorder may be difficult to clinically diagnose, because the patient may perceive some symptoms as adaptive (e.g., hypomania in the work environment) and other symptoms as nonpathological (e.g., euphoria, hyperactivity, hypersexuality). To confuse matters, the clinician's query about "highs" is frequently over-endorsed by patients, oftentimes with the misinterpretation of mood lability (i.e., vacillation from normal to dysphoric mood) for "highs and lows."

To add to the preceding diagnostic quagmires, as we have encountered, a number of patients actually have borderline personality and are misdiagnosed with bipolar disorder. Both disorders are characterized by impulsivity and affective instability. However, the impulsivity in bipolar disorder is typically expansive, grandiose, and hedonistically gratifying, whereas in borderline personality, the impulsivity is typically characterized by the need to contain a negative affect, the need to engage others, and/or intentful self-destructive behavior. As for further differences, bipolar patients have distinct euphoric and/or irritable moods that are punctuated by distinct depressed moods (i.e., demarcated or discrete episodes). Borderline patients typically experience fleeting normal moods that are overshadowed by ongoing dysphoria characterized by depression, anxiety, anger, and emptiness (i.e., stable instability). Despite these symptomatic differences, the two disorders can be difficult to differentiate from each other. In addition, both may coexist within the same individual.

Psychotherapy.   In most cases, psychotherapy treatment for eating pathology cannot be successfully undertaken in the bipolar patient until the mood symptoms have undergone reasonable stabilization. There are not any specific psychotherapy modifications in comorbid bipolar patients other than psychoeducation about the nature of this illness; identification of the early signs and symptoms of impending bipolar decompensation, including the development of methods for early detection of recurrent symptoms; and emphasis on the importance of medication compliance. Problem-solving work is frequently indicated in the aftermath of severe manic or depressive episodes along with supportive psychotherapy.

Medications.   Lithium, anticonvulsants, and atypical antipsychotics appear to be the current mainstays of medical treatment for bipolar disorder. In a critical meta-analysis of the literature, Bauer and Mitchner (2004) concluded that only lithium was effective for *both* manic and depressive episodes, and only valproate and olanzapine were effective for acute mania. Despite these evidence-based conclusions, other medications may be helpful in the treatment of bipolar disorder as well.

Lithium, the most effective mood stabilizer for bipolar disorder, is a risky undertaking in eating disorder patients. Any loss of sodium, which may occur with excessive sweating or elevations in body temperature from exercise, can precipitate lithium toxicity. Dehydration from self-induced vomiting, laxatives, and/or diuretics may result in increased lithium concentrations and toxicity as well. At therapeutic doses, lithium may cause abnormalities in the electrocardiogram and, on rare occasions, precipitate cardiac arrhythmias. Lithium is also known for causing weight gain as well as frank hypothyroidism. A potential unforeseen complication is that eating disorder patients with chronically low potassium levels due to weight-regulation efforts (e.g., vomiting, laxatives) may develop hypokalemic nephropathy. This development impairs the ability of the kidney to excrete lithium, and prescription requires careful monitoring of lithium levels to avoid toxicity. In summary, we generally avoid lithium in bipolar individuals with eating disorders.

Anticonvulsants appear to be plausible alternatives for the treatment of bipolar disorder, but their use may be complicated by limited or unknown efficacy with regard to either manic or depressed mood, weight gain, the need for serum levels and ongoing laboratory studies, and unusual side effects. We have summarized the characteristics of several anticonvulsants in Table 3–1 (Nemeroff 2003; Physicians' Desk Reference 2005; Singh et al. 2005; Velez and Selwa 2003). Note that eliminating those anticonvulsants with weight gain and/or unknown efficacy leaves only carbamazepine (difficult to work with because of drug interactions, autoinduction of its own metabolism, and the need for ongoing laboratory studies), topiramate, and lamotrigine. Interestingly, topiramate is a particularly attractive choice in eating disorder patients with bipolar disorder because it has been shown to have some efficacy in the treatment of binge eating in both bulimia nervosa and binge-eating disorder (Marx et al. 2003). However, *topiramate may impair the efficacy of oral contraceptives* (i.e., leading to lower serum levels), but only the ethinyl-estradiol component is affected (Bialer et al. 2004), and only at dosages above 200 mg/day (Bialer et al. 2004; Doose et al. 2003). Topiramate has been placed in pregnancy-risk category C. Lamotrigine is associated with skin rashes (10%) and, on occasion, skin exfoliation (i.e., Stevens-Johnson syndrome, which occurs in 1 in 6,000 patients with bipolar disorder; see Ghaemi 2006). Levetiracetam and zonisamide, both recently approved weight-neutral anticonvulsants, are presently under investigation for the treatment of bipolar disorder.

Table 3–1. Clinical characteristics of lithium and several anticonvulsants

Medication	Efficacy in bipolar disorder	Weight effects	Serum levels	Other
Lithium	+	↑	+	Ongoing laboratory studies
Valproate	+	↑	+	Ongoing laboratory studies
Carbamazepine	+	→	+	Ongoing laboratory studies Multiple drug interactions
Lamotrigine	+	→	?	Ongoing laboratory studies? Skin rashes/exfoliation
Topiramate	±	↓	?	Periodic serum bicarbonate levels
Gabapentin	?	↑	?	—
Tiagabine	?	→	?	Ongoing laboratory studies

Source. Collated from Nemeroff 2003; Physicians' Desk Reference 2005; Singh et al. 2005; Velez and Selwa 2003.

Finally, atypical antipsychotics have been increasingly examined and found to be effective as mood stabilizers in double-blind, placebo-controlled trials (McElroy et al. 2004). The most studied, olanzapine, is complicated by weight gain and potential metabolic abnormalities (i.e., elevations in serum levels of glucose, triglycerides, and cholesterol). The atypical antipsychotics and their respective properties are shown in Table 3–2.

On the basis of available data, topiramate and lamotrigine appear to be reasonable anticonvulsants of choice, given the limitations posed by the clinical characteristics noted in Table 3–1 (e.g., topiramate and oral contraceptives). Despite the availability of these two drugs, prescribers are in need of better anticonvulsant options. As for atypical antipsychotics, aripiprazole, ziprasidone, and risperidone appear to be the drugs of choice in the treatment of eating disorder patients with bipolar disorder. These particular drugs are relatively weight-neutral and are less likely to cause metabolic complications. Various combinations of these medications may be effectively used.

Hospitalization. Clinicians typically consider hospitalization for bipolar patients with psychosis, high-risk dyscontrol, suicidal or homicidal ideation,

Table 3–2.   Clinical characteristics of atypical antipsychotics

Medication	Weight effects	Other
Aripiprazole	None/minimal	Drug interactions
Ziprasidone	None/minimal	QT prolongation; twice-per-day dosing
Risperidone	Mild/moderate ↑	↑ Prolactin
Quetiapine	Mild/moderate ↑	Yearly ophthalmologic examination for cataracts?
Olanzapine	Moderate/high ↑	↑ Glucose, ↑ cholesterol, ↑ triglycerides
Clozapine	High ↑	↑ Glucose, ↑ cholesterol, ↑ triglycerides Sedation Tachycardia ↑ Risk of seizures Agranulocytosis (biweekly blood monitoring) Closed prescribing system (can be prescribed only by psychiatrists)

Source.   Collated from Fraunfelder 2004; Nasrallah and Newcomer 2004; Physicians' Desk Reference 2005; Volavka et al. 2004.

and/or an inability to effectively care for self. When a comorbid eating disorder is present, particularly one with purging behavior, the bipolar-driven impulsivity may exacerbate eating pathology such that acute metabolic compromise (e.g., hypokalemia) becomes a concern. Therefore, we tend to have *lower* symptom thresholds for the hospitalization of bipolar patients who are experiencing recalcitrant purging.

Anxiety Disorders

Assessment.   As described in the preceding section on mood disorders, anxiety symptoms, including acutely emerging panic attacks, tend to be exacerbated by nutritional and starvation effects. Assessment is probably most precise when eating disorder symptoms have improved and stabilized and when the patient's weight is within 10% of her healthy weight for height. However, regardless of weight status, symptoms of concern warrant treatment.

Psychotherapy.   As with mood disorders, we incorporate CBT for the anxiety disorders (i.e., GAD, panic disorder, social phobia), using the same techniques described in the previous section on mood disorders. In addition, like mood disorders, anxiety disorders may also be approached with various types of psychotherapy intervention (e.g., interpersonal therapy, psychodynamic therapy, problem-solving therapy, supportive psychotherapy). The same indications and caveats for these various types of psychotherapy that were discussed in the preceding section on mood disorders generally apply. For example, it might be very impractical to undertake psychodynamic psychotherapy with a 12-year-old patient, who may need more cognitive and supportive intervention. Likewise, most adult patients can potentially benefit from the aforementioned therapies, including psychodynamic intervention.

Medications. In the selection of medications for intervention, SSRIs are our first choices because of their broad therapeutic effects with anxiety symptoms, panic disorder, OCD, and social phobia. Regardless of the patient's weight status, we avoid those medications that cause weight gain (e.g., paroxetine), because it is not possible to strategize an ultimate weight outcome effectively. Buspirone is a possible alternative in individuals with GAD and may be dually helpful in patients with alcohol abuse (see subsection "Alcoholism and Substance Abuse" later in this section). Recently, in our anxiety patients, we have been successfully augmenting antidepressant therapy with gabapentin, which at low dosages (100–300 mg/day) has minimal effects on body weight. We generally avoid benzodiazepines in the treatment of anxiety disorders because of the risks of cognitive impairment (particularly problematic in low-weight patients) and physiological addiction. In addition, in patients with Cluster B personality disorders, the prescription of benzodiazepines may result in medication misuse and abuse as well as behavioral disinhibition.

Hospitalizaton. Surprisingly, we have rarely hospitalized eating disorder patients because of severe anxiety symptoms alone. Although these symptoms are common, they seem to rarely warrant hospitalization.

Obsessive-Compulsive Disorder

Psychotherapy. Because of the high prevalence of OCD in eating disorder populations, this anxiety disorder warrants specific mention. CBT is the recommended psychotherapy intervention for OCD (Clark 2004).

Medications. SSRIs are first-line medications in the treatment of OCD (Dougherty et al. 2004; Eddy et al. 2004). Doses are usually titrated to the recommended maximums, and drug trials are typically 12 weeks in duration. If SSRIs are ineffective, we undertake a drug trial with clomipramine, a TCA, despite the potential risk of weight gain. Again, we typically titrate doses to the recommended upper limit; drug trials are 12 weeks in duration. Interestingly, some data indicate that clomipramine may be more effective than SSRIs in the treatment of OCD; however, it remains unclear whether this advantage holds in head-to-head drug trials (Fineberg and Gale 2005).

Note that not all antidepressants are effective in the treatment of OCD; those with strong serotonergic effects appear most likely to be effective. For example, whereas bupropion, a noradrenergic-dopaminergic drug, is ineffective (Vulink et al. 2005), mirtazapine, a serotonergic-noradrenergic drug, may hold some promise (Koran et al. 2005).

When augmentation of a partially effective antidepressant is indicated, we recommend small doses of a weight-neutral atypical antipsychotic (Keuneman et al. 2005), such as aripiprazole, ziprasidone, or risperidone.

Alcoholism and Substance Abuse

Assessment.   In eating disorder patients with alcohol or substance abuse issues, which are more likely in individuals with impulsive eating pathology (i.e., binging, purging), we strongly recommend an adjunctive assessment for BPD. In a 1994 study comparing three study cells of women—those with eating disorder alone, substance abuse alone, and both disorders—we found, using a semistructured research interview, that the prevalence rates for BPD were 36%, 36%, and 94%, respectively (Sansone et al. 1994). This finding suggests that the presence of both impulsive eating pathology and alcohol/substance abuse heighten, to a considerable degree, the likelihood of comorbid BPD.

Psychotherapy.   Among eating disorder patients with comorbid alcohol or substance abuse, we generally favor the initial treatment of the alcohol/substance abuse, followed by eating disorder treatment (Sansone and Dennis 1996). A traditional 12-step approach is typically effective and reasonably compatible with subsequent eating disorder treatment.

After treatment for alcohol/substance abuse, the timing and components of eating disorder treatment are a consideration. Given the potentially regressive nature of a psychological treatment, we either 1) delay eating disorder treatment until the alcohol/substance abuse issues are under sustained control (e.g., the attainment of 6 months of sobriety) or 2) initiate eating disorder treatment in the immediate aftermath of alcohol/substance abuse treatment but focus on psychoeducation, cognitive-behavioral techniques, supportive psychotherapy, and nutritional management (i.e., we delay intensive psychological work because of the potential for psychological regression and a lapse in sobriety). In the latter scenario, only after stabilization of the alcohol/substance abuse is confirmed do we initiate intensive psychological work.

Medications for alcohol abuse. The U.S. Food and Drug Administration (FDA) has approved only three medications for the treatment of alcohol dependence: disulfiram, naltrexone, and acamprosate. Of these, only naltrexone has been studied in the treatment of eating disorders, and only in bulimia nervosa. Naltrexone, an opioid antagonist, does not appear to be superior to placebo in the treatment of bulimic symptoms ("Practice Guideline for the Treatment of Patients With Eating Disorders [Revision]" 2000). To date, we have not used naltrexone in these dually diagnosed patients.

As for nonapproved medications that might be efficacious in alcohol abuse, only topiramate and buspirone appear to be relevant candidates with regard to eating disorder treatment. Topiramate may decrease daily drinking as well as enhance abstinence (Johnson et al. 2003). Buspirone appears to decrease alcohol craving and other drinking behaviors (Bruno 1989) but may not affect overall alcohol consumption (Malec et al. 1996). Interestingly, buspirone was recently found to be effective in the treatment of opioid withdrawal as well (Buydens-Branchey et al. 2005). Both of these medications are used primarily for the augmentation of antidepressant therapy.

Medications for substance abuse. Psychostimulants, including cocaine, may be abused to control food intake and body weight in individuals with eating disorders. Although the FDA has approved no medication for cocaine addiction, several are currently under investigation (O'Brien 2005). These include disulfiram, modafinil, propranolol, topiramate, and vigabatrin. Again, topiramate may be cross-utilized in eating disorder patients to reduce binge-eating behavior. The remaining medications have undergone limited, if any, investigation with regard to their effects on eating pathology.

Hospitalization. The treatment locale for alcohol and/or substance abuse (e.g., inpatient, partial hospital, intensive outpatient) is determined on the basis of symptom severity. The exception to this general guideline is when, during inpatient treatment for alcohol/substance abuse, the eating disorder symptoms derail the intervention, which is less clinically common than the converse. Following acute inpatient alcohol/substance abuse treatment, we recommend continuing care in a 12-step program. Many women patients prefer 12-step meetings with a predominance of women. In some locales, women with both eating disorders and alcohol/substance abuse congregate at specific meetings.

Comorbid Axis II Disorders and Eating Disorders

The following vignette illustrates a not untypical patient who presents with a combination of eating disorders, other Axis I disorders, and a variety of Axis II disorders as well.

Clinical Vignette

Rachel was a 24-year-old single woman who had suffered from bipolar II disorder with several episodes of major depression from her early teens and bulimia nervosa since age 15. She was anxious in most situations and experienced frank panic attacks several times yearly. Her parents described her as having been "high-strung" and "thin-skinned" from early childhood, characteristics that her father acknowledged she shared with her well-intentioned but inconsistent mother. Her many romantic relationships had been stormy, occasionally violently physical, and dramatic and usually lasted no longer than 3 months. Although she had graduated from a good university with a degree in marketing, as a result of her marked irritability and temper she was fired from several jobs and impulsively quit several others. Easily frustrated, she sometimes cut or burned her skin for relief and shopped compulsively. In her late teens she had had several episodes of frequent "partying," including binge drinking, binge cocaine abuse, and impulsive sex, resulting in genital herpes. In addition to the Axis I disorders described above, her presentation met the criteria for mixed Cluster B disorders as well, with prominent borderline and narcissistic features.

Treatment included frequent individual therapy with elements derived from CBT, interpersonal therapy, some family and couples sessions, consultation with a registered dietician, and, intermittently, group therapy and meetings of Alcoholics Anonymous. Early in her treatment, in the pre-SSRI era, she benefited considerably from treatment with phenelzine 60 mg/day and initially followed the dietary requirements very closely. However, after she demonstrated serious indiscretion by abusing cocaine while taking the phenelzine, despite clear prior education about the dangers, and consequently experienced several days of delirium, the medication was discontinued. She subsequently benefited from a combination of fluoxetine 40 mg/day and trazodone 100 mg hs, and she continued in long-term psychotherapy. Subsequently in treatment she was also referred to a group program emphasizing dialectical behavior therapy (DBT). A 10-year follow-up revealed that Rachel had continued to take fluoxetine regularly, been able to sustain employment, married and had two children, and divorced after 6 years of marriage and, subsequently, seemed able with the assistance of her family to provide good care for her children and to resume other relationships with less turmoil than previously. Although she was still bothered by negative thoughts about her body, she no longer binged or purged.

Borderline Personality Disorder

Assessment.   BPD is the most common Axis II diagnosis among those with eating disorders, particularly among individuals with impulsive eating pathology. Because the diagnosis of BPD is potentially stigmatizing, we urge careful assessment in individuals with eating disorders. Vitousek and Stumpf (2005) describe the general difficulties with objective personality assessment in persons with eating disorders, including confusion about state versus trait symptoms (e.g., the intensifying effects of Axis I disorders on Axis II symptoms), the limited self-objectivity of adolescents, the misleading symptomatic effects of starvation (e.g., mood lability), and the psychological dynamics of denial and distortion in self-assessment. For these reasons, we strongly encourage detailed diagnostic assessment, with particular attention to those symptoms and behaviors that are not directly related to food, body, and weight issues (e.g., suicide attempts, self-cutting).

In our clinical assessment of BPD, we frequently augment the DSM (*Diagnostic and Statistical Manual of Mental Disorders*) diagnosis with findings from other diagnostic tools. These include a modified version of the original Diagnostic Interview for Borderlines (DIB; Kolb and Gunderson 1980), an interview strategy, and several self-report measures. In our modification of the DIB, we have rearranged the five diagnostic areas of assessment into the acronym PISIA (Table 3–3). Using these criteria for diagnosis via a semi-structured interview, there must be one type of psychotic or quasi-psychotic phenomenon, long-standing impulsivity characterized by both self-regulation difficulties *and* self-harm behavior, a reasonably intact social facade, chaotic and unfulfilling interpersonal relationships, and chronic affective disturbance with mood lability and/or dysphoria.

As for self-report measures, we suggest the Self-Harm Inventory (SHI; Sansone et al. 1998; Figure 3–4), the borderline personality scale of the Personality Diagnostic Questionnaire–4 (PDQ-4; S.E. Hyler, unpublished, 1994), or the McLean Screening Instrument for Borderline Personality Disorder (MSI-BPD; Zanarini et al. 2003). These measures are brief (one page in length), easily scored, and useful *adjuncts* to clinical diagnosis, albeit somewhat overly inclusive. On the SHI, the endorsement of five or more "yes" items is highly suggestive of BPD, with a diagnostic accuracy of 85% in relationship to the DIB (Sansone et al. 1998).

Psychotherapy.   According to the "Practice Guideline for the Treatment of Patients With Borderline Personality Disorder" (2001), "the primary treatment for borderline personality disorder is psychotherapy" (p. 4). The psychotherapy strategy in BPD focuses on enhancing overall self-regulation (including eating disorder symptomatology), reducing self-harm behavior, improving interpersonal relationships, and alleviating affective instability. Because BPD is a multidetermined and very heterogeneous disorder, a single psychotherapy approach is not likely to meet the needs of all eating disorder patients with this Axis II diagnosis. In addition, no treatment approach to BPD has been empirically proven to be superior to other approaches (i.e., there are no comparison trials in the literature).

It is our impression that most BPD treatment techniques consist of various components, frequently including contracting, psychoeducation, transference work, psychodynamic psychotherapy, and cognitive-behavioral strategies. We have elsewhere described our own eclectic psychotherapy approach to the treatment of eating disorder patients with BPD, which takes place on the individual psychotherapy level (Sansone and Johnson 1995; Sansone and Sansone 2006). Levitt (2005) has described an approach to treatment, the Self-Regulatory Approach (SRA), that takes place within both an individual and a group context.

In addition, there are several systematized or manualized approaches to treatment that are geared to institutional settings. The most well known of these, *dialectical behavior therapy* (DBT; Linehan 1993), is a combination treatment approach consisting of psychodynamic, cognitive-behavioral, supportive,

Table 3–3.   The PISIA criteria for borderline personality disorder

P   **Psychotic/quasi-psychotic episodes:** transient, fleeting, brief episodes that tend to emerge with stress and persist over the patient's lifetime; may include

Depersonalization

Derealization

Dissociation

Rage reactions

Paranoia (patient recognizes the illogical nature of his or her suspiciousness)

Fleeting or isolated hallucinations or delusions

Unusual reactions to drugs

I   **Impulsivity:** long-standing behaviors that may be stable over time, coexist with other behaviors, or replace each other over time (i.e., substitution);

Self-regulation difficulties (e.g., eating disorders such as anorexia and bulimia nervosa, binge-eating disorder, obesity; drug/alcohol/ prescription abuse; money management difficulties such as bankruptcies, credit card difficulties, uncontrolled gambling; promiscuity; mood regulation difficulties; chronic pain syndromes; somatic preoccupation)

Self-destructive behaviors (e.g., self-mutilation such as hitting, cutting, burning, or biting oneself; suicide attempts; sadomasochistic relationships; high-risk hobbies such as parachuting or racing cars; high-risk behaviors such as frequenting dangerous bars or jogging in parks at night)

S   **Social adaptation:** superficially intact social veneer; if the individual demonstrates high academic or professional performance, it is usually inconsistent and erratic.

I   **Interpersonal relationships:** chaotic and unsatisfying; the relationship style is characterized by "dichotomous relatedness," wherein social relationships tend to be very superficial and transient, and personal relationships tend to be extremely intense, manipulative, and dependent; intense fears of being alone; rage with the primary caretaker.

A   **Affect:** chronically dysphoric or labile; since adolescence, the majority of the mood experience has been dysphoric, with the predominant affects being anxiety, anger, depression, and/or emptiness.

Source.   Kolb and Gunderson 1980.

Instructions: Please answer the following questions by checking either "Yes" or "No." Check "yes" only to those items that you have done intentionally, or on purpose, to hurt yourself.

Yes   No   Have you ever intentionally, or on purpose,...

___ ___   1. Overdosed? (If yes, number of times____)
___ ___   2. Cut yourself on purpose? (If yes, number of times____)
___ ___   3. Burned yourself on purpose? (If yes, number of times____)
___ ___   4. Hit yourself? (If yes, number of times____)
___ ___   5. Banged your head on purpose? (If yes, number of times____)
___ ___   6. Abused alcohol?
___ ___   7. Driven recklessly on purpose? (If yes, number of times____)
___ ___   8. Scratched yourself on purpose? (If yes, number of times____)
___ ___   9. Prevented wounds from healing?
___ ___ 10. Made medical situations worse, on purpose (e.g., skipped medication)?
___ ___ 11. Been promiscuous (i.e., had many sexual partners)? (If yes, how many?____)
___ ___ 12. Set yourself up in a relationship to be rejected?
___ ___ 13. Abused prescription medication?
___ ___ 14. Distanced yourself from God as punishment?
___ ___ 15. Engaged in emotionally abusive relationships? (If yes, number of relationships____)
___ ___ 16. Engaged in sexually abusive relationships? (If yes, number of relationships____)
___ ___ 17. Lost a job on purpose? (If yes, number of times____)

Figure 3–4.   The Self-Harm Inventory.
Source.   Reprinted from Sansone RA, Wiederman MW, Sansone LA: "The Self-Harm Inventory (SHI): Development of a Scale for Identifying Self-Destructive Behaviors and Borderline Personality Disorder." *Journal of Clinical Psychology* 54:973–983, 1998. Copyright 1995, R.A. Sansone, L.A. Sansone, M.W. Wiederman. Used with permission.

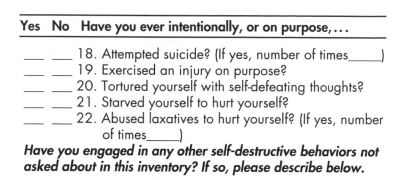

Yes	No	Have you ever intentionally, or on purpose,...
___	___	18. Attempted suicide? (If yes, number of times___)
___	___	19. Exercised an injury on purpose?
___	___	20. Tortured yourself with self-defeating thoughts?
___	___	21. Starved yourself to hurt yourself?
___	___	22. Abused laxatives to hurt yourself? (If yes, number of times___)

Have you engaged in any other self-destructive behaviors not asked about in this inventory? If so, please describe below.

Figure 3–4. The Self-Harm Inventory *(continued).*

and educational elements that are provided in both a group and an individual format. Originally developed for BPD, DBT can be modified for patients with eating disorders with the addition of specific modules (Wisniewski and Kelly 2003). Another approach, *Systems Training for Emotional Predictability and Problem Solving* (STEPPS; Blum et al. 2002), is a cognitive-behavioral group treatment for BPD that includes both family members and significant others. This manual-based treatment consists of twenty 2-hour weekly treatment sessions. Although STEPPS is used in the treatment of BPD, there are no current data on its use in patients with eating disorders, but an adaptation is surely inevitable. A third approach is *integrative cognitive therapy* (ICT; Wonderlich et al. 2002), which is a personality-centered approach to the treatment of eating disorders that can be modified for individuals with BPD. Like most of the preceding treatments, ICT is a multicomponent endeavor with cognitive-behavioral, motivational, interpersonal, emotion-focused, and feminist elements.

To summarize, regardless of psychotherapy approach, BPD patients require additional and specialized psychotherapy intervention beyond that offered through eating disorder treatment. In addition, a number of these individuals will require specialized psychotherapeutic work in the area of childhood trauma.

While beyond the scope of this chapter, a small number of eating disorder individuals with PTSD. It is known that BPD heightens the risk for subsequent victimization in adulthood and, therefore, the risk of PTSD. When present, PTSD is approached in the traditional manner (i.e., cognitive-behavioral intervention, exposure/desensitization, SSRIs). However, in large inpatient treatment programs, it may be essential to develop a "trauma track."

Medications.   According to the "Practice Guideline for the Treatment of Patients with Borderline Personality Disorder" (2001), intervention in BPD should be "complemented by symptom-targeted pharmacotherapy" (p. 4). Given this recommendation, the only modification in the pharmacotherapy of eating disorder patients with BPD is the *avoidance* of medications with 1) high frequencies of weight gain (e.g., paroxetine, lithium, valproate, most TCAs, several atypical antipsychotics, such as olanzapine and clozapine), as patients with BPD tend to have higher body weights than the general psychiatric patient (Sansone et al. 2001); 2) a greater risk of death in overdose (e.g., TCAs, lithium, citalopram), as BPD patients typically have a high frequency of suicide attempts; and 3) addiction potential (e.g., benzodiazepines, benzodiazepine-receptor hypnotics), as BPD patients have chronic self-regulation difficulties.

We typically initiate treatment with an SSRI because the broad clinical efficacy of this class effectively addresses the polysymptomatic concerns of BPD patients. While the American Psychiatric Association's practice guideline recommends next a low-dose atypical antipsychotic, we frequently precede this with a trial of anticonvulsants to control anxiety and impulsivity.

Hospitalization.   When dramatic self-harm behavior or suicidal ideation is present, hospitalization may be a consideration. We carefully use the word *may* for several reasons. First, self-harm behavior and/or suicidal ideation are often *chronic* themes in borderline patients; to our knowledge, there is no *acute* treatment for either of these symptoms. While it can be successfully argued that immediate protection of the patient is indicated, we perceive distinct differences in the management of acute versus chronic suicidal ideation (Sansone 2004). To complicate matters, there are distinct risks with the hospitalization of borderline patients. These include inpatient regression, use of re-emergent "suicidal ideation" to prolong an unproductive hospitalization, risk of assimilating new self-destructive behaviors from other patients (i.e., contagion), and difficulties in maintaining a healthy treatment environment for patients who continually split treatment team members. Therefore, we believe that the decision to hospitalize a borderline patient must be undertaken with some care, rather than reflexively, with careful attention to the potential risks and benefits in each individual case. In considering hospitalization, we typically attempt to elicit a specific treatment goal from the patient that can reasonably be accomplished within a 2- to 3-day time frame (e.g., reevaluation of medication, acute relationship work), rather than using the resolution of suicidal ideation as the discharge focus.

Obsessive-Compulsive Personality Disorder

Assessment.   Obsessive-compulsive personality disorder (OCPD) is commonly encountered in patients with restricting anorexia nervosa. During assessment, this Axis II disorder may be difficult to detect, because the preoccupation with order and detail, perfectionism, inflexibility, and rigidity may predominate in the areas of food, body, and weight management. In addition, starvation may intensify the thoughts and behaviors related to obsessionalism (Keys et al. 1950). Therefore, we suggest scrutinizing other areas of life functioning, such as academics, sports activities, and environmental management (i.e., the patient's level of tidiness with his or her bedroom), to fully evaluate for OCPD. An additional quagmire is the occasional difficulty differentiating OCD from OCPD.

Psychotherapy.   Many of the cognitive-behavioral interventions used in treating anorexia nervosa can be used to address obsessive-compulsive personality symptomatology. The only modification that we recommend is broadening these techniques to address other areas of life functioning (e.g., academics, sports achievement, bedroom organization).

Medications.   SSRIs are known to exert a therapeutic effect on obsessive thinking and worry. Although they are not indicated by the FDA for OCPD, we
typically prescribe these drugs to curb the symptom domain of anxiety and the
related symptoms of rumination and worry. On occasion, we have augmented
SSRIs with low-dose buspirone (e.g., 20 mg/day), with excellent clinical results.

Hospitalization.   As with the other Axis I anxiety disorders, we have rarely
hospitalized individuals because of symptoms related to OCPD.

Conclusion

Eating disorder patients appear to have high levels of psychiatric comorbidity,
both on Axis I and on Axis II. On Axis I, common comorbid disorders include
mood and anxiety disorders, as well as alcohol and substance abuse. Common
comorbid Axis II disorders include borderline personality disorder in those
patients with impulsive eating pathology (i.e., binge eating, purging) and obsessive-compulsive personality disorder, which is oftentimes encountered in
patients with restricting anorexia nervosa. These comorbid disorders require
some treatment modifications, and for each, we have described the major
treatment adjustments in terms of assessment, psychotherapy, and medications.

How these comorbid conditions affect overall treatment outcome remains
empirically unclear. Unfortunately, outcome studies examining the intersec-
tion of eating disorders and other Axis I disorders and Axis II disorders are relatively scant, but we believe that these comorbid disorders tend to hamper eating disorder treatment.

We also believe that active assessment and intervention will result in a better overall outcome with the eating disorder as well as the comorbid psychiatric condition. Only additional research will confirm these clinical impressions. From our experience, however, eating disorder patients with comorbid
psychiatric conditions can be effectively treated and experience favorable outcomes.

References

Bauer MS, Mitchner L: What is a "mood stabilizer"? An evidence-based response. Am J Psychiatry 161:3–18, 2004

Bialer M, Doose DR, Murthy B, et al: Pharmacokinetic interactions of topiramate. Clin Pharmacokinet 43:763–780, 2004

Blum N, Pfohl B, St. John D, et al: STEPPS: a cognitive-behavioral systems-based group treatment for outpatients with borderline personality—a preliminary report. Compr Psychiatry 43:301–310, 2002

Brewerton TD, Lydiard RB, Herzog DB, et al: Comorbidity of Axis I psychiatric disorders in bulimia nervosa. J Clin Psychiatry 56:77–80, 1995

Bruno F: Buspirone in the treatment of alcohol patients. Psychopathol 22:49–59, 1989

Bulik CM, Sullivan PF, Fear JL, et al: Eating disorders and antecedent anxiety disorders: a controlled study. Acta Psychiatr Scand 96:101–107, 1997

Bulik CM, Klump KL, Thornton L, et al: Alcohol use disorder comorbidity in eating disorders: a multicenter study. J Clin Psychiatry 65:1000–1006, 2004

Buydens-Branchey L, Branchey M, Reel-Brander C: Efficacy of buspirone in the treatment of opioid withdrawal. J Clin Psychopharmacol 25:230–236, 2005

Clark DA: Cognitive-Behavioral Therapy for OCD. New York, Guilford, 2004

Compton SN, March JS, Brent D, et al: Cognitive-behavioral psychotherapy for anxiety and depressive disorders in children and adolescents: an evidence-based medicine review. J Am Acad Child Adolesc Psychiatry 43:930–959, 2004

De Mello MF, de Jesus Mari J, Bacaltchuk J, et al: A systematic review of research findings on the efficacy of interpersonal therapy for depressive disorders. Eur Arch Psychiatry Clin Neurosci 255:75–82, 2005

Doose DR, Wang SS, Padmanabhan M, et al: Effect of topiramate or carbamazepine on the pharmacokinetics of an oral contraceptive containing norethindrone and ethinyl estradiol in healthy obese and nonobese female subjects. Epilepsia 44:540–549, 2003

Dougherty DD, Rauch SL, Jenike MA: Pharmacotherapy for obsessive-compulsive disorder. J Clin Psychol 60:1195–1202, 2004

Eddy KT, Dutra L, Bradley R, et al: A multidimensional meta-analysis of psychotherapy and pharmacotherapy for obsessive-compulsive disorder. Clin Psychol Rev 24:1011–1030, 2004

Fineberg NA, Gale TM: Evidence-based pharmacotherapy of obsessive-compulsive disorder. Int J Neuropsychopharmacol 8:107–129, 2005

Fraunfelder FW: Twice-yearly exams unnecessary for patients taking quetiapine. Am J Ophthalmol 138:870–871, 2004

Ghaemi SN: Hippocratic psychopharmacology for bipolar disorder: an expert's opinion. Psychiatry 3:30–39, 2006

Godart NT, Flament MF, Perdereau F, et al: Comorbidity between eating disorders and anxiety disorders: a review. Int J Eat Disord 32:253–270, 2002

Hudson JI, Hudson RA, Pope HG: Psychiatric comorbidity and eating disorders, in Eating Disorders Review, Part I. Edited by Wonderlich S, Mitchell JE, de Zwaan M, et al. Seattle, WA, Radcliffe Publishing, 2005, pp 43–57

Hudson JI, Hiripi E, Pope Jr HG, et al: The prevalence and correlates of eating disorders in the National Comorbidity Survey Replication. Biol Psychiatry 61:348–358, 2007

Iwasaki Y, Kiriike N, Matsunaga H, et al: Comorbidity of anxiety disorders in patients with eating disorders. Seishin Igaku 41:855–859, 1999

Johnson BA, Ait-Daoud N, Bowden CL, et al: Oral topiramate for treatment of alcohol dependence: a randomised controlled trial. Lancet 361:1677–1685, 2003

Jordan J, Joyce PR, Carter FA, et al: Anxiety and psychoactive substance use disorder comorbidity in anorexia nervosa or depression. Int J Eat Disord 34:211–219, 2003

Kawa I, Carter JD, Joyce PR, et al: Gender differences in bipolar disorder: age of onset, course, comorbidity, and symptom presentation. Bipolar Disord 7:119–125, 2005

Kaye WH, Bulik CM, Thornton L, et al: Comorbidity of anxiety disorders with anorexia and bulimia nervosa. Am J Psychiatry 161:2215–2221, 2004

Keuneman RJ, Pokos V, Weerasundera R, et al: Antipsychotic treatment in obsessive-compulsive disorder: a literature review. Aus N Z J Psychiatry 39:336–343, 2005

Keys A, Brozek J, Henschel A, et al (eds): The Biology of Human Starvation. Minneapolis, University of Minnesota Press, 1950, pp 819–853

Kolb JE, Gunderson JG: Diagnosing borderline patients with a semi-structured interview. Arch Gen Psychiatry 37:37–41, 1980

Koran LM, Gamel NN, Choung HW, et al: Mirtazapine for obsessive-compulsive disorder: an open trial followed by a double-blind discontinuation. J Clin Psychiatry 66:515–520, 2005

Krishnan KRR: Psychiatric and medical comorbidities of bipolar disorder. Psychosom Med 67:1–8, 2005

Levitt JL: A therapeutic approach to treating the eating disorder/borderline personality disorder patient. Eat Disord 13:109–121, 2005

Lilenfeld LR, Kaye WH, Greeno CG, et al: A controlled family study of anorexia nervosa and bulimia nervosa: psychiatric disorders in first-degree relatives and effects of proband comorbidity. Arch Gen Psychiatry 55:603–610, 1998

Linehan MM: Cognitive-Behavioral Treatment of Borderline Personality Disorder. New York, Guilford, 1993

Malec E, Malec T, Gagne MA, et al: Buspirone in the treatment of alcohol dependence: a placebo-controlled trial. Alcohol Clin Exp Res 20:307–312, 1996

Marx RD, Kotwal R, McElroy SL, et al: What treatment data support topiramate in bulimia nervosa and binge eating disorder? What is the drug's safety profile? How is it used in these conditions? Eat Disord 11:71–75, 2003

McElroy SL, Kotwal R, Malhotra S: Comorbidity of bipolar disorder and eating disorders: what can the clinician do? Prim Psychiatry 11:36–41, 2004

McElroy SL, Kotwal R, Keck PE, et al: Comorbidity of bipolar and eating disorders: distinct or related disorders with shared dysregulations? J Affect Disord 86:107–127, 2005

Milos G, Spindler A, Ruggiero G, et al: Comorbidity of obsessive-compulsive disorders and duration of eating disorders. Int J Eat Disord 31:284–289, 2002

Milos GF, Spindler AM, Buddeberg C, et al: Axes I and II comorbidity and treatment experiences in eating disorder subjects. Psychother Psychosom 72:276–285, 2003

Mufson L, Dorta KP, Moreau D, et al: Interpersonal Psychotherapy for Depressed Adolescents, 2nd Edition. New York, Guilford, 2004

Nasrallah HA, Newcomer JW: Atypical antipsychotics and metabolic dysregulation. J Clin Psychopharmacol 24 (5, suppl):S7-S14, 2004

Nemeroff CB: Safety of available agents used to treat bipolar disorder: focus on weight gain. J Clin Psychiatry 64:532–539, 2003

O'Brien CP: Anticraving medications for relapse prevention: a possible new class of psychoactive medications. Am J Psychiatry 162:1423–1431, 2005

Pearlstein T: Eating disorders and comorbidity. Arch Womens Ment Health 4:67–78, 2002

Physicians' Desk Reference, 59th Edition. Montvale, NJ, Thomson PDR, 2005

Practice guideline for the treatment of patients with borderline personality disorder. American Psychiatric Association. Am J Psychiatry 158 (10, suppl):1–52, 2001

Practice guideline for the treatment of patients with eating disorders (revision). Am J Psychiatry 157 (1, suppl):1–39, 2000

Roelofs J, Muris P: Psychological treatments of depression, in Mood Disorders: Clinical Management and Research Issues. Edited by Griez EJL, Faravelli C, Nutt DJ, et al. New York, Wiley, 2005, pp 352–371

Sansone RA: Chronic suicidality and borderline personality. J Personal Disord 18:215–225, 2004

Sansone RA, Dennis AB: The treatment of eating disorder patients with substance abuse and borderline personality. Eat Disord 4:180–186, 1996

Sansone RA, Johnson CL: Treating the eating disorder patient with borderline personality disorder: theory and technique, in Dynamic Therapies for Psychiatric Disorders (Axis I). Edited by Barber J, Crits-Christoph P. New York, Basic Books, 1995, pp 230–266

Sansone RA, Sansone LA: Borderline personality and eating disorders: an eclectic approach to treatment, in Personality Disorders and Eating Disorders: Exploring the Frontier. Edited by Sansone RA, Levitt JL. New York, Routledge, 2006, pp 197–212

Sansone RA, Fine MA, Nunn JL: A comparison of borderline personality symptomatology and self-destructive behavior in women with eating, substance abuse, and both eating and substance abuse disorders. J Personal Disord 8:219–228, 1994

Sansone RA, Wiederman MW, Sansone LA: The Self-Harm Inventory (SHI): development of a scale for identifying self-destructive behaviors and borderline personality disorder. J Clin Psychol 54:973–983, 1998

Sansone RA, Wiederman MW, Monteith D: Obesity, borderline personality symptomatology, and body image among women in a psychiatric outpatient setting. Int J Eat Disord 29:76–79, 2001

Sansone RA, Levitt JL, Sansone LA: The prevalence of personality disorders among those with eating disorders. Eat Disord 13:7–21, 2005

Singh V, Muzina DJ, Calabrese JR: Anticonvulsants in bipolar disorder. Psychiatr Clin N Am 28:301–323, 2005

Speranza M, Corcos M, Godart N, et al: Obsessive compulsive disorders in eating disorders. Eat Behav 2:193–207, 2001

Striegel-Moore RH, Garvin V, Dohm F-A, et al: Eating disorders in a national sample of hospitalized female and male veterans: detection rates and psychiatric comorbidity. Int J Eat Disord 25:405–414, 1999

Turnbull SJ, Troop NA, Treasure JL: The prevalence of post-traumatic stress disorder and its relation to childhood adversity in subjects with eating disorders. Eur Eat Disord Rev 5:270–277, 1997

Velez L, Selwa LM: Seizure disorders in the elderly. Am Fam Physician 67:325–332, 2003

Vitousek KM, Stumpf RE: Difficulties in the assessment of personality traits and disorders in eating-disordered individuals. Eat Disord 13:37–60, 2005

Volavka J, Czobor P, Cooper TB, et al: Prolactin levels in schizophrenia and schizoaffective disorder patients treated with clozapine, olanzapine, risperidone, or haloperidol. J Clin Psychiatry 65:57–61, 2004

Vulink NCC, Denys D, Westenberg HGM: Bupropion for patients with obsessive-compulsive disorder: an open-label, fixed-dose study. J Clin Psychiatry 66:228–230, 2005

Wisniewski L, Kelly E: The application of dialectical behavior therapy to the treatment of eating disorders. Cogn Behav Pract 10:131–138, 2003

Wonderlich S, Myers T, Norton M, et al: Self-harm and bulimia nervosa: a complex connection. Eating Disord 10:257–267, 2002

Zanarini MC, Vujanovic A, Parachini EA, et al: A screening measure for BPD: the McLean Screening Instrument for Borderline Personality Disorder (MSI-BPD). J Personal Disord 17:568–573, 2003

4

Management of Anorexia Nervosa in Inpatient and Partial Hospitalization Settings

Katherine A. Halmi, M.D.

Severity of symptoms is the basis of guidelines for partial hospitalization or inpatient treatment for eating disorder patients. Although, unfortunately, the length of hospitalization is now primarily determined by managed care companies and health maintenance organizations, guidelines based on expert clinical consensus are ordinarily far more preferable for patients and families. There are no randomized controlled studies to determine the evidence-based criteria for either hospitalization or discharge from the hospital. Subjecting severely medically ill patients with anorexia nervosa to randomized controlled treatment studies has been nearly impossible. However, open studies have shown that a multifaceted treatment approach is most effective. This treatment includes medical management, psychoeducation, and individual therapy that involves both cognitive and behavior therapy principles. If the patient is under the age of 18, family counseling or therapy is essential and depending on the individual case may be highly desirable for those over age 18. Nutritional counseling is often part of the ward milieu program, and pharmacological intervention may be necessary in specific cases. This chapter reviews criteria for hospitalization and partial hospital programs for patients with anorexia nervosa and gives specific treatment information for each of these intensive therapies.

Inpatient Hospitalization for Anorexia Nervosa: Inclusion Criteria

Several different guidelines for determining if a patient with anorexia nervosa requires hospitalization have been proposed. Often, the most compelling reasons for hospitalization of an anorexia nervosa patient are the medical indications listed in Table 4–1. However, there are patients who have relapsed from previous treatment and/or have a history of repeated hospitalizations for anorexia nervosa who may benefit from a period of brief hospitalization in a structured environment. Existing comorbid psychiatric disorders may require the patient to be hospitalized. For example, patients with psychotic depression or serious suicidal ideation may require hospitalization. Some patients are uncooperative with outpatient treatment and need a highly structured setting to initiate an effective treatment. Significant environmental psychosocial stressors with inadequate social support may facilitate an impairment of function, and removal from this environment may be beneficial to the patient. Incapacitating obsessions and compulsions related and/or not related to the eating disorder are another reason for hospitalization. Uncontrolled vomiting or severe disabling episodes of binge eating often necessitate a structured environment for initial effective treatment. This includes a need for supervision during and after all meals and in bathrooms. Severe co-occurring substance abuse disorder may require a combined withdrawal treatment plan in addition to nutritional rehabilitation in an inpatient unit. The following is an example of a patient requiring a lengthy hospitalization.

> Susan began losing weight at age 13 after being teased by her brother. She was initially 5 feet, 2 inches in height and 120 pounds. She lost 20 pounds in

3 months and developed amenorrhea. After her primary care physician referred her for therapy, she was seen in family therapy weekly, met with the nutritionist weekly, and saw the psychiatrist, who weighed her every other week. However, she continued to lose weight (albeit more slowly) down to 78 pounds and would consent to eat only fruits, vegetables, and diet sodas. She fainted once at school and had trouble completing her schoolwork. She developed bradycardia (pulse=43 bpm), orthostatic hypotension, hypothermia (96.4°F), hypocomplementemia, and abnormalities on her electrocardiogram (ST depression, T-wave flattening, U wave). She was admitted to the hospital, and her weight the next morning after voiding was 74 pounds. She acknowledged she had been drinking large quantities of water before being weighed as an outpatient.

Inpatient brief hospitalization (7–14 days) is sometimes possible for patients with the following: 1) relapse from previous treatment or duration of illness of less than 6 months; 2) weight loss of 10%–15% from normal weight if relapsed, or 16%–20% if first episode; 3) hypokalemic alkalosis with serum potassium < 2.5 mEq/L; and 4) cardiac arrhythmias. However, such patients may need extended hospitalization.

Extended hospital treatment (14–60 days) is often necessary for patients who have 1) weight loss >20% of normal for age, height, and bone structure; 2) a history of repeated hospitalizations for anorexia nervosa or being underweight for more than 6 months; 3) psychotic depression or a serious suicide attempt; 4) incapacitating obsessions and compulsions related or not related to eating disorders; or 5) serious comorbid medical conditions such as edema, hypoproteinemia, and severe anemia. The following is an example of a patient with comorbid alcohol dependence and bipolar disorder who required hospitalization.

Sarah is a 23-year-old woman who developed anorexia nervosa at age 17. She lost weight—from 130 pounds at 5 feet, 6 inches in height down to 98 pounds—and had amenorrhea for 6 months. She was hospitalized briefly at age 20 for a cardiac arrhythmia and subsequently gained weight, to 108 pounds, in outpatient treatment. However, at age 22, she began losing weight again down to 95 pounds and started inducing vomiting whenever she ate. She also developed insomnia, was restless, complained she could not concentrate, and had multiple projects she could not complete. She began using alcohol to try to sleep and gradually increased her daily consumption to a bottle of wine every evening. She gained 5 pounds and her purging by vomiting increased. These behaviors continued for nearly a year. She was admitted to the hospital after she received a DUI citation after narrowly missing a child riding a bicycle. One day after admission, her temperature increased, she became shaky, and she had visual misperceptions. A chlordiazepoxide withdrawal program was started, with the withdrawal taking place over the course of 2 weeks. Concurrently a weight restoration program was started, with an initial focus on weight maintenance until the withdrawal was complete, at which time weight gain was encouraged. She became progressively more irritable and restless and complained of racing thoughts and insomnia. Her family revealed that several members of the family had alcohol dependence and bipolar disorder. She was diagnosed with bipolar I disorder, mixed state, and began taking a mood stabilizer (aripiprazole was chosen, since it is usually weight-neutral).

Inpatient Treatment of Anorexia Nervosa

There is little research concerning the effectiveness of intensive treatments in eating disorders. A significant number of anorexia nervosa patients refuse to participate in hospitalization treatment, and others leave prematurely. Dropout rates for inpatient treatment range from 20% (Surgenor et al. 2004) to 51% (Woodside et al. 2004). Patients with the binge-eating/purge subtype of anorexia nervosa are more likely to dropout of inpatient treatment (Woodside et al. 2004). Other predictors of dropout are high levels of depression and more severe eating disorder psychopathology at admission and higher levels of maturity fears (Zeeck et al. 2004). Case series studies of inpatient treatment of anorexia nervosa have shown consistently that it is effective in achieving short-term weight restoration (Bowers and Anderson 1994; Lowe et al. 2003).

Involuntary admission may be necessary to manage a life-threatening emergency or when the patient is at an acute risk for serious medical deterioration and is unwilling to take any steps to cooperate in treatment. In this situation, nasal gastric tube feeding may be necessary for involuntary feeding and should be administered by an experienced staff. Follow-up studies have shown that involuntary admission and feeding is often effective and that patients treated under these circumstances subsequently often express gratitude to those who have intervened (Russell 2001).

Because of the complexities and special knowledge required to promote effective treatment of anorexia nervosa, hospitalized patients are best treated in a specialized inpatient eating disorder setting, which provides a team of individuals highly skilled in the multidisciplinary management of anorexic patients. Medical

Table 4–1. Common medical indications for inpatient hospitalization for anorexia nervosa

1. Generally, weight <85% of individually estimated healthy body weight or acute weight decline with food refusal

2. For adults:
   Heart rate <40 beats per minute (bpm)
   Blood pressure <90/60 mmHg or orthostatic hypotension (with an increase in pulse of >20 bpm or a drop in blood pressure of >10–20 mmHg/minute from lying to standing)

3. For children:
   Heart rate near 40 bpm
   Orthostatic changes of >20 bpm increase in heart rate or >10–20 mmHg drop in blood pressure
   Blood pressure <80/50 mmHg

4. Blood glucose levels <60 mg/dL

5. Potassium <3 mEq/L

6. Electrolyte imbalance (hypo- or hypernatremia, hypophosphatemia, hypomagnesemia, hypokalcmia)

7. Body temperature <97.0°F

8. Dehydration

9. Hepatic, renal, or cardiovascular organ compromise requiring acute treatment

10. Poorly controlled diabetes

11. Edema, hypoproteinemia, and severe anemia

Source. Birmingham and Beumont 2004: "Practice Guideline for the Treatment of Patients With Eating Disorders, Third Edition" 2006.

management involves weight restoration, nutritional rehabilitation, rehydration, and correction of serum electrolytes. This management requires daily monitoring of weight, food and calorie intake, and urine output. In the patient who is vomiting, frequent assessment of serum electrolytes is necessary. Patients must be closely monitored for attempts to vomit. The staff may help patients by means of response prevention of purging, staying with them after meals to prevent access to a bathroom for purging, and until the urge to vomit subsides.

Medical Management and Nutritional Rehabilitation

An appropriate weight range should be established for the patient. In establishing the range, the treatment team should consider the patient's height, bone structure, and weight at the time of onset of menses. Because weight often fluctuates with fluid shifts, placing a target weight within a 5-pound range may be physiologically more sensible than having one specific number. However, this range should be set so that the lower end of the range is in the healthy target area, not "discounted" simply for psychological acceptability.

In addition to a physical examination, the following laboratory tests should be obtained: a complete blood cell count, liver function test, serum creatinine level, serum electrolytes, calcium, magnesium, and phosphate. An electrocardiogram is necessary, since electrolyte abnormalities can cause T-wave flattening, ST depression, and a variety of arrhythmias. Early assessment of bone mineral density is important to appraise the extent of initial bone loss and to provide a baseline against which to evaluate potential improvement consequent to nutritional rehabilitation. Vomiting, laxative abuse, and diuretics can result in metabolic alkalosis (elevated serum bicarbonate), and all forms of purging can lead to hypokalemia and, less frequently, hypomagnesemia and hypocalcemia. Elevated serum salivary amylase is a strong indicator that the patient is self-inducing vomiting, because amylase is released when the parotid glands are stimulated. A complete list of recommended laboratory tests is presented in Table 2–1 in Chapter 2, "Assessment and Determination of Initial Treatment Approaches for Patients With Eating Disorders," in this volume.

Nutritional rehabilitation should usually begin with an intake of 30–40 kcal/kg per day (approximately 1,000–1,600 kcal/day); intake may be increased to as high as 70–100 kcal/kg per day after it is determined that the patient is tolerating the calorie load well. This means there is no evidence of peripheral edema or cardiac failure. Severely emaciated patients given a liquid formula in six equal feedings throughout the day can very efficiently digest the necessary fluid, electrolytes, and calories for the patients. A randomly assigned, controlled treatment study in a Japanese inpatient setting (Okamoto et al. 2002) showed that a liquid formula with activity restriction was the most effective program with regard to both the amount and the rate of increase of body mass index measured at the end of hospitalization and 6 months after discharge. The liquid formula was given only in the early stages of hospitalization, and after a period of some weight gain patients were transferred to monitored food intake. Adding vitamin and mineral supplements when the patients are on food is particularly useful to prevent serum hypophosphatemia and to facilitate adequate nutritional rehabilitation. Patients may eat together as a group but must be supervised carefully by staff.

For symptom control and weight gain, it is necessary to create a milieu that incorporates emotional nurturance and a combination of reinforcers that link exercise, bed rest, and privileges to weight gain and desired behaviors. Feedback concerning other observable parameters is also helpful. It is necessary to help the patient limit physical activity and caloric expenditure according to food intake and fitness requirements.

After the liquid formula phase, devising individual meal plans with food served on trays for each patient is helpful in allowing the patient to have a cognitive recognition of the amount of food she is eating and the rate of weight gain. A short time before discharge the patient can then be given the opportunity to choose her own foods and practice determining an intake that will promote either a necessary continued weight gain or weight maintenance. It is desirable for each patient to receive nutritional counseling individually as well as nutritional education in group therapy. Patients can be helped with devising meal plans to follow after they are discharged from the hospital. Several studies have shown that the patient's target weight should be within a BMI equivalent range of 19–21 (Commerford et al. 1997; Howard et al. 1999).

Psychosocial Treatments Within an Inpatient Setting

Individual, family, and group therapy are all advisable for the inpatient setting. Individual therapy can deal with the patient's unique problem, which often concerns maturity fears, family difficulties, and interpersonal problems. The cognitive distortions of anorexia nervosa patients may be dealt with during individual cognitive therapy, which can proceed after some initial weight gain. The anorexic patient's extreme and rigid thinking style, distorted thoughts around self-esteem and self-concept (with pervasive feelings of ineffectiveness), and often a drive for perfectionism can respond to cognitive therapy techniques such as cognitive restructuring and problem solving (Kleifield et al. 1996).

A family analysis should be done on all anorexic patients who are living with their families. On the basis of this analysis, the type of family therapy or counseling that is likely to be helpful can be chosen. Family therapy or counseling is necessary for all children under age 18 (Eisler et al. 1997). When family therapy is not possible, issues of family relationships can be addressed in individual therapy or in brief counseling sessions with immediate family members. The family counseling can begin during the hospitalization phase and continue through partial hospitalization and outpatient treatment.

Group therapy can occur frequently and cover a variety of topics. It is a useful format for, to give only one example, psychoeducation in which the patients are informed about nutrition and medical complications, as well as for relapse prevention, assertiveness training, self-control strategies, maturing and autonomy issues, and limit-setting problems. Patients may be given homework assignments of intensive self-monitoring. An example of this kind of homework is keeping a daily diary that includes a record of all foods eaten, symptoms, symptom urges, and feelings. In a group format patients can discuss their symptoms and have increased awareness of their eating behavior, symptom triggers, and coping strategies.

A cognitive-behavioral framework is useful for the overall ward milieu. Exposure and response prevention techniques are used when patients are asked to have their meals at regular intervals and are prevented from exercising or vomiting. In these techniques, patients may be "exposed" to a reasonable amount of exercise or food, for example, but then prevented from continuing on to excessive exercise or compensatory purging. Patients may receive regular feedback about their weight every morning and deal with interpersonal conflict on the inpatient unit in the context of group therapy. Preparing eating plans for after hospital discharge can also be done in a group format. Therapists must remember, both in the individual and the group therapy format, that the patient's symptoms and interpersonal behavior are serving a function or a need in the patient's life. Open discussions of the advantages and disadvantages of specific symptoms, having an eating disorder, and recovery are helpful in alerting patients to the problem they have had in the past and are likely to have in the future.

Discharge From the Inpatient Setting

Ideal discharge criteria include the following:

1. Attainment of ideal body weight
2. Medical stability (e.g., a normal electrocardiogram and serum electrolytes), together with identification and appropriate treatment for any unresolved physiological complications due to the eating disorder
3. No suicide risk

4. Ability to maintain ideal body weight and normal nutritional intake during passes outside the structured environment
5. Ability to select foods in family style servings
6. Ability to avoid binge eating, purging, and overexercise
7. No incapacitating impairment from comorbid conditions such as psychosis or severe obsessions and compulsions
8. Identification of existing comorbid psychiatric conditions and initiation of appropriate treatment
9. Family educated about the eating disorder and prepared to assist the patient during the outpatient recovery process
10. Identification of associated and underlying interpersonal, social psychological, and psychodynamic issues and a plan for addressing them
11. Identification of an outpatient team, and placement of appropriate referrals, with all treatment team members and other involved health care personnel prepared to proceed with outpatient treatment

Medications may be useful adjuncts in the inpatient treatment of anorexia nervosa. If effective, the medication can be continued when the patient is transferred to outpatient status. Cyproheptadine at high dosages (up to 24 mg/day) can facilitate weight gain in restricting anorexic patients and also provide a mild antidepressant effect (Halmi et al. 1986). Chlorpromazine was the first drug used to treat anorexia nervosa; however, no double-blind, controlled studies are available to show the efficacy of this drug for inducing weight gain and reducing agitation in patients with anorexia nervosa. In open trial observations, the medication was especially helpful in the anorexic patients with severely obsessive-compulsive behavior and agitation. It may be necessary to start at a low dosage (10 mg tid) and gradually increase the dosage. Newer antipsychotics, such as olanzapine, are also useful for severely obsessive-compulsive and very agitated anorexic patients (Powers et al. 2002). Tricyclic antidepressants and serotonin reuptake inhibitors are not effective and have undesirable side effects for emaciated anorexic patients (Kaye et al. 2001). In addition, many patients have comorbid Axis I psychiatric disorders that require treatment with medications.

Summary

A multifaceted treatment approach is effective for hospitalized anorexia nervosa patients. Behavioral contingencies are useful for inducing weight gain and changing the medical condition of the patient by response prevention techniques. As medical rehabilitation proceeds, an associated improvement in psychological state occurs. Patients can benefit from individual cognitive psychotherapy, psychoeducation, and group therapy that addresses specific issues of anorexia nervosa. Family therapy or counseling should begin with all patients younger than age 18 in the inpatient setting and continue after discharge.

Partial Hospitalization for Anorexia Nervosa

Inclusion and Exclusion Criteria

Partial hospitalization programs for anorexia nervosa patients usually involve transitioning of patients from an inpatient program. The patients most suitable for partial hospitalization are those who have a history of repeated hospitalization and who have severe chronic anorexia nervosa. It is unlikely these patients can transition directly from an inpatient program to outpatient visits solely. Outpatients who have had a recent relapse of weight loss and have returned to core anorectic behaviors causing severe impairment of function may also benefit from a partial hospitalization program.

If a patient has a weight loss >20% from a normal weight for age, height, and bone structure, and if there is a suicide risk or medical instability such as an abnormal electrolyte profile or abnormal electrocardiogram, partial hospitalization should be excluded and the patient should be admitted for inpatient treatment.

Dropout rates for partial hospitalization are not as high as those for inpatient treatment reported in the literature. Rates of 18.8% and 13.5% were reported for 4-day and 5-day treatment programs (Olmsted et al. 2003) and 15.2% for a 4-month day-treatment program (Franzen et al. 2004). In the latter study, dropout was associated with more severe bulimic symptoms, higher levels of aggression and extroversion, and lower levels of inhibition.

Treatment

For partial hospitalization, a multifaceted program with a cognitive-behavioral focus on symptom change is recommended. Such programs have reported weight gain in anorexia nervosa patients and improvements in eating disorder attitude and depressive symptoms (Dancyger et al. 2003; Heinberg et al. 2003;

Zipfel et al. 2002). A partial hospitalization program using only supportive and interpersonal group therapy reported that among the first 23 patients with anorexia nervosa, 95% lost weight during the program and 64% required admission to an inpatient unit (Piran et al. 1989).

The intensity of a partial hospitalization program required for effectiveness is unknown. Programs of varying intensity (3-, 4-, 5-, and 6-day) have been described, but no randomized controlled trials have been conducted. Some data suggest that outcomes improve with the intensity of the partial hospitalization program—that is, as the number of days per week and number of hours per day increase. There is some indication that the patient's level of motivation is associated with response to the partial hospitalization program (Thornton et al. 2005). Most reports on partial hospitalization programs describe transferring patients from inpatient units to the partial hospitalization program (Gaurda and Heinberg 1999; Howard et al. 1999). In a study by Howard et al. (1999), patients with a BMI < 19 at the time of transfer were less likely to do well. Another study showed that patients who rapidly responded to the partial hospitalization treatment and achieved control of their symptoms in the first 4 weeks of treatment had lower relapse rates (16%) than patients who managed symptom control only at the end of the treatment (57%) (Olmsted et al. 1996).

At least one structured meal is advisable in the context of a partial hospitalization program. Nutritional counseling and meal planning can occur in the context of group therapy or in specific individual counseling sessions. Multiple group therapies addressing issues such as social skills training, social anxiety, body image distortion, or maturity fears are effective ways of continuing themes developed during inpatient treatment.

Discharge Criteria

There are no studies to provide evidence-based criteria for discharge. In the partial hospitalization studies referred to in the previous subsection, most centers discharged patients from partial hospitalization to an outpatient setting when their weight was within 5%–10% of normal weight and when patients had demonstrated improved functional behavior with a significant decrease of core anorectic symptoms. Verbalization of intent to continue cognitive-behavioral skills learned to reduce the core anorectic behavior is also a valuable criterion for transitioning a patient to outpatient treatment alone.

Anorexia nervosa patients have a very difficult time accepting treatment and being motivated to give up their illness and follow through with treatment recommendations. Future research must deal with the problems of resistance to treatment and develop innovative techniques to address this issue.

References

Birmingham CL, Beumont PJV: Medical Management of Eating Disorders. London, Cambridge University Press, 2004

Bowers WA, Anderson AE: Inpatient treatment of anorexia nervosa: review and recommendations. Harv Rev Psychiatry 2:193–203, 1994

Commerford MC, Licinio J, Halmi KA: Guidelines for discharging eating disorder patients. Eat Disord 5:69–74, 1997

Dancyger I, Fornari V, Schneider M, et al: Adolescents and eating disorders: an examination of a day treatment program. Eat Weight Disord 8:242–248, 2003

Eisler I, Dare C, Hodes M, et al: Family therapy for adolescent anorexia nervosa: the results of a controlled comparison of two family interventions. J Child Psychol Psychiatry 41:727–736, 2000

Franzen U, Blackmund H, Gerlinghoff M: Day treatment group program for eating disorders: reasons for dropout. European Eating Disorders Review 12:153–158, 2004

Gaurda AS, Heinberg L: Effective weight gain in a step-down partial hospitalization program for eating disorders. Poster presented at the annual meeting of the Academy for Eating Disorders, San Diego, CA, May 1999

Halmi KA, Eckert E, Ladu T: Anorexia nervosa: treatment efficacy of cyproheptadine and amitriptyline. Arch Gen Psychiatry 43:177–181, 1986

Heinberg AL, Haug N, Freeman Y, et al: Clinical course and short-term outcome of hospitalized adolescents with eating disorders: the success of combining adolescents and adults on an eating disorder unit. Eat Weight Disord 8:326–331, 2003

Howard W, Evans K, Quintero C, et al: Predictors of success or failure of transition to day hospital treatment for inpatients with anorexia nervosa. Am J Psychiatry 156:1697–1702, 1999

Kaye W, Nagata T, Weltzin T, et al: Double-blind placebo controlled administration of fluoxetine in restricting and restricting-purging-type anorexia nervosa. Biol Psychiatry 49:644–652, 2001

Kleifield E, Wagner S, Halmi KA: Cognitive-behavioral treatment of anorexia nervosa. Psychiatr Clin North Am 19:715–735, 1996

Lowe MR, Davis WN, Annunziato RA, et al: Inpatient treatment for eating disorders: outcome at discharge and 3-month follow-up. Eat Behav 4:385–397, 2003

Okamoto A, Yamashita T, Nagoshi Y: A behavior therapy program combined with liquid nutrition designed for anorexia nervosa. Psychiatry Clin Neurosci 56:515–522, 2002

Olmsted M, Kaplan A, Rockert W, et al: Rapid responders to intensive treatment of bulimia nervosa. Int J Eat Disord 19:279–285, 1996

Olmsted M, Kaplan A, Rockert W: Relative efficacy of a 4-day vs a 5-day hospital day program. Int J Eat Disord 34:441–449, 2003

Piran N, Kaplan A, Garfinkel PE: Evaluation of a day hospital program for eating disorders. Int J Eat Disord 8:523–532, 1989

Powers PS, Santana CA, Bannon YS: Olanzapine in the treatment of anorexia nervosa: an open label trial. Int J Eat Disord 32:146–154, 2002

Russell GF: Involuntary treatment in anorexia nervosa. Psychiatr Clin North Am 24:337–349, 2001

Surgenor LJ, Maguire S, Beumont PJV: Dropouts and inpatient treatment for anorexia nervosa: can risk factors be identified at point of admission? European Eating Disorders Review 12:94–100, 2004

Thornton C, George L, Touyz S: The Wellesley Hospital Eating Disorder Day Programs, in Selected Papers From the First Asian Pacific Eating Disorders Congress. Edited by Burrow GD, Bosanac P, Beumont PJV. Victoria, University of Melbourne, 2005, pp 47–61

Woodside DB, Carter JC, Blackmore E: Predictors of premature termination of inpatient treatment for anorexia nervosa. Am J Psychiatry 161:2277–2281, 2004

Zeeck A, Herzog T, Hartmann A: Day clinic or inpatient care for severe bulimia nervosa? European Eating Disorders Review 12:79–86, 2004

Zipfel S, Reas DL, Thornton C, et al: Day hospitalization programs for eating disorders: a systematic review of the literature. Int J Eat Disord 31:105–117, 2002

5

Management of Anorexia Nervosa in an Ambulatory Setting

Allan S. Kaplan, M.Sc., M.D., FRCPC

Sarah Noble, M.D.

Clinical Vignette

Ms. A. is a 24-year-old single woman who lives alone and works part-time as a receptionist in a beauty spa. She presents with an 8-year history of anorexia nervosa. She currently weighs 90 pounds, and her height is 5 feet, 6 inches. Her weight prior to the onset of her eating disorder at age 16 was 145 pounds; her highest weight ever was 165 pounds at age 18, before she began to purge regularly; her lowest weight ever was 80 pounds, 6 months prior to her present treatment, around the time she collapsed at school, lost consciousness, had a grand mal seizure, and was brought to the emergency room and hospitalized briefly.

Ms. A. currently consumes nothing during the day but black coffee and spends her evenings binge eating and vomiting. When she is not working, she spends her time walking compulsively, on average 4–5 miles per day. Twice a week she takes 40–60 Ex-Lax, usually after a particularly large binge. She also takes an ephedrine-containing compound daily that she purchases from friends since it was taken off the market some time ago. She used to take her brother's methylphenidate, claiming that this helped curtail her appetite.

In addition to her eating disorder, Ms. A. also struggles with obsessive-compulsive disorder (OCD), which predates her anorexia nervosa; she spends upwards of 3 hours a day engaged in cleaning rituals, including washing her hands 20 times each day. As a result, the skin on her hands has been denuded. She also cannot use any public washroom, a fact that has caused her to develop significant gastrointestinal and genitourinary difficulties, including severe constipation, edema, and recurrent urinary tract infections.

Ms. A. has experienced several medical complications. She has been amenorrheic for the past 5 years, and bone density studies reveal significant osteoporosis. On two occasions she fractured ribs without any physical trauma. She is cold much of the time, has complained of thinning of her scalp hair, is severely constipated, and has completely lost her libido. She complains of dizziness and on one occasion experienced a loss in consciousness, which was accompanied by a questionable seizure. Periodically she complains of chest pain and palpitations. She has been briefly hospitalized several times for medical management of fluid and electrolyte imbalance and cardiac complications related to her malnutrition and purging behaviors.

Despite repeated recommendations, she has refused hospitalization in a specialized eating disorder inpatient unit, claiming she is not ill enough to warrant such intervention and feeling shame at being admitted to a psychiatric ward. Her only other hospitalization was at age 22, when she underwent cosmetic breast augmentation surgery. She is currently taking sertraline 200 mg/day, which is primarily prescribed for the OCD; zopiclone 7.5 mg hs for initial and middle insomnia; and oral potassium supplements.

Ms. A.'s family history is significant for a history of an eating disorder in her mother and OCD in her father, a cosmetic surgeon. Her younger, 18-year-old sister recently began self-inducing vomiting. A maternal grandfather had bipolar disorder. Regarding personal history, at age 10 the patient was molested on several occasions by a male babysitter. Shortly thereafter she developed symptoms of OCD, which eventually interfered with her school performance. After high school, she worked for several years as a waitress and hostess and eventually enrolled in a community college, where she is studying to become an aesthetician. She is currently on a leave of absence because of her inability to concentrate as a result of her symptoms.

She is socially isolated, since most of her former high school friends have finished college and left her city for careers elsewhere. She has never had a boyfriend and attributes this to her poor body image, which she feels most men would find unacceptable. Although her body image has improved somewhat since her recent breast surgery, she feels that she still needs to lose more weight from her hips and thighs before she can consider dating.

Ms. A. is currently seen once per week for treatment by a psychiatrist experienced in the treatment of eating disorders.

Treatment Goals

The treatment goals in treating Ms. A. and others like her with anorexia nervosa include the following:

1. **Assuring medical stability by regular assessment (at least monthly) of the patient's medical status** (Kaplan and Garfinkel 1993). The treatment goals are medical stability with normal fluid and electrolyte balance, renal function, menses, and cardiac functioning. Medical monitoring should include the regular assessment of blood pressure, pulse rate, core body temperature, serum electrolytes, blood urea nitrogen and serum creatinine, and cardiovascular status by regular electrocardiograms (ECGs). If the patient is judged medically unstable, such monitoring may be required monthly. If there are reasons to suspect abnormalities, consideration should be given to periodically assessing blood glucose, liver function, calcium, phosphate, and serum proteins. A DEXA (dual-energy X-ray absorptiometry) scan to assess for the presence of osteopenia or osteoporosis should be considered, especially if the patient develops pathological fractures or complains of bone pain. The presence of abnormal bone density studies may help motivate patients to tolerate a weight that can once again support normal menses.

    In Ms. A. dehydration and hypokalemia with associated electrocardiographic abnormalities were common medical complications. When her serum potassium levels fell below 2.5 mEq/L, which occurred every 6–8 weeks, brief stays in the emergency room for intravenous rehydration and potassium chloride infused over an 8- to 12-hour period were arranged. This intervention usually normalized her fluid and electrolyte abnormalities and ECG and avoided unnecessary hospital admissions. She was otherwise maintained on oral potassium supplements.

2. **Targeting behavioral symptoms of binge eating, vomiting, and compulsive exercising through cognitive-behavioral strategies that have proven to be effective in the management of such bulimic symptoms.** These interventions include strategies that can be implemented in an outpatient setting, such as

- Self-monitoring of eating behavior and associated feeling states.
- Leisure and time management strategies so that time alone is limited.
- Distraction and relaxation techniques that help facilitate affect tolerance and reduce responding maladaptively to negative feeling states. Helpful techniques that can be taught to outpatients include yoga, meditation, and mindfulness.
- Imposing structures that prevent immediate capitulation to urges to binge eat or vomit, such as eating in a public place (e.g., restaurant, cafeteria), to facilitate response prevention.
- Teaching healthy exercise as opposed to compulsive, pathological exercise. Pathological exercise is not enjoyable, is performed in isolation, is not constrained by the amount of time spent (but may be limited by feelings of utter depletion), and is driven primarily by the desire to burn calories, so it tends to be carefully titrated against the amount of food consumed. In contrast, healthy exercise tends to be social and enjoyable, such as in a sport or game in which built-in constraints limit the time spent exercising (e.g., games such as basketball, soccer, or tennis that end when one individual or team wins the match) and in which the time spent exercising is independent of the amount eaten.

3. **Normalization of eating and weight through nutritional rehabilitation.** The treatment goals are to establish a normal healthy body weight, which usually means a body mass index (BMI) of greater than 20 for adults. Such a weight should approximate the patient's premorbid weight (i.e., the

weight the patient was able to maintain in a healthy state prior to the on-set of disordered eating behavior). For most patients this weight is usually within the normal range of weight for age and height. Some patients, like Ms. A., may need to accept a weight that is higher than desired and higher than the statistical mean for their age and height. A meal plan should be developed that incorporates adequate amounts of carbohydrates, fats, and proteins; most patients can tolerate an initial caloric intake of 1,500 kcal/day (30–40 kcal/kg/day), and intake should be increased to up to 70–80 kcal/kg/day for weight gain. Liquid supplements can be useful in the re-feeding process during the period of initial weight gain in helping patients who experience significant postprandial bloating following the intake of solid foods. Keeping a diary of food intake, disordered eating behavior (e.g., binge eating and purging), and feeling states associated with eating and reviewing these diaries during weekly sessions can be helpful.

4. **Treating psychiatric comorbidity.** Comorbidity is the rule rather than the exception in patients with anorexia nervosa. As with Ms. A., the comorbid symptoms often complicate the treatment of the eating disorder. This pa-tient's rituals and compulsions involved both food-related and non-food-related behaviors and significantly interfered with attempts to normalize eating. Ms. A. spent so many hours engaged in ritualistic behaviors or be-ing consumed by anxiety about them that it was difficult for her to try to adhere to any kind of normal meal plan. Treatment of the OCD was nec-essary to maximize the possibility that her eating disorder symptoms would be amenable to treatment. This patient was given a selective sero-tonin reuptake inhibitor (SSRI), which controlled her OCD symptoms to the point that she could subsequently actively attempt to normalize her eating to some extent. As with Ms. A., specific psychosocial treatments for the comorbid disorder should be instituted, either by the clinician treating the eating disorder or by another clinician expert in the treatment of the co-morbid condition. In Ms. A.'s case, she was referred to a clinic specializing in OCD for a brief course of cognitive-behavioral therapy (CBT) specifi-cally targeting the non-food-related and eating-related obsessions and com-pulsions while she continued seeing her eating disorder specialist. We also suggested that she attend an outpatient substance use facility to help her stop taking amphetamines, but she refused to do so.

5. Treating the underlying psychosocial issues that both contribute to the development of an eating disorder and perpetuate the ongoing symptoms. These psychosocial variables are often not the same; for example, factors that predispose to the development of an eating disorder are not always the same as those that maintain disordered eating. Clinicians need to have many psychotherapeutic techniques in their treatment "toolboxes" to competently treat patients with anorexia nervosa. Adherence to one single theoretical framework is insufficient to effectively treat these patients. In the absence of established effective evidence-based psychotherapeutic approaches to anorexia nervosa, working knowledge of psychotherapeutic paradigms that embrace self psychological, cognitive, behavioral, interpersonal, motivational, and psychodynamically informed principles is necessary to provide optimum outpatient management for patients with anorexia nervosa. In addition, for younger patients under the age of 16 who have been ill for a short period of time, a small but respectable evidence base supports family therapy as the preferred psychotherapeutic approach. Both separated and conjoint forms of family therapy may be beneficial.

Psychosocial Approaches to the Outpatient Treatment of Anorexia Nervosa

In the absence of a clear and cogent understanding of the pathophysiology of anorexia nervosa, psychosocial approaches remain the cornerstone of ambulatory management for this disorder. Despite a relative dearth of evidence-based support and little guidance from the literature regarding which modality may be superior, psychotherapy is a central facet of ongoing care. In clinical practice, clinicians usually need to employ several different psychotherapeutic techniques to maximize their ability to be effective when treating patients with anorexia nervosa. The so-called nonspecific factors that ordinarily permeate all psychotherapeutic approaches—that is, unconditional acceptance, accurate empathy, positive regard, and support—are particularly salient in establishing therapeutic alliances with patients who have anorexia nervosa. Psychotherapeutic approaches can be safely utilized in the outpatient treatment of moderately ill patients with anorexia nervosa. However, very starved and emaciated patients, usually with a BMI of under 16, are generally neither psychologically nor cognitively available for psychotherapeutic engagement.

Adolescent Populations

As discussed in detail in Chapter 6 ("Family Treatment of Eating Disorders") in this volume, reasonable evidence exists for the role of family therapy in the treatment of younger adolescents with anorexia nervosa who have been ill for relatively short periods of time. Clearly, more research is needed regarding the potential utility of individual psychotherapy and other psychosocial approaches for outpatient adolescents, particularly when family therapy has failed or is not feasible.

Underweight Adults

Historically, psychoanalytically or psychodynamically informed therapies have been utilized by therapists for decades in the treatment of anorexia nervosa (Bruch 1970), but their effectiveness for these conditions has never been subjected to rigorous study. Although helpful in elucidating the psychological underpinnings of these disorders, the insights achieved through these therapies do not usually lead to behavioral change and a normalization of eating behaviors and weight. Rather the psychotherapy of patients with anorexia nervosa usually requires a "two track" approach to care (Garner et al. 1986). One track focuses on specific behaviors associated with weight loss and disordered eating, such as caloric restriction, compulsive exercising, and binge eating and purging. Cognitive behavioral techniques can be useful in normalizing eating and weight in such patients (Wilson 2001). The other track focuses on the underlying deficits in psychological functioning with which virtually all patients with anorexia nervosa struggle, such as deficits in affect awareness and affect regulation and self-esteem; maturity fears; and interpersonal mistrust. These deficits are best dealt with psychotherapeutically by using self psychological, interpersonal, and psychodynamically informed approaches.

Overall, very few systematic clinical trials have been published comparing different psychotherapies for anorexia nervosa. Early studies examining the role of shorter-term, focused therapies were compromised by small sample sizes and nonspecific results. For example, Channon and colleagues (1989) randomly assigned 24 adult patients to either CBT, behavior therapy, or routine care consisting of support and medical monitoring. All interventions demonstrated equal and only modest efficacy, but the small group sizes and restricted number of 24 sessions limited the power of the study. A larger trial by Crisp and colleagues (1991) randomly assigned 90 patients to one of four different interventions: 1) inpatient treatment followed by 12 outpatient sessions; 2) 12 outpatient sessions combining individual and family work with some incorporation of dietary counseling; 3) 10 sessions of an outpatient group, again with some dietary counseling; or 4) an assessment only. Despite a high dropout rate (18 of 30) in the inpatient group, all treatments were equally as effective in terms of weight gain at 1 year, and all were superior to no treatment. In a subsequent report following the outpatient individual/family therapy group (Gowers et al. 1994), 12 of the 20 original participants continued to do well at 2 years. Although the results are impressive, the value of this study is limited by several factors. The described intervention was a complicated one, combining elements of CBT and psychodynamic approaches, with the addition of family meetings as clinically indicated. Additionally, both therapists involved in the study had considerable experience in treating eating disorders with psychotherapy; thus, their results may not be readily reproducible.

Cognitive analytic therapy is a potential treatment for anorexia nervosa that incorporates elements of cognitive therapy with brief, focused psychodynamic psychotherapy. The patient and therapist develop a visual diagram of how the patient's illness is linked to how she experiences herself, as well as to her past and present relationships. The treatment goal is to enhance the patient's insight regarding her feelings and behaviors, theoretically minimizing the need for anorectic coping behaviors. Educational behavioral treatment is a more didactic intervention comprising nutritional education, discussion of eating disorders, and behavioral monitoring of food intake and exercise. Treasure and colleagues (1995) compared these two treatments in a trial of 30 patients with anorexia nervosa. Results were relatively positive for both groups, with 63% overall displaying good or intermediate nutritional outcome after 5 months and 37% achieving recovery after 1 year. But no differences were noted between the groups.

In a large, multitreatment study, Dare and colleagues (2001) compared outcomes for 84 patients randomly assigned to one of four short-term psychotherapy interventions: 1) a focal psychotherapy treatment (with the therapist adopting a nondirective stance, while exploring the conscious and unconscious meanings of the eating disorder pathology, the effects of these symptoms, and elements of transference), 2) a family therapy treatment addressing the manner in which a patient's eating disorder might control family relationships and methods through which its influence may be diminished, 3) cognitive analytic therapy as described in the previous paragraph, and 4) a routine treatment program in which patients received 30-minute weekly sessions with a resident in training, consisting of information regarding anorexia, medical monitoring, and encouragement. All three treatment interventions were more likely than the routine intervention to retain subjects over 1 year. Patients treated in the focal psychotherapy and family therapy interventions fared better than those receiving routine treatment in terms of weight gain, and there was a trend toward significance for those treated with cognitive analytic therapy.

In a recent randomized controlled trial of outpatient psychotherapy in anorexia nervosa (McIntosh et al. 2005), a group of 56 women with anorexia nervosa were randomly assigned to receive 20 sessions of manualized CBT, interpersonal psychotherapy (IPT), or nonspecific supportive clinical management (NSCM). The nonspecific clinical management intervention combined elements of psychoeducation, fostering of a therapeutic alliance to promote treatment adherence, and supportive psychotherapeutic techniques such as praise, reassurance, and advice. In the intent-to-treat analysis, the NSCM group had higher global ratings of much improved or minimal symptoms compared with the CBT and IPT groups, but these differences were significant only in comparison to IPT. In the analysis of completers, the NSCM group performed significantly better than both the CBT and IPT groups. The authors argued that NSCM might be particularly appropriate for acute, underweight patients. Certainly, the detailed emphasis on normalized eating and weight gain ought to be an important component of acute care. Moreover, much of the supportive content was patient-driven, thus allowing patients to attain a sense of autonomy and control. Conversely, IPT may be limited by factors such as a lack of symptom focus and a pattern of interpersonal avoidance in the acutely ill patient with anorexia nervosa. The cognitive rigidity and ego-syntonic nature of symptoms in more severely ill patients may at least partly explain the poor outcome with CBT in this study. The authors hypothesized that NSCM may thus be an appropriate initial-phase treatment in a stepwise approach to the treatment of anorexia nervosa.

Weight-Restored Adults

In the only controlled study of this population to date, Pike and colleagues (2003) examined the efficacy of outpatient CBT in a group of weight-restored patients after discharge from the hospital. Their manualized CBT intervention addressed cognitive and behavioral features linked to eating disorder pathology and examined cognitive schemas in relation to self-esteem and interpersonal functioning. Thirty-three patients were randomly assigned to 50 sessions over 1 year of CBT or nutritional counseling, which was largely psychoeducational and supportive. When relapse and dropout rates were combined, the results showed that 73% of the nutritional counseling group versus 22% of those receiving CBT experienced a treatment failure. Furthermore, 44% of the CBT group versus 7% of the nutritional counseling group met the criteria for "good outcome." Although, given its small sample size, this study must be considered quite preliminary, this was one of the first studies to provide empirical support for the utility of posthospitalization psychotherapeutic treatment of anorexia nervosa.

A single randomized controlled study of weight-restored patients with adolescent onset anorexia nervosa compared family therapy and individual therapy. This study found family therapy to be more effective than individual therapy in preventing relapse, but only in the younger patients with shorter duration of illness.

Of note, many patients with anorexia nervosa participate in group therapies led by professionals or advocacy groups. To date, there have been no systematic studies evaluating the efficacy of group therapies for anorexia nervosa. However, several published clinical descriptions of group treatment for anorexia nervosa (e.g., Kerr et al. 1992) have emphasized the difficulties inherent in using this approach with anorexia nervosa patients.

Novel Approaches: Third-Generation Psychotherapies

The patient's denial and rationalization of symptoms accompanied by significant resistance to change and extreme ambivalence often frustrate psychotherapeutic attempts and create significant therapeutic "disconnects" as patients enter treatments that are generally focused on modifying ego-syntonic behaviors. Since patients usually view their maladaptive eating behaviors as a means to an end they desire and admire (i.e., weight loss), they are frequently fearful of efforts aimed at getting them to change their ways. This barrier has lead investigators to examine more client-centered approaches for treating anorexia nervosa that focus not primarily on symptoms but on underlying attitudes. One prominent approach is motivational enhancement therapy (MET), based on a model used successfully in the field of substance abuse, where denial, ambivalence, and resistance to change are also significant treatment issues. The addictions field successfully incorporated the *trans-theoretical model of change* (Prochaska and DiClemente 1983) to help move patients' attitudes from denial through willing engagement in treatment—or, in the terms of this model, from the stage of precontemplation through contemplation, preparation, action, and maintenance—by means of several consciousness-raising processes that allow an individual to move from one stage to the next. The model argues that treatment is most effective when tailored to the patient's stage of change. The addictions field has adopted motivational interviewing to help patients who are ambivalent regarding treatment find intrinsic motivation, particularly in the early stages of precontemplation and contemplation.

This approach has now been applied to patients with eating disorders (Treasure et al. 1999). In a pilot study, Feld and colleagues (2001) demonstrated that four group sessions of MET over 4 weeks produced a statistically significant increase in motivation to change in a group with anorexia nervosa. However, no controlled trials regarding the efficacy of MET in terms of actual treatment outcomes for anorexia nervosa have yet been reported.

Other psychosocial approaches that may be helpful in the outpatient management of anorexia nervosa, especially for the core body image disturbance that often resists more traditional interventions, include experiential nonverbal therapies such as dance movement therapy and expressive art therapy, as well as mindfulness-based cognitive therapy. Although no published systematic evidence exists to support the effectiveness of these techniques, clinically they are often useful as adjunct interventions for patients who struggle mightily with recognizing, labeling, and verbalizing internal emotional states.

Summary

In summary, since few data exist to guide treatment choices regarding psychosocial interventions in the outpatient management of anorexia nervosa, there are currently no substitutes for thoughtful clinical experience, a longitudinal view of the disorder, and common sense in deciding on the optimal outpatient management for these patients. Although it seems that many patients in the non-weight-restored population can benefit from outpatient psychotherapy, it is wise to assess the individual patient's readiness to change before choosing a particular approach. Interventions such as nonspecific clinical management, MET, and even more traditional psychodynamic approaches may all directly or indirectly address resistance to change while strengthening the therapeutic alliance. More formally structured psychotherapies, such as CBT, may be more appropriate for weight-restored patients. It is likely that nonspecific therapeutic factors such as empathy, authenticity, and support are integral to any therapeutic approach, and astute clinicians must always remain attuned to the quality of the therapeutic alliance.

Pharmacological Approaches to the Outpatient Treatment of Anorexia Nervosa

In reviewing the literature and available treatment guidelines for eating disorders, we found notable disconnects between clinical practice and the paucity of empirical support for pharmacotherapy for eating disorders. Unfortunately, clear, strong, evidence-based support for the effectiveness of pharmacotherapy in underweight or weight-restored patients with anorexia nervosa simply does not exist at the present time. Much of the available research has focused on either reducing anxiety or alleviating mood-related symptoms in attempts to facilitate refeeding; increasing hunger (even though there is no evidence to support that hunger cues are disturbed in anorexia nervosa); inducing weight gain as a side effect of a particular agent; or treating a medical complication. None of these strategies have proven fruitful, and no drug as yet exists that effectively treats the core features of the disorder: body image disturbance, obsessionality and perfectionism, and extreme anticipatory anxiety.

Antidepressants

Early reports indicated that trials of tricyclic antidepressants (TCAs) neither addressed the core symptoms of anorexia nor resulted in significant weight gain. In addition, both TCAs and low weight may increase underweight patients' susceptibility to hypotension and cardiac arrhythmias (most notably prolongation of the QTc interval) in potentially additive fashion. Thus, the limited efficacy and safety concerns have militated against the use of this class of medications.

More recently, investigators have examined the role of SSRIs in anorexia nervosa, for both acutely ill and weight-restored populations. At present, no controlled trials of outpatient treatment with SSRIs in patients with low BMIs have been published. Clinical reports suggest that very low-weight anorexia nervosa patients are relatively unresponsive to the antidepressant, antiobsessional, and anxiolytic effects of SSRIs. This unresponsiveness may relate to the relative hyposerotonergic state of the brains of starved anorexia nervosa patients secondary to the nutritional effects of a diet low in tryptophan, making in vivo serotonin substrate unavailable for SSRIs to act on. A recently published retrospective study (Holtkamp et al. 2005) found that a group of patients receiving SSRI treatment did not differ from a group of patients not receiving SSRIs regarding the course of illness, including BMI and eating disorder psychopathology, during acute inpatient treatment and at 6 months post-discharge.

Better data exist regarding the potential role of SSRIs in preventing relapse in weight-restored individuals. A preliminary study by Kaye and colleagues (2001) randomly assigned 35 patients with anorexia nervosa who had successfully completed an inpatient program to fluoxetine maintenance treatment (average dosage=40 mg/day) versus placebo. Over the 1-year study, 84% of the placebo group versus 37% of the fluoxetine treated group experienced relapse. Of particular significance, the weight loss and appetite suppression occasionally associated with the short-term use of fluoxetine were not reported in these patients. More recently, in a large randomized controlled trial (Walsh et al. 2006), 93 weight-restored adults with anorexia nervosa were randomly assigned to receive either fluoxetine (up to 80 mg/day) or placebo, in addition to manualized CBT over 1 year. Both groups experienced similar rates of relapse over 1 year. This study suggests that even in the weight-restored state, patients with anorexia nervosa are resistant to the effects of SSRIs. Having said that, we must point out that clinically there are individual weight-restored patients with AN who clearly benefit from SSRI therapy, particularly for treatment of comorbid anxiety, depression, or OCD symptoms. No published research exists on the use of serotonin-norepinephrine reuptake inhibitors such as venlafaxine for anorexia nervosa. Bupropion is contraindicated in this population because of an increased risk of seizures, and mirtazapine has been associated with neutropenia and should therefore not be used in patients already at risk for this blood dyscrasia.

Antipsychotic Medications

Given the near-delusional intensity of body image distortion associated with anorexia nervosa, investigators have historically examined the efficacy of antipsychotic medications in the treatment of anorexia nervosa. Early trials of typical antipsychotics such as chlorpromazine (Dally and Sargant 1966), pimozide (Vandereycken et al. 1982), and sulpiride (Vandereycken 1984) yielded conflicting results. Moreover, the problematic adverse effects of reduced seizure threshold and QTc prolongation have limited the utility of these agents. Greater interest exists in the newer class of atypical antipsychotics because of their demonstrated propensity for inducing weight gain, their antiobsessional and anxiolytic properties, and their more favorable adverse-effect profile. Several groups have specifically examined the efficacy of olanzapine in anorexia nervosa, and case reports have described risperidone as helpful. Several case studies of inpatients treated with olanzapine at a dosage of 5–10 mg/day have reported weight increases, a decreased fear of fatness, and reduced agitation and resistance to treatment (Hansen 1999; La Via et al. 2000). In a series of five hospitalized adolescent patients with anorexia nervosa, olanzapine (at 2.5–10 mg/day) did not accelerate rates of weight gain but did lead both to a decline in anorectic symptoms such as fear of gaining weight and rigidity of thinking and to adequate sedation (Mehler et al. 2001). In an open-label study, Powers and colleagues (2002) treated 18 outpatients with olanzapine 10 mg/day over 10 weeks. In this series, 10 of the 14 patients completing the study gained an average of 8.75 pounds, and the medication was well tolerated, with only mild and transient sedation noted. However, the apparent effectiveness of medication in this study may have been confounded by the concurrent use of a weekly medication adherence group and phone check-ins for all subjects. Regardless, these results suggest that the combination of medication and an active "disease management" program may improve both adherence and outcomes. A National Institute of Mental Health–supported randomized controlled trial examining the role of olanzapine in the outpatient treatment of underweight patients with anorexia nervosa (Attia et al. 2005) is currently under way at two sites. Clearly, although definitive evidence of effectiveness does not yet exist, atypical antipsychotics may be helpful in the ongoing management of individual cases. In using this class of medications for off-label indications such as anorexia nervosa, however, it is important to be aware of risks and inform patients and their families accordingly. For example, the extent to which these patients treated with these medications might develop metabolic disturbances, including hyperlipidemia and insulin resistance, is unknown.

Mood Stabilizers

There is no evidence to support the efficacy of mood stabilizers for the core symptoms of anorexia nervosa. In the presence of a bipolar illness, these medications, especially lithium, should be used with considerable caution in anorexia nervosa patients, who may be dehydrated and whose renal function may be compromised.

Prokinetic Agents

Patients with anorexia nervosa typically report early satiety and bloating with refeeding. Furthermore, these patients may objectively have delayed gastric emptying, although a strong relationship between the two has not been observed (Domstad et al. 1987). Early studies examined the efficacy of prokinetic drugs such as metoclopramide (Domstad et al. 1987), domperidone (Stacher et al. 1986), or intravenous cisapride (Stacher et al. 1987; Szmukler et al. 1995) in early refeeding, generally by short-term parenteral administration. Since those trials were published, cisapride has been removed from the market because of potentially fatal cardiac effects, and there have been no publications of alternative prokinetic interventions. Oral domperidone 10–20 mg before meals is still employed in countries other than the United States, and patients do clinically report an alleviation of their gastrointestinal complaints with this agent. One must be aware, however, of the risk of extrapyramidal side effects associated with this medication and monitor patients carefully.

Hormone Replacement Therapy for Osteoporosis

Anorexia nervosa is associated with a high prevalence of osteoporosis (38%) and osteopenia (92%) (Grinspoon et al. 2000). These potentially devastating complications, which can be present even in young patients, interfere with growth and increase patients' risks of pathological fracture (Rigotti et al. 1991). The pathophysiology of osteopenia/osteoporosis seen in anorexia nervosa is more complex than that seen in postmenopausal women. Estrogen deficiency results in decreased new bone formation, but the hypercortisolism associated with starvation contributes to increased bone resorption in anorexia nervosa as well. Moreover, measures of insulin-like growth factor–1 (IGF-1), a nutritionally dependent hormone and important regulator of skeletal growth and mineralization, are consistently lower in patients with anorexia nervosa (Grinspoon et al. 2002). Thus, a combination of anabolic and catabolic mechanisms likely underlies the diminished bone density commonly found in anorexia nervosa.

Despite widespread use of hormone treatment, generally in the form of oral contraceptive pills, there is no evidence that this intervention is effective in preventing osteopenia/osteoporosis in anorexia nervosa. In a randomized, placebo-controlled trial of adults, estrogen replacement had no effect on bone mineral density (Klibanski et al. 1995). Similarly, two groups (Golden et al. 2002; Munoz et al. 2002) have examined the role of estrogen-progestin oral contraceptives in adolescent outpatients. Despite some weight gain in both groups, there was no observed effect of the estrogen-progestin on bone mineral density. It has been hypothesized that estrogen administration does not address the ongoing destructive effects of variables such as insulin-like growth factor (IGF) deficiency and hypercortisolism, and that estrogen therapy alone is therefore insufficient. Furthermore, many clinicians feel that the use of hormone replacement and the monthly pseudo-menstrual cycle induced by the oral contraceptives may provide a false sense of reassurance to patients with ongoing symptoms of anorexia nervosa.

More recent studies have examined the impact of novel treatments on preserving or improving bone mineral density in individuals with anorexia nervosa. For example, an oral contraceptive was combined with subcutaneous recombinant human (rh) IGF (Grinspoon et al. 2002) in a small group of adult outpatients, with some promising results. Although interesting, this intervention demands further study and is not yet clinically available. Additionally, Miller and colleagues (2004) administered risedronate 5 mg/day to 10 women with a persistently low BMI and found increased bone density of the AP spine at both 6 and 9 months when compared with a placebo group. Although the intervention was well tolerated, the safety of long-term bisphosphonates has not been established, nor are they approved for use in premenopausal women. Furthermore, these medications are teratogenic and may be stored in bone for years posttreatment, with the risk that they might be mobilized from bone during pregnancy. Therefore, they should be used with great caution in women of childbearing age.

Long-Term Monitoring and Follow-Up: Indications for Hospitalization and Management of the Chronic Patient

The majority of patients who develop anorexia nervosa will at one point in the course of their illness require some form of inpatient treatment. Reasons for admission to the hospital usually fall into three categories: treatment for the core symptoms of the illness, which usually involves an extended admission in a specialized residential or inpatient unit and which includes nutritional rehabilitation; a brief admission, often on a medical unit, for treatment of the medical complications of the illness; and treatment of psychiatric comorbidity, including suicidality. Indications for the first two reasons have not been absolutely clearly established; clinical judgment and experience play an important role in making these decisions (see Table 4–1 in Chapter 4, "Management of Anorexia Nervosa in Inpatient and Partial Hospitalization Settings," in this volume for a listing of the common physiological reasons for hospital admission). Generally speaking, acute rapid weight loss is more dangerous than chronic slow weight loss. Rapid weight loss is often associated with several medical reasons for hospitalization. Binge eating and purging in an underweight state are ominous symptoms and are more likely to lead to serious medical complications and the need for hospitalization. Younger patients are more susceptible to the acute effects of nutritional deprivation and weight loss and are more likely to require hospitalization sooner than older patients with similar levels of symptoms.

Once weight has been restored, patients require ongoing close outpatient follow-up, since relapse is the rule rather than the exception in weight-restored patients with anorexia nervosa. Patients should be seen at least weekly for the first several months after weight restoration, although the risk of relapse extends for at least 18 months posthospitalization (Carter et al. 2004). Relapse prevention strategies that have been examined include family therapy, CBT, and pharmacotherapy, as reviewed earlier in this chapter. Clinical judgment should be used in deciding the appropriate use of these approaches in weight-restored patients. The patient should be weighed periodically (once a month) unless there is evidence that her condition is unstable and she is losing weight, in which case weekly weights are appropriate. This process usually requires a negotiation with the patient, first not to compulsively weigh herself outside the office, second to agree to be weighed in the office, and third to be told what her weight actually is so that reactions to it can be examined and discussed in a therapeutic context. Assessment of medical status through regularly monitoring blood work and ECGs also needs to be part of ongoing care. The ideal approach to ambulatory treatment is based on close interdisciplinary collaboration in outpatient care, with input from a dietitian, psychologist, and/or social worker who may be assessing or treating the family and/or providing the psychotherapy, and the primary care physician and psychiatrist who are medically monitoring the patient and providing appropriate pharmacotherapy.

The specific management of chronically ill treatment-resistant patients is covered in detail in Chapter 16 ("Management of Patients With Chronic, Intractable Eating Disorders"). Suffice it to say that the treatment of such patients raises many difficult clinical and ethical issues, including that of involuntary admission to the hospital and forced feeding. In determining whether to impose treatment, the clinician must always consider the basic principles of ethical treatment, which include respect for the patient's autonomy and assessment of competence, nonmaleficence, and beneficence. Sometimes, in dealing with such patients' disordered eating and weight, less is better; the clinician's main focus should be on keeping patients alive through ongoing medical monitoring and on improving quality of life rather than eradication of symptoms. The provision of hope, genuine respect, warmth, and unconditional acceptance within a therapeutic context is critical to the long-term management of such patients. With this in mind, we have recently developed an innovative, modified eating disorder assertive community treatment (ED ACT) approach to chronically ill treatment-resistant eating disorder patients (Kaplan et al. 2005). This approach adapts the ACT model, typically applied to patients with schizophrenia, to patients with chronic eating disorders, usually anorexia nervosa. This client-centered, community-based multidisciplinary approach focuses on three main goals in this patient population: 1) to improve quality of life, 2) to facilitate medical stabilization, and 3) to reduce recidivism rates and hospitalization. Initial response in the first cohort of ED ACT patients supports the application of this model to this group of seriously ill patients. Time will tell the extent to which this program will be realized.

References

Attia E, Kaplan AS, Schroeder L, et al: Atypical antipsychotic medication in anorexia nervosa. Presentation at the annual meeting of the Eating Disorders Research Society, Toronto, ON, September 29, 2005

Bruch H: Psychotherapy in primary anorexia nervosa. J Nerv Ment Dis 150:51–67, 1970

Carter JC, Blackmore E, Sutandar-Pinnock K, et al: Relapse in anorexia nervosa: a survival analysis. Psychol Med 34:671–679, 2004

Channon S, de Silva P, Hemsley D, et al: A controlled trial of cognitive-behavioural and behavioural treatment of anorexia nervosa. Behav Res Ther 27:529–535, 1989

Crisp AH, Norton K, Gowers S, et al: A controlled study of the effect of therapies aimed at adolescent and family psychopathology in anorexia nervosa. Br J Psychiatry 159:325–331, 1991

Dally P, Sargant W: Treatment and outcome of anorexia nervosa. Br Med J 2(5517):793–795, 1966

Dare C, Eisler I, Russell G, et al: Psychological therapies for adults with anorexia nervosa: randomised controlled trial of out-patient treatments. Br J Psychiatry 78:216–221, 2001

Domstad PA, Shih WJ, Humphries L, et al: Radionuclide gastric emptying studies in patients with anorexia nervosa. J Nucl Med 28:816–819, 1987

Feld R, Woodside DB, Kaplan AS, et al: Pretreatment motivational enhancement therapy for eating disorders: a pilot study. Int J Eat Disord 29:393–400, 2001

Garner DM, Garfinkel PE, Irvine MJ: Integration and sequencing of treatment approaches for eating disorders. Psychother Psychosom 46:67–75, 1986

Golden NH, Lanzkowsky L, Schebendach J, et al: The effect of estrogen-progestin treatment on bone mineral density in anorexia nervosa. J Pediatr Adolesc Gynecol 15:135–143, 2002

Gowers S, Norton K, Haiek C, et al: Outcome of outpatient psychotherapy for adults with anorexia nervosa. Int J Eat Disord 15:165–177, 1994

Grinspoon S, Thomas E, Pitts S, et al: Prevalence and predictive factors for regional osteopenia in women with anorexia nervosa. Ann Intern Med 133:790–794, 2000

Grinspoon S, Thomas L, Miller K, et al: Effects of recombinant human IGF-I and oral contraceptive administration on bone density in anorexia nervosa. J Clin Endocrinol Metab 87:2883–2891, 2002

Hansen L: Olanzapine in the treatment of anorexia nervosa (letter). Br J Psychiatry 175:592, 1999

Holtkamp K, Konrad K, Kaiser N, et al: A retrospective study of SSRI treatment in adolescent anorexia nervosa: insufficient evidence for efficacy. J Psychiatr Res 39:303–310, 2005

Kaplan AS, Garfinkel PE (eds): Medical Issues and the Eating Disorders: The Interface. New York, Brunner/Mazel, 1993

Kaplan A, Colton P, Cavanaugh P, et al: A new community-based approach to the care of the chronically ill eating disorder patient: an Assertive Eating Disorder Community Treatment Team (ACTT) for eating disorders. Presentation at the annual meeting of the Eating Disorders Research Society, Toronto, ON, September 30, 2005

Kaye W, Nagata T, Weltzin TE, et al: Double-blind placebo-controlled administration of fluoxetine in restricting type anorexia nervosa. Biol Psychiatry 49:644–652, 2001

Kerr A, Leszcz M, Kaplan A: Continuing care groups for chronic anorexia nervosa, in Group Psychotherapy for Eating Disorders. Edited by Harper-Guiffre H, MacKenzie KR. Washington, DC, American Psychiatric Press, 1992, pp 261–272

Klibanski A, Biller BM, Schoenfeld DA, et al: The effects of estrogen administration on trabecular bone loss in young women with anorexia nervosa. J Clin Endocrinol Metab 80:898–904, 1995

La Via MC, Gray N, Kaye WH: Case reports of olanzapine treatment of anorexia nervosa. Int J Eat Disord 27:363–366, 2000

McIntosh V, Jordan J, Luty S, et al: Three psychotherapies for anorexia nervosa: a randomized controlled trial. Am J Psychiatry 162:741–747, 2005

Mehler C, Wewetzer CH, Schulze V, et al: Olanzapine in children and adolescents with chronic anorexia nervosa: a study of five cases. Eur Child Adolesc Psychiatry 10:151–157, 2001

Miller KK, Grieco KA, Mulder J, et al: Effects of risedronate on bone density in anorexia nervosa. J Clin Endocrinol Metab 89:3903–3906, 2004

Munoz MT, Morande G, Garcia-Centenera JA, et al: The effects of estrogen administration on bone mineral density in adolescents with anorexia nervosa. Eur J Endocrinol 146:45–50, 2002

Pike KM, Walsh BT, Vitousek K, et al: Cognitive therapy in the posthospitalization treatment of anorexia nervosa. Am J Psychiatry 160:2046–2049, 2003

Powers PS, Santana CA, Bannon YS: Olanzapine in the treatment of anorexia nervosa: an open label trial. Int J Eat Disord 32:146–154, 2002

Prochaska JO, DiClemente CC: Stages and processes of self-change of smoking: toward an integrative model of change. J Consult Clin Psychol 51:390–395, 1983

Rigotti NA, Neer RM, Skates SJ, et al: The clinical course of osteoporosis in anorexia nervosa: a longitudinal study of cortical bone mass. JAMA 265:1133–1138, 1991

Stacher G, Kiss A, Wiesnagrotzki S, et al: Oesophageal and gastric motility disorders in patients categorised as having primary anorexia nervosa. Gut 27:1120–1126, 1986

Stacher G, Bergmann H, Wiesnagrotzki S, et al: Intravenous cisapride accelerates delayed gastric emptying and increases antral contraction amplitude in patients with primary anorexia nervosa. Gastroenterology 92:1000–1006, 1987

Szmukler GI, Young GP, Miller G, et al: A controlled trial of cisapride in anorexia nervosa. Int J Eat Disord 17:347–357, 1995

Treasure J, Todd G, Brolly M, et al: A pilot study of a randomised trial of cognitive analytical therapy vs educational behavioral therapy for adult anorexia nervosa. Behav Res Ther 33:363–367, 1995

Treasure J, Katzman M, Schmidt U, et al: Engagement and outcome in the treatment of bulimia nervosa. Behav Res Ther 37:405–418, 1999

Vandereycken W: Neuroleptics in the short-term treatment of anorexia nervosa: a double-blind placebo-controlled study with sulpiride. Br J Psychiatry 144:288–292, 1984

Vandereycken W, Pierloot R: Pimozide combined with behavior therapy in the short-term treatment of anorexia nervosa: a double-blind placebo-controlled cross-over study. Acta Psychiatr Scand 66:445–450, 1982

Walsh BT, Kaplan AS, Attia E, et al: Fluoxetine after weight restoration in anorexia nervosa: a randomized, placebo-controlled trial. JAMA 295:2605–2612, 2006

Wilson GT: Cognitive-behavioral and interpersonal therapies for eating disorders, in Treatments of Psychiatric Disorders, Vol 2. Gabbard GO, Editor-in-Chief. Washington, DC, American Psychiatric Press, 2001, pp 2139–2158

Family Treatment of Eating Disorders

James D. Lock, M.D., Ph.D.

Daniel le Grange, Ph.D.

Family treatments for eating disorders have long been recommended, starting with the earliest medical descriptions of anorexia nervosa, when Charles Lasegue (1883) suggested that the family and patient should both be subjects of treatment. However, Lasegue's view was not widely endorsed even at the time, as both William Gull (1874) and Jean-Martin Charcot suggested that separation from family members was necessary for treatment (Silverman 1997). As a result, it was left to the pioneering work of Salvador Minuchin and colleagues to revive an interest in family approaches to eating disorders (Liebman et al. 1974). In this chapter, we describe a range of family approaches to eating disorders and review the rationale and empirical support for them.

Why Families Have Been Targeted for Treatment

There has been much speculation and some research into family processes and eating disorders (Lock 2002). Although a number of genetic predispositions are likely to shape eating preferences and behaviors, parents also influence the development of eating patterns (Birch and Fisher 1998). Decisions about types of foods, style of eating (e.g., snacking and fast food, mealtimes), and the availability of foods establish a milieu around food that informs much of the child's experience of eating. A few studies suggest that some family eating processes can increase the risk for disordered eating (Marchi and Cohen 1990). In relation to eating disorders themselves, data suggest that parents, particularly mothers, may contribute to their children's (particularly daughters') decision to lose weight (Pike and Rodin 1991). In addition, general family functioning may contribute to the development of bulimia, particularly in families that are conflicted, disorganized, critical, and less cohesive (Johnson and Flach 1985). Modeling behavior by parents with unhealthy eating behaviors may also influence their children to adopt similar attitudes and behaviors (Fairburn et al. 1998). A family's placing undue importance on thinness also appears to be correlated with increased bulimic symptoms and beliefs (Stice 2002). Studies of anorexia nervosa suggest that highly critical parents may contribute to poorer outcome in treatment (Hodes and le Grange 1993). In sum, most of the data available on the role of families and parents in the development and maintenance of eating disorders are correlational rather than experimental, and most are more clearly applicable to bulimia nervosa. Nonetheless, the evidence that does exist has contributed to the development of treatments that focus on parents and families, with the aim of correcting or minimizing perceived problems in order to help with eating disorders.

A range of family-based therapies, including structural family therapy, strategic family therapy, narrative family therapy, and family-based treatment (FBT; i.e., the Maudsley approach), have emerged to treat eating disorders (Dare and Eisler 1997). Although it is beyond the scope of this chapter to review all types of family therapy, a summary of the principal components of major approaches and their main targets is presented in Table 6–1. We cover structural family therapy as practiced by Minuchin and the Maudsley approach in detail below because these approaches are the best known and probably best represent the most prominent types of family therapy currently provided in community service.

Table 6–1. Types of family therapy for eating disorders

Type	Main therapeutic targets	Main characteristics of method
Traditional	Increases the protective factors for the vulnerable individual by increasing family support and skill	Educates parents to reduce the impacts of external stresses or separation of parents from child if they are the main source of stress ("parentectomy")
Structural	Encourages appropriate family hierarchies and roles; decreases enmeshment and rigidity	Alters family organization through limiting some patterns and encouraging others
Strategic	Views symptoms as influencing family functioning, and families are not blamed (atheoretical stance)	Uses paradoxical prescriptions to diminish symptoms' impact on patient and family
Milan	Indirectly confronts the role of symptoms in the maintenance of family structure and process in order to manage a theoretical self-protective homeostatic mechanism in families	Encourages therapist to take a neutral stance and promote self-examination through circular questioning and end-of-session reviews
Narrative	Views family in nonpathological way; specific techniques are developed to encourage change (e.g., externalization)	Uses externalization and co-generation of a shared story to unite family in struggle against illness
Maudsley approach (family-based treatment)	Remains agnostic as to cause of anorexia nervosa; focuses on symptom management by parents; adopts neutral stance	Uses circular questioning, therapist consultant, externalization; adopts nonconfrontational approach

Family Treatment for Adolescent Anorexia Nervosa

Minuchin: Psychosomatic Approach to Treatment of Families

Minuchin and colleagues at the Philadelphia Child Guidance Center began examining family therapy as a strategy for assisting in the treatment of psychosomatic illnesses in children and adolescents. Anorexia nervosa became the paradigmatic exemplar for their conceptualization of ways that family processes contribute to the development and maintenance of behavioral and psychological symptoms. Specifically, these researchers identified four major problems in "psychosomatic families" (Minuchin et al. 1978): enmeshment, conflict avoidance, overprotectiveness, and rigidity. *Enmeshment* was characterized as a failure to maintain adequate personal boundaries among family members, sometimes leading to what these researchers called "structural problems in the family," wherein the roles of parents and siblings were reversed or inadequately differentiated. *Conflict avoidance* in these families led to suppression of anger or other difficult emotions that contributed to a failure to address significant problems. At the same time, these families tended to be inwardly directed and viewed the outside world as potentially threatening to the equilibrium of the family. Hence, they developed an *overly protective attitude and set of behaviors* toward their children. Finally, these families were characterized as being *limited in the range of problem-solving strategies they could imagine or use.* In addition, they often responded defensively to new ideas and suggestions, thereby effectively limiting their ability to use new information. This rigidity made integration of the developmental needs of the family as it changed over time challenging to manage.

Taken together, these family characteristics were seen as particularly important in contributing to the development of anorexia nervosa. Enmeshment made it difficult for the emerging adolescent to disentangle herself from the family as she found increasing need to be more independent. Her independent strivings in turn needed to be suppressed in order to avoid conflict and disappointment or other strong feelings. This problem was further exacerbated by the tendency of the family to be overprotective just when the adolescent needed to turn to resources outside the family to support her burgeoning identity. Finally, the inflexibility of the family made responding to these dilemmas rigid and ineffective (Minuchin et al. 1978).

Minuchin's approach to these dilemmas as posed in particular by anorexia nervosa is well described in his classic book *Psychosomatic Families: Anorexia Nervosa in Context* (Minuchin et al. 1978). The overall approach is one that aims to address the problems attendant on psychosomatic family process. There is an attempt to modify structural problems that result largely from enmeshment by challenging inappropriate alliances between a parent and a child, most particularly the patient. There are attempts to reinforce more appropriate structural hierarchies by insisting that parents take up the parental role and work together in achieving change. On the other hand, sibling subsystems are also encouraged, so as to oppose dyads between a parent and child as well as to link siblings more closely together when they are facing their particular family dilemmas. Overprotectiveness and rigidity are challenged by the therapeutic process itself, which is both intrusive and at times frankly confrontational (Liebman et al. 1974).

Dare and Eisler: Family Empowerment

Minuchin and his colleagues' work was seen as both highly innovative and provocative at the time. Their published account of a case series of 53 subjects, in which about 80% recovered powerfully, motivated the field of family therapy, particularly for anorexia nervosa. Subsequent work by Haley, Mandanes, and Selvini Palazzoli enriched the armamentarium of family therapists considerably, and for a time these approaches to family therapy were routinely recommended for the care of adolescents with anorexia nervosa (Haley 1973; Mandanes 1981; Palazzoli 1974). However, a major adjustment to the psychosomatic approach to family treatment began to emerge in the mid-1980s at the Maudsley Hospital in London, where Christopher Dare and Ivan Eisler, working in the laboratory of Gerald Russell, began to reconfigure family therapy for adolescent anorexia nervosa. The changes they made were based on three factors: their clinical experience on an inpatient ward where adolescents were routinely refed by nurses; a strongly held view that inpatient care was in many ways a corrosive experience for adolescents that should be avoided if possible; and observations that the families in which anorexia nervosa developed seemed more structurally and psychodynamically divergent than those described by Minuchin as psychosomatic. In addition, Dare and Eisler incorporated into their thinking new models of family therapy, particularly narrative therapy and feminist challenges to authoritarian therapeutic maneuvers (Mandanes 1981; White and Epston 1990). The result of these influences was a particular form of family therapy that was specific for anorexia nervosa (Dare and Eisler 1992).

Dare and Eisler's family approach is described as "agnostic" as to the cause of the disorder. In contrast to Minuchin et al.'s model, no presumption is made about disrupted family processes either causing or maintaining the symptoms. Rather, the family is viewed as a resource for the therapist and patient, and the family is held in continuous positive regard in order to facilitate and enhance feelings of efficacy. Suggestions of guilt and blame are assiduously avoided by the therapist and are challenged when brought up by the parents themselves or other family members. As in structural therapy, the approach supports proper alignment of parental resources that may have been set awry by the challenges of having a daughter or son with a life threatening illness. Thus, parents are asked to work together to find agreed-on solutions; siblings are asked to refrain from trying to parent the sibling with anorexia nervosa and instead to align with her as she struggles with the demands the parents place on her. To reduce blame and guilt on the part of the parents and the patient, the therapist attempts to externalize the illness based on narrative techniques that separate the illness from the patient. This allows parents to use the full measure of their abilities to fight the illness per se rather than to feel that they are struggling against their emaciated child. Furthermore, this strategy lays the groundwork for helping the patient to see herself as being different from, and more complex than, simply a case of anorexia nervosa, by illustrating the many ways she has been damaged and distorted by the illness. Perhaps most importantly, the approach is highly focused on disrupting the disordered eating behaviors, particularly self-starvation and overexercise, that lead to the behavioral, psychological, and physiological reinforcements of anorexia nervosa. Finally, the therapist takes the stance of an expert consultant who is joining the family in their dilemma to help them rather than to direct them in finding solutions. This stance encourages both empowerment and autonomy.

Family-Based Treatment

The family approach developed by Dare and Eisler has been manualized (Lock and le Grange 2001; Lock et al. 2001). In this formulation, the treatment is called *family-based treatment* and is structured in three distinct phases replicating the design of Dare et al. (Table 6–2). Phase 1 is designed to help the family and particularly the parents confront the symptoms of anorexia nervosa and begin refeeding their child. The initial session is designed to adjust parental anxiety to a level that makes the use of therapy possible. In some cases, when families have become inured to the effects of starvation on their child, the aim is to raise anxiety and generate a sense of alarm and need for action. In other cases, families are paralyzed by their anxieties to the extent that they are afraid to take any action. In these cases, the therapist aims to modulate the anxiety so that it can become productive. The therapist is seen as both warm and caring but also the bearer of very bad news insofar as anorexia nervosa is threatening the life of their child. The balance of these two stances is measured in relation to the unique needs of the family. In the first session, the therapist attempts to align with the family in their plight and then to take a history focused on how the disorder emerged and what its effects have been on the family, with the aim of establishing a shared story about these events.

Next, the therapist aims to help the family separate the illness from their child by asking each family member, including the patient, to identify how he or she has changed since the anorexia nervosa began. Typically, these changes include becoming isolated, irritable, depressed, and obsessive. The therapist then describes in great detail and with deliberate effect the debilitating impact of anorexia nervosa medically, psychologically, and socially over a lifetime, and emphasizes the need for immediate and decisive action to change the current course to prevent these dire outcomes.

This process is illustrated in the treatment of Susan, a 14-year-old competitive runner with an 8-month history of anorexia nervosa.

> The therapist explained to Susan's parents that it was imperative that something be done to avert the ongoing slow heart rate, loss of mineralized bone as a result of persistent amenorrhea, and extreme social and psychological withdrawal that now characterized their previously healthy young daughter. The therapist added that it was clear that unless the parents took charge of this situation, medical

Table 6–2. Family-based treatment: phases and interventions

Phase	Aims	Main interventions	End point
Parental refeeding	To promote taking charge of eating and weight-loss behaviors	Modulate parental anxieties to encourage taking action; support and educate parents in their activities; assist siblings in supporting their ill sibling; support patient in her efforts to tolerate refeeding	Weight is near normal and eating occurs without undo conflict or distress under parental supervision.
Adolescent control of eating and weight processes	To transition the control of eating and weight to the adolescent under parental guidance	Assist family in identifying patient's readiness to begin to take up control of eating and weight behaviors appropriate for age; manage parental anxiety about this transition; problem-solve around issues specifically related to food and weight in the adolescent's life	Adolescent is under full control of eating and weight-related behaviors; is gaining or maintaining weight at level appropriate for height, and is able to manage eating in social settings outside the family.
Addressing of adolescent issues and termination	To promote an understanding of adolescence and to support family in identifying issues that may require attention (no focus on eating disorder symptoms)	Conduct a psychoeducational review of adolescent development; examine implications for the patient and family; identify any other emotional or developmental issues with which the patient and family need assistance	Patient and family are on track, and the patient is ready for full reentry into adolescence; other psychological issues not specific to anorexia that need treatment (e.g., obsessive-compulsive disorder, depression) have been identified and recommendations for treatment have been made.

hospitalization would occur imminently, and ultimately Susan's risk of death due to either cardiac arrest or suicide would increase markedly. After these dire warnings, the therapist ended the session by asking the parents to bring a meal for the next session that they believed would help restore their child's health so they could begin the process of averting these dire outcomes.

The second session built on the concept of the family meal first initiated by Minuchin et al. (1978). The aim of the meal in FBT is primarily to learn about how the family is currently trying to help their child eat. Thus, the family is interviewed about food shopping, meal preparation, mealtime processes, and the current dilemmas they are facing in these regards. The therapist observes the family during the meal and notes in what ways, if any, the family attempts to change the eating behavior of their child. This allows the therapist to join in a very specific way with the family around the problematic behaviors and adds to the therapist's credibility. A secondary aim of the session is to help the family try to assist their child to eat a bit more than she planned. This involves coaching the parents to work together and be persistent and insistent in their demands, while at the same time controlling their tempers, criticism, and blame. Whether or not the child eats more at this meal is less important than what the parents and therapist learn about these processes.

> Susan's parents, Susan, and her 9-year-old sister arrived with a meal that con-
> sisted of baked chicken, mashed potatoes, green beans, rolls and butter, and a
> cherry pie. The therapist observed that Susan's mother served the meal by
> placing the dishes at the center of the table. Each family member served them-
> selves. In response to the therapist's question about who usually made the
> meals, Susan's mother replied that she did and that Susan's father often arrived
> home too late to eat with the family. Susan made her own breakfast and
> lunches. The therapist asked the parents if they were certain that Susan ate her
> breakfast and lunch. They replied that they were sometimes dubious because
> Susan continued to lose weight. When it appeared that Susan stopped eating
> after only eating a small amount of chicken and some green beans, the ther-
> apist asked her parents if they felt she had eaten enough to begin to gain
> weight. They replied that they did not think so. Susan looked down and
> pushed her plate away. The therapist asked her parents to sit on either side of
> Susan. They asked her to eat some more chicken. She shook her head, indi-
> cating she would not. The therapist noted to the parents that Susan had cho-
> sen only a small amount of food and had served herself, and suggested that
> perhaps the parents needed to make their suggestion more specific by choos-

ing a food for Susan to eat. Susan's mother put some green beans on the plate. The therapist asked why she chose green beans. Susan's mother said she thought it more likely Susan would eat them than anything else. "Do you think that a roll and butter or more chicken would be better for her?" the therapist asked. "Yes, I do, but I don't want to make her angry." "It may be necessary to face that anger, though, if you are going to help her," replied the therapist. The therapist turned to Susan's father and asked him if he agreed with his wife about what Susan should eat. "Yes. She needs to eat something besides vegetables," he replied. "So you are both in agreement. Can you both now together tell Susan that she needs to eat the roll and butter?" the therapist asked. At this point, Susan tried to push her chair back and murmured under her breath, "You can't make me." Still, for another 10 minutes, Susan's parents persisted in their insistence that she eat. The therapist continued to support them in these efforts, Finally, Susan relented and ate a small bite. She said, "Anything to get out of here. I hate all of you!" The therapist congratulated the parents on helping Susan and told Susan that she appreciated that anorexia nervosa had made her angry and that she respected Susan for all her strength and determination. She explained to the parents that this was a big step forward and that they needed to build on this success. The therapist told the parents that she would be there to help them figure out how to proceed each step of the way, though she was confident in their judgment.

The remainder of the first phase of FBT is a weekly detailed examination of parents' attempts at refeeding their child. These sessions begin with a review of a weight chart that allows them access to information about how their child is doing and what ways their efforts at refeeding are effective (Figure 6–1). For example, parents are asked about each meal and snack: what was prepared, what was eaten, who prepared it, how it could be more nutritionally robust, and what the emotional tone of the meals was. In this way the therapist helps the parents make persistent and consistent changes to support the reversal of self-starvation and, at the same time, attempts to minimize blame and criticism.

Susan's parents made a number of changes in the week after the family meal. Susan's mother made her breakfast and her lunch. Further, both parents stayed with her while she ate breakfast. If she did not eat, she had to return to her room and miss school until she did. Susan's father changed his work schedule so that he could be home to help with monitoring Susan's dinner. At lunch, Susan's mother came to eat with her; this approach, though embarrassing for Susan, did help Susan make weight progress she otherwise would have avoided. All the while, Susan+'s parents were evenhanded but unrelenting in their expec-

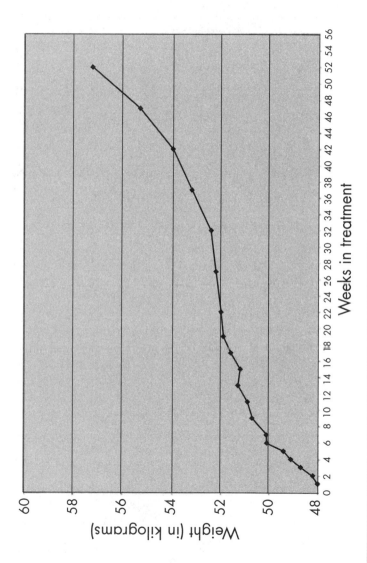

Figure 6–1.   Typical weight chart (12 months) for use in family-based treatment of patients with anorexia nervosa.

tations. On numerous occasions Susan tried to pick a fight with them, but they did not take the bait. Instead, they simply ignored her tantrums and waited until she realized they were not going to relent in their expectations.

The second phase of treatment begins when the patient has regained most of her weight and is eating under parental supervision without protest. The mood of the family is generally much improved at this point, and there is usually an atmosphere of hope that previously was not apparent. The aim of the second phase is to return full control of eating and weight-related behaviors (e.g., exercise) to the adolescent as would be appropriate for her age. Parents are sometimes understandably reluctant to hand control back. It has usually been an unpleasant battle for them to get the control in the first place, and they are often worried that symptoms will return. At the same time, the therapist needs to help the family evaluate the readiness of the adolescent to take charge of feeding herself and help them to develop safe strategies to test her readiness. Often, meals will be returned in a sequence starting with snacks and lunches at school. Return to sport activities, especially for the competitive athletes, is another challenge that the family faces. Sometimes it is necessary to take this transition very slowly, while in other cases the transition occurs rather quickly. Often during this phase weight gain slows, but in many cases it begins to pick up again as the adolescent and family become more confident that the problem is mastered.

> The biggest challenge during the second phase of Susan's treatment was her desire to return to competitive running. Both the therapist and the parents felt running was a challenging sport to return to at this point and encouraged her to take up a more team-oriented sport. Susan struggled with this advice, but she ultimately decided that she would play basketball, and if that went well and her parents agreed, she could consider track in the spring. Susan lost some weight when she began playing basketball, but she appreciated the comradeship of the team and picked her weight up again.

The third and final phase of FBT is aimed at promoting increased autonomy in the family, examining how the adolescent process has been affected by anorexia nervosa, and terminating treatment. In some ways, the third phase of treatment resembles what might be done initially in many other forms of family treatment, because it is in this phase that there is a first attempt to look at how anorexia nervosa relates to adolescent processes as a whole. The principal aim is to make sure that the anorexia nervosa has not disrupted school, social, and family processes or, when it has, to identify ways that any problems can be addressed. For example, in early adolescence, it is not uncommon for anorexia nervosa to lead to increased difficulties in developing a peer group at school; in later adolescence, anorexia nervosa may make it more difficult to develop more intimate romantic relationships or to leave home.

Family Treatment for Adults With Anorexia Nervosa

Family therapy has also been used in treating adults with anorexia nervosa. The overall program is very similar to that used in adolescence, although the role of the parents and other significant relationships is by necessity more negotiated, since the adult with anorexia nervosa is not legally as dependent on these other adults as is the adolescent patient. Although this decreased legal leverage may make behavioral control of self-starvation and related behaviors more challenging, it is possible in many cases to negotiate these formal family programs with the patient and family, especially when the general relationship with the parents is good. Even with adults, the three phases are similar, but the emphasis in the third phase is usually more clearly on the tasks of adolescence that remain to be completed even in adulthood.

Nonetheless, most adults with eating disorders present with a greater variety of living arrangements—for example, many adults live on their own, with their family of origin, or with a spouse, partner, or friend. Although some reports suggest that an increasing number of adult patients are married or live in committed relationships (Woodside et al. 2000), our understanding about these relationships and their potential role in maintaining or helping with an eating disorder is quite limited (e.g., Van den Broucke and Vandereycken 1985; Woodside and Shekter-Wolfson 1991). Some research on adult patients and their families has examined the quality of the marital relationship (e.g., Van den Broucke and Vandereycken 1989; Van den Broucke et al. 1995, 1997; Woodside et al. 1993). Reports on these marriages document difficult relationships due to the eating disorder or suggest that the eating disorder has emerged in response to the troubled relationships. The prognosis appears to be poor for marital relationships unless the eating disorder is resolved (Woodside et al. 2000). It is noteworthy that many young adults with anorexia nervosa continue to live with their parents while struggling with their disorder, but these families are relatively unexamined.

In terms of marital therapy, it appears that the marital relationship is potentially an important target for therapy that might affect the course of the disorder. Van den Broucke and Vandereycken (1989) suggest that examination of the relationship between the initiation of anorexia nervosa and the decision to marry, as it relates to symptom development and progression, can be helpful in identifying how the marriage can impact symptoms for good and ill. It also appears important to evaluate the levels of interdependency in the relationship, the ways conflicts are resolved (or avoided), and the strategies used to support partners during stressful periods. These patterns should be examined specifically in relation to their effects on eating disordered thoughts and behaviors (Van den Broucke and Vandereycken 1989).

Family Therapy for Bulimia Nervosa and Eating Disorder Not Otherwise Specified

The use of family therapy for bulimia nervosa is considerably more limited than for anorexia nervosa, although, as we suggested earlier in the chapter, data indicating problematic family relationships and various family problems are more available for bulimia nervosa than for anorexia nervosa. The applicability of Maudsley-type family therapy for bulimia nervosa is being explored. The overall principles of the family-based approach described for patients with anorexia nervosa—in particular, empowering parents and giving them responsibility for helping their child improve without blaming the parents or families—apply for this clinical group as well. A published case study illustrates how an adolescent with bulimia nervosa and her family progressed through this treatment (le Grange et al. 2003). Some important differences for FBT for adolescent bulimia nervosa include

1. Treatment emphasizes regulation of eating and curtailing of purging as opposed to weight restoration.
2. Parents and adolescent collaborate more actively and directly, in contrast to the full parental control established with anorexia nervosa. Adolescents

with bulimia nervosa compared with their counterparts with anorexia nervosa are usually more "advanced" developmentally, more readily permitting the collaborative approach for bulimia nervosa.

3. Attempts are made to address the shame and guilt associated with bulimia nervosa. Because bulimia nervosa is generally ego-dystonic (in contrast to anorexia nervosa, which is frequently ego-syntonic), a collaborative effort in bulimia nervosa treatment is more feasible.

4. Frequently, a greater number of comorbid psychiatric disorders complicate early treatment, in that these illnesses can distract not only the family but also the therapist from retaining a focus on the eating disorder symptoms.

5. In eating disorder not otherwise specified, binge and purge frequency can be irregular, and the challenge for the therapist is often to highlight preventive work instead of actively focusing on curtailing these behaviors. Again, "losing" treatment focus under these circumstances is a common pitfall.

Many adolescents with bulimia nervosa report that parental involvement is helpful to them when it is supportive rather than judgmental and critical. It is possible that FBT may contribute to a reduction of the shame and guilt that commonly accompany bulimia nervosa by highlighting that symptomatic behaviors are due to an illness rather than to indulgent and willful adolescents.

Empirical Support for Family Therapy for Eating Disorders

Family therapy for anorexia nervosa is the most studied treatment modality at this point, although the evidence supporting this approach is still quite limited. The data in Table 6–3 document that only a small number of subjects have been studied in randomized clinical trials of family therapy for anorexia nervosa. On the whole the data suggest that family therapy is superior to both no treatment and routine care (Crisp et al. 1991; Dare et al. 2001) as well as to specified treatments such as dietary advice (Hall and Crisp 1987) and supportive individual therapy for younger patients with short-duration illness (Russell et al. 1987). However, it is unclear whether family therapy is superior to a more active form of individual therapy, as longer-term outcomes appear similar for adolescents who receive these treatments (Robin et al. 1999). It is also unclear whether family therapy is superior to individual therapy for adults with anorexia nervosa or bulimia nervosa (Russell et al. 1987). One study found a nonsignificant tendency to favor individual treatment for this older age group, while another found no difference (Dare et al. 2001; Russell et al. 1987). In both cases, the small numbers in the trial limit the power to detect differences, so definitive conclusions are not possible. Finally, it appears that family therapy may work well in a relatively small dose, with 6 months of therapy, comprising about 10 sessions, being as effective as longer-term therapy (i.e., 12 months) (le Grange et al. 1992; Lock et al. 2005).

Researchers have been interested in, but also somewhat skeptical of, the feasibility of FBT, given the high demands the approach places on families and the possibility that many adolescents may be highly resistant to this approach. The first qualitative descriptions by le Grange and Gelman (1998) suggested that this form of family treatment was acceptable to adolescents and parents. A more recent, larger study found that adolescents and parents alike rated the effectiveness of the treatment and the therapeutic alliance with the therapists very highly, but 30% expressed a desire for individual therapy in conjunction with family therapy (Krautter and Lock 2004). Finally, a recent study examining the therapeutic alliance in FBT suggests that both patients and parents have high ratings of the therapeutic relationship in this form of treatment (Pereira et al. 2006).

Several important qualifications to the available data related to family therapy for eating disorders bear mention. For example, only two controlled studies have been published of family therapy that are not of the type developed at the Maudsley Hospital (Crisp et al. 1991; Hall and Crisp 1987). Both of these studies focused primarily on adults. On the whole, the superiority of family therapy to other treatments was uncertain, because in one study family therapy was combined with individual therapy (Hall and Crisp 1987), and in the other family therapy was superior only to no treatment (Crisp et al. 1991). These qualifications suggest that the empirical support available is limited to a single approach to family therapy and not family therapy in general.

In addition, available research data provide no systematic support for family therapy for bulimia nervosa, although a small case series suggests that FBT may be helpful for adolescents with this disorder (Dodge et al. 1995). However, it has been argued that because binge-eating and purging subtypes of an-

Table 6–3. Evidence supporting family therapy for eating disorders

Study	Population (N)	Comparison groups	End-of-treatment outcomes
Russell et al. 1987	Adults and adolescents (80)	Family therapy and individual therapy	Family therapy superior to individual therapy in adolescents with anorexia nervosa of short duration; no difference for adolescents with chronic anorexia nervosa or adults with anorexia nervosa or bulimia nervosa
Hall and Crisp 1987	Adults (30)	Family therapy and dietary advice	Family therapy superior to dietary advice
le Grange et al. 1992	Adolescents (18)	Family therapy with and without the patient	No difference between groups
Crisp et al. 1991	Adolescents and adults (90)	No treatment, family therapy, individual therapy, inpatient treatment, and group therapy	All treatments superior to no treatment
Robin et al. 1999	Adolescents (37)	Family therapy and individual therapy	Family therapy superior to individual treatment at end of treatment; no differences on follow-up
Eisler et al. 2000	Adolescents (40)	Family therapy with and without the patient	No differences between groups
Dare et al. 2001	Adults (84)	Focal, family, and cognitive analytic therapy; routine care	All treatments superior to routine care
Lock et al. 2005	Adolescents (86)	Family therapy for 6 months or 12 months	No differences between groups

orexia nervosa have been effectively treated by using FBT, and since considerable overlap in symptoms exists between adolescent anorexia nervosa and bulimia nervosa (le Grange and Lock 2002; le Grange et al. 2004), this treatment is likely useful in adolescents with bulimia nervosa (Eisler et al. 2000; Lock and le Grange 2005). This paucity of systematic research shows that the routine practice of recommending family therapy for adolescents, especially given that the type of family therapy is seldom specified, rests largely on clinical impressions and not on firm evidence. A few single case reports of family therapy for adults with bulimia nervosa have been published (Mandanes 1981; Roberto 1986; Root et al. 1986; Wynne 1980), as well as two studies of family therapy that describe how this treatment was devised (Russell et al. 1987; Schwartz et al. 1985). However, findings in both of these studies were inconclusive.

Future Directions in Family Therapy for Eating Disorders

Among the many gaps in our knowledge are answers to the following pressing questions:

- To what extent, under what circumstances, and for what types of patients are family therapies helpful for adults with anorexia nervosa?
- To what extent, under what circumstances, and for what types of patients are family therapies helpful in adults and adolescents with bulimia nervosa?
- To what extent, under what circumstances, and for what types of patients are family therapies other than those based on the Maudsley approach helpful for anorexia nervosa or bulimia nervosa?
- To what extent, under what circumstances, and for what types of patients is it beneficial to combine family and individual approaches for anorexia nervosa and bulimia nervosa?

In addition, we lack a deep understanding of how and why family treatments might work, and we know little about how best to specifically tailor family treatments for patients on factors other than age and chronicity. It will also be of interest to examine how family involvement might enhance other known treatments, such as cognitive-behavioral therapy (CBT), especially for bulimia nervosa. Some preliminary evidence suggests that involving parents in CBT for adolescents with bulimia nervosa leads to outcomes similar to those expected in adults treated with CBT (Lock 2005; Schapman and Lock 2006).

More intensive forms of family therapy are also being proposed, designed in part for those patients who do not respond to usual family therapy alone. These include *multiple-family groups* (Dare and Eisler 2000), an approach that involves several families at the same time and attempts to replicate in an intensive 3-day forum much of the early program of the first phase of FBT. Current research on this approach is promising but preliminary (Dare and Eisler 2000; Scholz and Asen 2001).

The overall assessment of the role of family therapy for eating disorders is that family approaches are likely to be important in all aspects of treatment, particularly for adolescents with anorexia nervosa. But family therapies may also contribute innovative approaches to treating adults with more chronic forms of anorexia nervosa and adolescents with bulimia nervosa. In these circumstances, adding innovative parental and familial components might help bring new hope for prevention and recovery.

References

Birch L, Fisher J: Development of eating behaviors among children and adolescents. Pediatrics 101:539–549, 1998

Crisp AH, Norton K, Gowers S, et al: A controlled study of the effect of therapies aimed at adolescent and family psychopathology in anorexia nervosa. Br J Psychiatry 159:325–333, 1991

Dare C, Eisler I: Family therapy for anorexia nervosa, in The Nature and Management of Feeding Problems in Young People. Edited by Cooper I, Stein A. New York, Harwood Academics, 1992, pp 146–160

Dare C, Eisler I: Family therapy for anorexia nervosa, in Handbook of Treatment for Eating Disorders. Edited by Garner DM, Garfinkel P. New York, Guilford, 1997, pp 307–324

Dare C, Eisler I: A multi-family group day treatment programme for adolescent eating disorders. European Eating Disorders Review 8:4–18, 2000

Dare C, Eisler I, Russell G, et al: Psychological therapies for adults with anorexia nervosa: randomized controlled trial of outpatient treatments. Br J Psychiatry 178:216–221, 2001

Dodge E, Hodes M, Eisler I, et al: Family therapy for bulimia nervosa in adolescents: an exploratory study. Journal of Family Therapy 17:59–77, 1995

Eisler I, Dare C, Hodes M, et al: Family therapy for adolescent anorexia nervosa: the results of a controlled comparison of two family interventions. J Child Psychol Psychiatry 41:727–736, 2000

Fairburn CG, Doll HA, Welch SL, et al: Risk factors for binge eating disorder: a community-based, case-control study. Arch Gen Psychiatry 55:425–432, 1998

Gull W: Anorexia nervosa (apepsia hysterica, anorexia hysterica). Transactions of the Clinical Society of London 7:222–228, 1874

Haley J: Uncommon Therapy: The Psychiatric Techniques of Milton H Erickson. New York, WW Norton, 1973

Hall A, Crisp AH: Brief psychotherapy in the treatment of anorexia nervosa: outcome at one year. Br J Psychiatry 151:185–191, 1987

Hodes M, le Grange D: Expressed emotion in the investigation of eating disorders: a review. Int J Eat Disord 13:279–288, 1993

Johnson C, Flach A: Family characteristics of 105 patients with bulimia. Am J Psychiatry 142:1321–1324, 1985

Krautter T, Lock J: Is manualized family based treatment for adolescent anorexia nervosa acceptable to patients? Patient satisfaction at end of treatment. Journal of Family Therapy 26:65–81, 2004

Lasegue E: De l'anorexie hystérique. Archives Générales de Médécine 21:384–403, 1883

le Grange D, Gelman T: The patient's perspective of treatment in eating disorders: a preliminary study. S Afr J Psychol 28:182–186, 1998

le Grange D, Lock J: Bulimia nervosa in adolescents: treatment, eating pathology, and comorbidity. South African Psychiatry Review, August, 2002, pp 19–22

le Grange D, Eisler I, Dare C, et al: Evaluation of family treatments in adolescent anorexia nervosa: a pilot study. Int J Eat Disord 12:347–357, 1992

le Grange D, Lock J, Dymek M: Family-based therapy for adolescents with bulimia nervosa. Am J Psychother 57:237–251, 2003

le Grange D, Loeb KL, Orman S, et al: Bulimia nervosa: a disorder in evolution? Arch Pediatr Adolesc Med 158:478–482, 2004

Liebman R, Minuchin S, Baker L: An integrated treatment program for anorexia nervosa. Am J Psychiatry 131:432–436, 1974

Lock J: Treating adolescents with eating disorders in the family context: empirical and theoretical considerations. Child Adolesc Psychiatr Clin N Am 11:331–342, 2002

Lock J: Adjusting cognitive behavioral therapy for adolescent bulimia nervosa: results of a case series. Am J Psychother 59:267–281, 2005

Lock J, le Grange D: Can family-based treatment of anorexia nervosa be manualized? J Psychother Pract Res 10:253–261, 2001

Lock J, le Grange D: Family-based treatment of eating disorders. Int J Eat Disord 38(suppl):S64–S67, 2005

Lock J, le Grange D, Agras WS, et al: Treatment Manual for Anorexia Nervosa: A Family-Based Approach. New York, Guilford, 2001

Lock J, Agras WS, Bryson S, et al: Comparison of short- and long-term family therapy for adolescent anorexia nervosa. J Am Acad Child Adolesc Psychiatry 44:632–639, 2005

Mandanes C: Strategic Family Therapy. San Francisco, CA, Jossey-Bass, 1981

Marchi M, Cohen P: Early childhood eating behaviors and adolescent eating disorders. J Am Acad Child Adolesc Psychiatry 29:112–117, 1990

Minuchin S, Rosman B, Baker L: Psychosomatic Families: Anorexia Nervosa in Context. Cambridge, MA, Harvard University Press, 1978

Palazzoli M: Self-Starvation: From the Intrapsychic to the Transpersonal Approach to Anorexia Nervosa. London, Chaucer Publishing, 1974

Pereira T, Lock J, Oggins J: Role of therapeutic alliance in family therapy for adolescent anorexia nervosa. Int J Eat Disord 39:677–684, 2006

Pike K, Rodin J: Mothers, daughers, and disordered eating. J Abnorm Psychol 100:198–204, 1991

Practice guideline for the treatment of patients with eating disorders (revision). American Psychiatric Association Work Group on Eating Disorders. Am J Psychiatry 157 (1, suppl):1–39, 2000

Roberto L: Bulimia: the transgenerational view. J Marital Fam Ther 12:231–240, 1986

Robin A, Siegal P, Moye A, et al: A controlled comparison of family versus individual therapy for adolescents with anorexia nervosa. J Am Acad Child Adolesc Psychiatry 38:1482–1489, 1999

Root MPP, Fallon P, Friedrich WN: Bulimia: A Systems Approach to Treatment. New York, WW Norton, 1986

Russell GF, Szmukler GI, Dare S, et al: An evaluation of family therapy in anorexia nervosa and bulimia nervosa. Arch Gen Psychiatry 44:1047–1056, 1987

Schapman A, Lock J: Cognitive-behavioral therapy for adolescent bulimia. Int J Eat Disord 39:252–255, 2006

Scholz M, Asen KE: Multiple family therapy with eating disordered adolescents. European Eating Disorders Review 9:33–42, 2001

Schwartz R, Barrett M, Saba G: Family therapy for bulimia, in Handbook of Psychotherapy for Anorexia Nervosa and Bulimia. Edited by Garner D, Garfinkel P. New York, Guilford, 1985, pp 280–310

Silverman J: Charcot's comments on the therapeutic role of isolation in the treatment of anorexia nervosa. Int J Eat Disord 21:295–298, 1997

Stice E: Sociocultural influences on body image and eating disturbance, in Eating and Weight Disorders and Obesity: A Comprehensive Handbook. Edited by Fairburn CG, Brownell K. New York, Guilford, 2002, pp 103–107

Van den Broucke S, Vandereycken W: Eating disorders in married patients: theory and therapy, in The Family Approach to Eating Disorders. Edited by Vandereycken W, Kog E, Vanderlinden J. New York, PMA Publishing, 1985, pp 333–345

Van den Broucke S, Vandereycken W: The marital relationship of patients with an eating disorder: a questionnaire study. Int J Eat Disord 8:541–556, 1989

Van den Broucke S, Vandereycken W, Vertommen H: Marital intimacy in patients with an eating disorder: a controlled self-report study. Br J Clin Psychol 34 (pt 1): 67–78, 1995

Van den Broucke S, Vandereycken W, Norré J: Eating Disorders and Marital Relationships. New York, Routledge, 1997

White M, Epston D: Narrative Means to Therapeutic Ends. New York, WW Norton, 1990

Woodside DB, Shekter-Wolfson L: Family treatment in the day hospital, in Family Approaches in Treatment of Eating Disorders. Edited by Woodside D, Shekter-Wolfson L. Washington, DC, American Psychiatric Press, 1991, pp 87–106

Woodside DB, Shekter-Wolfson L, Brandes JS, et al (eds): Eating Disorders and Marriage. New York, Brunner/Mazel, 1993

Woodside DB, Lackstrom J, et al: Marriage and eating disorders: comparisons between patients and spouses and changes over the course of treatment. J Psychosom Res 49:165–168, 2000

Wynne L: Paradoxical interventions: leverage for therapeutic change in individual and family systems, in The Psychotherapy of Schizophrenia. Edited by Strauss T, Bowers S, Downey S, et al. New York, Plenum, 1980

7

Management of Bulimia Nervosa

James E. Mitchell, M.D.
Kristine J. Steffen, Pharm.D.
James L. Roerig, Pharm.D.

Both pharmacological and psychotherapeutic treatments have been developed for bulimia nervosa. As we describe in this chapter, both have a role in the treatment of patients with these disorders, particularly the use of cognitive-behavioral therapy (CBT) as a psychotherapy approach and the use of selective serotonin reuptake inhibitors (SSRIs) as pharmacotherapy. However, the literature suggests that the remission rates are higher among those who receive CBT, and thus this treatment should be considered the treatment of choice for most patients.

Generally patients with bulimia nervosa can be managed successfully out of the hospital, although at times a brief hospitalization can be useful in helping treatment-resistant patients gain control of their eating symptoms. Often in clinical practice patients see a dietitian for nutritional counseling, a psychotherapist for psychotherapy, and a physician for medication management. Therefore, coordination of care among these team members is clearly important.

Clinical Vignette

A.L., a 23-year-old white woman, presented to the outpatient clinic with a 5-year history of problems with bulimia nervosa. She had been very concerned about her weight throughout high school and following graduation. Under the stress of beginning college, she started having problems with binge eating and then compensatory vomiting. At the time of her evaluation she was binge eating and purging several times a day and was developing symptoms of depression. She denied having suicidal ideas. Following outpatient evaluation she was referred for nutritional counseling with the program's dietitian. In nutritional counseling she received detailed information as to how to meal plan and was instructed that beginning to eat regular meals would impact significantly on the binge eating and purging. At the same time she was also seen by the family practitioner who worked with the program, who conducted a physical examination and ordered some screening laboratory tests, including serum electrolytes. Although A.L. had slight alkalosis and had a slightly decreased serum chloride level, these changes were thought not to be clinically significant. She also initiated outpatient CBT twice a week with one of the program's psychologists. Although she seemed to be profiting from the therapy, after 4 weeks she was still quite symptomatic, and because her depressive symptoms persisted as well, she was seen by the program's psychiatrist, who initiated treatment with fluoxetine hydrochloride. She initially received 20 mg/day, but the dosage was rapidly increased to 60 mg/day over a 2-week period. This combination seemed to provide the added help she needed, and by the end of the eighth week of treatment she was free of binge-eating and purging symptoms and was beginning to work meaningfully on underlying cognitions about weight and shape concerns. Her mood brightened considerably, and she reported better social functioning and indicated she was doing better in school as well. Following 20 sessions of CBT, she was instructed to return for follow-up at monthly intervals, and she continued to be followed up in medication management for another 12 months.

Target Symptoms and Treatment Goals

The target symptoms include those that directly result in the diagnosis, such as the presence of binge-eating episodes and compensatory behaviors, as well as associated clinical symptoms of depression and anxiety. The treatment goals should be elimination of binge-eating and purging behaviors and reductions in depressive and anxious features. Reducing the frequency of bulimic symptoms but not entirely eliminating them usually results in relapse to full syndromal status after treatment.

Nutritional Issues

Even when they are not binge eating, patients with bulimia nervosa generally are not eating normally. Many fast for extended periods of time, make unwise food choices, and/or are overly restrictive in their diets when not binge eating. For this reason it is usually helpful for them to meet with a dietitian on a regular basis, particularly early in the course of treatment.

Psychosocial Approaches

CBT is the form of psychotherapy that has been studied most intensively for the treatment of patients with bulimia nervosa. This psychosocial intervention specifically addresses eating disorder symptoms and the underlying cognitions that are common in patients with bulimia nervosa (Agras et al. 2000; Bulik et al. 1998; Garner et al. 1993; Mitchell et al. 1993; Wilson et al. 2002; Yager et al. 1989). CBT is applied in both group and individual formats. In the most commonly used version, 20 psychotherapy sessions are administered over 16 weeks, with 2 scheduled sessions each week for the first 4 weeks (Fairburn 1981; Wilson et al. 2002). Although many patients respond quite well to CBT, and most have significant improvement in the frequency of their target symptoms such as binge eating and purging, in many of the studies the majority of subjects are still symptomatic at the end of treatment (Hay et al. 2004). The CBT format usually employed with patients with bulimia nervosa focuses early on the use of self-monitoring techniques and regular meal planning, with an examination of cues and consequences associated with bulimic behavior and underlying cognitions that seem to fuel the disorder. In controlled trials CBT has been shown to be superior to minimal interventions, nutritional counseling, nondirective therapies, and waiting list controls, as well as specific forms of psychodynamic psychotherapy.

Behavior therapy using exposure and response prevention (ERP) has also been studied, but the results have been mixed, with some studies finding enhanced improvement (Leitenberg et al. 1988) and others finding reductions in the rate of improvement (Agras et al. 1989) with the addition of ERP. In a recent meta-analysis, Hay and colleagues (2004) concluded that there does not appear to be substantial evidence of additive benefit from concurrently administering ERP. Two other therapies have been shown to be effective in randomized trials: interpersonal psychotherapy (IPT) (although CBT worked more rapidly) (Agras et al. 2000; Wilson et al. 2002) and dialectical behavior therapy (in one study) (Safer et al. 2001).

Studies have also shown that including dietary counseling as part of treatment programs seems to increase their efficacy, and that scheduling treatment visits more frequently than weekly, particularly early in the course of treatment, results in improved outcome (Mitchell et al. 1993). A direct comparison of individual and group CBT failed to find evidence of substantial differences at follow-up (Chen et al. 2003). Family therapy has been recommended as a treatment for adolescents with bulimia nervosa (Schwartz et al. 1985), and a trial of such an approach for bulimic adolescents is currently being conducted (le Grange et al. 2003) (see Chapter 6, "Family Treatment of Eating Disorders," this volume).

Medication and Other Somatic Treatments

The pharmacotherapy of bulimia nervosa has been extensively researched. Agents that have been found to have greater efficacy than placebo include antidepressants such as tricyclic antidepressants (TCAs), SSRIs, serotonin-norepinephrine reuptake inhibitors (SNRIs), and a variety of other antidepressant compounds. In addition, multiple other agents, including high-dose narcotic antagonists, serotonin$_3$ receptor (5-HT$_3$) antagonists, and an anticonvulsant compound, topiramate, have been reported to be helpful. Combination therapy involving CBT and pharmacotherapy has, in some studies, been found to be beneficial, but in other studies the benefit was less evident. In this section, we review the various aspects of pharmacotherapy, including the efficacy of different drug groups, comparison of medications with CBT, combination of medications with CBT, sequential paradigms, and switch studies. We also review issues of outcome, response versus remission, and maintenance treatments.

Antidepressants

Antidepressants Versus Placebo

Antidepressant medications have received the most extensive investigation among pharmacological treatments for bulimia nervosa. Since more than 50% of bulimia nervosa patients have a lifetime diagnosis of major depressive disorder, it was logical to investigate antidepressant efficacy for this condition. Interestingly, however, the efficacy of these agents appears to be independent of whether or not patients have comorbid preexisting depression (Goldstein et al. 1999; Walsh and Devlin 2000). Further, it appears that efficacy does not differ substantially between classes of antidepressants, including the TCAs, SSRIs, monoamine oxidase inhibitors (MAOIs), and other antidepressant agents (Bacaltchuk and Hay 2005). The efficacy of antidepressants in bulimia nervosa is attributable to two concurrent effects: they contribute to reductions in the core symptoms of binge eating and vomiting and improve the mood and anxiety aberrations that often accompany the eating disorder (Mitchell et al. 2001).

While the efficacy of these agents has been fairly consistently demonstrated in several randomized, placebo-controlled bulimia nervosa treatment trials, there is ample room for therapeutic improvement. Short-term abstinence rates (average of 8 weeks) are around 30%, and bulimic behaviors tend to decrease by about 70% (Agras et al. 1992; Bacaltchuk and Hay 2005; Leitenberg et al. 1994). Despite these reductions, however, relapse rates are reportedly high. Agras and colleagues (1992) found that the use of a single antidepressant resulted in the full recovery of only 25% of patients entering treatment; over time, with continued treatment, one-third of those patients relapsed. Published relapse prevention studies, although limited in number, have shown an effect for continuing therapy (Fichter et al. 1996; Romano et al. 2002).

Tricyclic Antidepressants and Monoamine Oxidase Inhibitors

TCAs have been studied relatively extensively for the treatment of bulimia nervosa. The efficacy of TCAs in comparison with placebo has been substantiated in the treatment of bulimia nervosa (Agras et al. 1987; Alger et al. 1991; Barlow et al. 1998; Blouin et al. 1988; Hughes et al. 1986; Mitchell and Groat 1984; Pope et al. 1983; Rothschild et al. 1994). Similarly, the MAOIs have been demonstrated to be superior in efficacy to placebo at reducing depressive symptoms as well as reducing bingeing and purging behaviors (Carruba et al. 2001; Kennedy et al. 1988, 1993; Walsh et al. 1985, 1988). Table 7–1 provides further descriptions of these trials.

Although the TCAs and MAOIs have a record of established efficacy in the treatment of bulimia nervosa and remain historically interesting, their clinical application in bulimia nervosa pharmacotherapy has been largely supplanted by the SSRI medications, because the SSRIs have shown efficacy coupled with markedly improved adverse-effect profiles (Fichter et al. 1996; "Fluoxetine in the Treatment of Bulimia Nervosa" 1992; Goldstein et al. 1995, 1999; Romano 1999; Romano et al. 2002).

Selective Serotonin Reuptake Inhibitors

The SSRI antidepressant medication fluoxetine has U.S. Food and Drug Administration (FDA) approval for the treatment indication of bulimia nervosa at a dosage of 60 mg/day. The trial that was instrumental in leading to this FDA approval was carried out by the Fluoxetine Bulimia Nervosa Collaborative Study Group ("Fluoxetine in the Treatment of Bulimia Nervosa" 1992). In this multicenter study, 387 subjects with bulimia nervosa were enrolled in an 8-week trial to examine the efficacy of fluoxetine at dosages of 20 mg/day and 60 mg/day in comparison with placebo. Enrolled subjects had had a minimum of three binge episodes per week for at least 6 months. Subjects who responded to placebo were excluded from the trial prior to randomization. Participants were randomly assigned to receive fluoxetine 20 mg/day, fluoxetine 60 mg/day, or placebo. Those who received fluoxetine 60 mg/day demonstrated the greatest reduction in binge-eating frequency and vomiting episodes at end point. Following the Fluoxetine Bulimia Nervosa Collaborative Study Group trial, Goldstein et al. (1995) randomly assigned 225 subjects to fluoxetine 60 mg/day or to placebo. The authors concluded that at 16 weeks, the fluoxetine treatment had resulted in significant decreases in vomiting and binge eating. Several other SSRI trials have also documented the efficacy of these agents. A review of these studies is presented in Table 7–1.

Other Medications

Bupropion

Several miscellaneous agents have been evaluated in the quest for effective treatment for bulimia nervosa. In 1988, the noradrenergic and dopaminergic antidepressant compound bupropion was examined in a controlled study of bulimia nervosa subjects and was found to be superior to placebo at reducing episodes of binge eating and purging (Horne et al. 1988). Despite the promising results, 4 of 55 participants in the bupropion group experienced grand mal seizures, leading to bupropion's contraindication in the treatment of anorexia nervosa and bulimia nervosa.

Ondansetron

The peripherally active 5-HT$_3$ antagonist ondansetron has been evaluated as a potential treatment for bulimia nervosa (Faris et al. 2000; Hartman et al. 1997). The research group that has led these investigations proposes that patients with bulimia nervosa have defects in satiety that can be attributed to post–binge vomit vagal activity. Useful for the prevention of vagally mediated emesis, ondansetron decreases afferent vagal activity and therefore has a theoretical rationale for application in the treatment of bulimia nervosa. Hartman et al. (1997) first completed an open-label trial, involving five participants with bulimia nervosa, that demonstrated reduced binge-vomit frequency. Subsequently, this research group completed a randomized, double-blind trial to evaluate the effects of ondansetron versus placebo in a group of 25 participants with severe bulimia nervosa. During the double-blind phase of the study, participants were instructed to take one 4-mg capsule of ondansetron (or matching placebo) whenever they felt an urge to binge eat or to vomit, and then to try to restrain themselves for 30 minutes. If the urges were ill-defined or constant, the participants were instructed to take the dose 30 minutes before consuming food. They were instructed to take a total of six capsules per day (to equal a dosage of 24 mg/day), but they were allowed flexibility to vary the timings of administration. During the 4-week double-blind treatment phase, the placebo group binge-vomit mean frequency decreased from 13.4±9.9 coupled episodes per week at baseline to 13.2±11.6 per week at the end of treatment. The ondansetron group demonstrated a decrease from 12.8±5 coupled episodes per week to 6.5±3.9 per week—an estimated reduction of 6.8 episodes per week

Table 7–1. Randomized controlled trials of antidepressants versus placebo for bulimia nervosa treatment

Author	N	Maximum dosage (mg/day)	Duration (weeks)	Treatment	Outcome		Comment
					% Abstinent	% Reduction in binge eating	
Pope et al. 1983	22	200	6	Imipramine		70	Greater reduction in depression scores (Ham-D) with imipramine than with placebo
				Placebo		2	
Agras et al. 1987	22	300	16	Imipramine	30	73	No change in depression scores (BDI) between groups
				Placebo	10	43	
Mitchell et al. 1990	85	300	10	Imipramine	10	49	Greater reduction in depression and anxiety scores (Ham-D, Ham-A) with imipramine than with placebo
				Placebo	16	2.5	
Alger et al. 1991	55[a]	200	8	Imipramine		22	Reduction in bingeing with both imipramine and naltrexone, but reduction was not significantly different from that seen with placebo
		150		Naltrexone		30	
				Placebo		30	
Mitchell and Groat 1984	38	150	8	Amitriptyline		72	Significantly greater reduction in depression scores (Ham-D) with amitriptyline than with placebo
				Placebo		52	
Hughes et al. 1986	22	200	6	Desipramine		91	Patients originally receiving placebo and crossed over to desipramine experienced an 84% decrease in binge frequency
				Placebo		+19 (%↑)	

Table 7–1. Randomized controlled trials of antidepressants versus placebo for bulimia nervosa treatment *(continued)*

Author	N	Maximum dosage (mg/day)	Duration (weeks)	Treatment	Outcome % Abstinent	Outcome % Reduction in binge eating	Comment
Barlow et al. 1988[b]	47	150	6	Desipramine Placebo	4	62 2.5	Antibulimic effects of desipramine were not associated with antidepressant effects
Blouin et al. 1988[c]	36	150 60	6	Desipramine Fenfluramine Placebo			Both drugs superior to placebo in reducing bingeing and vomiting frequency; fenfluramine superior to desipramine
Walsh et al. 1991	78	300	6	Desipramine Placebo	13 8	47 +7 (%↑)	No reduction in depression scores (Ham-D) relative to placebo
Sabine et al. 1983	50	60	8	Mianserin Placebo	0 0	0 0	No difference in reduction in depression scores (Ham-D) between groups
Horne et al. 1988	81	450	8	Bupropion Placebo	30 0	66 23	Study terminated early because of seizures; no difference in reduction in depression scores (Ham-D) between groups
Pope et al. 1989	46	400	6	Trazodone Placebo	10 0	31 +21 (%↑)	No difference in reduction in depression scores (Ham-D) between groups

Table 7–1. Randomized controlled trials of antidepressants versus placebo for bulimia nervosa treatment (*continued*)

Author	N	Maximum dosage (mg/day)	Duration (weeks)	Treatment	Outcome % Abstinent	Outcome % Reduction in binge eating	Comment
Walsh et al. 1985	38	90	8	Phenelzine Placebo	43 0	66 6	May be some benefit of phenelzine even in nondepressed patients with bulimia (based on preliminary data only)
Walsh et al. 1988	62	90	8	Phenelzine Placebo	35 4	64 5.5	Greater reduction in depression scores (Ham-D) with phenelzine than with placebo; benefit of phenelzine not limited to depressed participants
Kennedy et al. 1988[c]	29	60	6	Isocarboxazid Placebo	33		Greater reduction in depression (Ham-D) and anxiety (Ham-A) scores with isocarboxazid than with placebo
Kennedy et al. 1993	36	200	8	Brofaromine Placebo	19 13	62 50	Significantly greater decrease in vomiting with brofaromine than with placebo, but change in depression scores (Ham-D) not significant between groups
Carruba et al. 2001[d]	77	600	6	Moclobemide Placebo	22 44		Moclobemide not useful in bulimia treatment; no serious side effects occurred during trial

Table 7–1. Randomized controlled trials of antidepressants versus placebo for bulimia nervosa treatment *(continued)*

Author	N	Maximum dosage (mg/day)	Duration (weeks)	Treatment	Outcome		
					% Abstinent	% Reduction in binge eating	Comment
FBNCSG ("Fluoxetine in Treatment of Bulimia Nervosa" 1992)	387	60 20	8	Fluoxetine Fluoxetine Placebo	23 11 11	67 45 33	Greater reduction in depression scores (Ham-D) with fluoxetine than with placebo
Goldstein et al. 1995	398	60	16	Fluoxetine Placebo	18 12	50 18	Significant reduction in binge eating and vomiting with fluoxetine compared with placebo[e]
Romano et al. 2002	150	60	52	Fluoxetine Placebo			Frequency of vomiting and binge-eating episodes reduced, and CGI-Severity and -Improvement scores and YBCEDS scores improved, with fluoxetine compared with placebo[f]

Note. BDI = Beck Depression Inventory; CGI = Clinical Global Impression; FBNCSG = Fluoxetine Bulimia Nervosa Collaborative Study Group; Ham-A = Hamilton Rating Scale for Anxiety; Ham-D = Hamilton Rating Scale for Depression; YBCEDS = Yale-Brown–Cornell Eating Disorder Scale.
[a]Study enrolled 22 subjects with bulimia and 33 subjects with obesity and binge-eating.
[b]Crossover study; 23 of 47 patients dropped out prior to study completion. [c]Crossover study. [d]29% dropout rate.
[e]Randomization was 3:1 fluoxetine:placebo; 225 participants (57% of those randomly assigned) completed the trial.
[f]High dropout rate (61.3%).

(P<0.0001). Despite some encouraging research results, the feasibility of prescribing ondansetron clinically for the maintenance treatment of bulimia nervosa remains questionable. Ondansetron, as well as the other 5-HT$_3$ antagonists (granisetron and dolasetron), is typically used for the short-term prevention and management of nausea and vomiting associated with the postoperative period, as well as with chemotherapy and radiation therapy. Currently, the cost to purchase these medications from a retail pharmacy (e.g., generally over $30 per tablet for ondansetron) is likely to be prohibitive for most patients.

Topiramate

The anticonvulsant topiramate has been associated with weight loss and has received preliminary study in bulimia nervosa. In an open-label case series with five patients, almost complete resolution of bingeing and purging was observed in three patients, and this effect was sustained throughout an 18-month follow-up period (Barbee 2003). A two-part subsequent double-blind, placebo-controlled study also supported the efficacy of topiramate (Hedges et al. 2003; Hoopes et al. 2003). Subjects with bulimia nervosa who were between the ages of 16 and 50 years were randomly assigned to 10 weeks of treatment with placebo or a titrated dose of topiramate up to a maximum dosage of 400 mg/day (median dosage = 100 mg/day, range = 25–400 mg/day). Patients in the topiramate group demonstrated a 44.8% reduction in mean weekly number of binge and/or purge days, whereas those in the placebo group experienced a 10.7% reduction (P = 0.004). Mean weekly number of binge days and mean weekly number of purge days were also significantly reduced with topiramate compared with placebo. Topiramate-treated patients had a decrease in mean body weight of 1.8 kg, whereas the placebo group had a mean increase of 0.2 kg (P = 0.004).

Most recently, a 10-week, double-blind trial evaluating the effects of topiramate versus placebo in bulimia nervosa was conducted by Nickel et al. (2005). Thirty participants were randomly assigned to each treatment group. Topiramate was titrated up over the first 6 weeks of the trial to a final dosage of 250 mg/day. In the topiramate group, 36.7% of the participants, versus 3.3% of the placebo participants, experienced a greater than 50% reduction in bingeing/purging (P<0.001). Topiramate also demonstrated a significant reduction in body weight compared with placebo and was associated with significant improvement on the Social Function–36 (SF-36) measure of health-related quality of life. Topiramate was reportedly well tolerated in this trial.

Flutamide

A placebo-controlled, double-blind pilot study on the efficacy of the androgen antagonist flutamide in bulimia nervosa was recently published (Sundblad et al. 2005). These authors cited literature suggesting that women with bulimia may have elevated serum levels of androgens that may be caused by polycystic ovaries (Cotrufo et al. 2000; Dumoulin et al. 1996; Morgan et al. 2002; Sundblad et al. 1994). They further supported their rationale for testing an androgen antagonist by suggesting the possibility that androgens promote bulimic behavior, perhaps through influencing food craving or affecting impulse control. Subjects (ages 21–45 years) with the bulimia nervosa purging subtype were randomly assigned to one of four treatment groups for 3 months: flutamide ($n=9$), citalopram ($n=15$), flutamide plus citalopram ($n=10$), or placebo ($n=12$). Dosages were escalated to 500 mg/day of flutamide and 40 mg/day of citalopram. The results suggested that flutamide significantly decreased binge eating in both groups that were given the drug. This effect was not seen in the groups given only citalopram or placebo. The effect of flutamide on purging was not significant.

Reboxetine

The SNRI reboxetine, which is not approved for use in the United States, has also received preliminary study in bulimia nervosa. Seven outpatients (ages 19–53 years) with DSM-IV-diagnosed bulimia nervosa were treated in an open-label paradigm with 8 mg/day of reboxetine over 12 weeks (El-Giamal et al. 2000). Monthly binge frequency was decreased by 73%, and the monthly frequency of vomiting was decreased by 67%. Depression ratings were also decreased. Subsequently, Fassino et al. (2004) assessed the efficacy of reboxetine (4 mg/day) in 28 outpatients who had bulimia nervosa without Axis I comorbidity. Sixty percent of the patients treated experienced at least a 50% decrease in bulimic behaviors. By 3 months of treatment, depressive symptoms, as well as global function scores, had significantly improved. Although the FDA has declined to approve reboxetine, other SNRI medications, such as atomoxetine, may be worth investigating for the treatment of bulimia nervosa.

Miscellaneous Agents

Several other drug modalities have been explored, including D-fenfluramine (Fahy et al. 1993; Russell et al. 1988), lithium (Hsu et al. 1999), phenytoin (Wermuth et al. 1977), methylphenidate (in bulimia nervosa patients with Cluster B personality disorders) (Sokol et al. 1999), milnacipran (El-Giamal et al. 2002), and naltrexone (Ingoin-Apfelbaum and Apfelbaum 1987; Mitchell et al. 1989). Naltrexone has been associated with conflicting results in clinical trials. Mitchell et al. (1989) reported that in their crossover study of 16 normal-weight women with bulimia, low-dose naltrexone was not associated with a clinically significant reduction in bingeing or vomiting frequency. Conversely, Marrazzi et al. (1995) found significant reductions in binge/purge symptoms during naltrexone treatment in 18 of 19 patients with bulimic symptoms (either anorexia nervosa of the bulimic subtype or bulimia nervosa) during a double-blind placebo crossover study.

Combination CBT and Pharmacotherapy Trials

In light of the efficacy of CBT, two obvious question arise: 1) What results can be obtained with the combination of CBT and pharmacotherapy? and 2) What is the relative efficacy of CBT versus pharmacotherapy? Table 7–2 lists six trials that have compared CBT and pharmacotherapy alone and in combination. The trials were short-term (ranging from 10 to 32 weeks). The pharmacotherapy consisted of imipramine, desipramine, or fluoxetine. In reviewing these data, it is relevant to consider two markers of outcome: percent reduction of binge symptoms and percentage of the population that became abstinent.

The results vary considerably across these trials. One common result, however, is that the drug alone was never the most efficacious treatment in terms of percent abstinence or percent reduction in bulimia nervosa symptoms. In addition, the drug groups consistently had high dropout rates (range= 25%–57.1%).

Table 7–2. Comparison of trials of medication and psychotherapy alone and in combination

Author	N	Maximum dosage (mg/day)	Duration (weeks)	Treatment	% Abstinence	Outcome	Comment
Mitchell et al. 1990	39/52		10	Combination	51	91.7	Combined treatment superior only in reducing depression and anxiety; high dropout rate with imipramine alone
	29/34			CBT	45	89.1	
	31/54	300		Imipramine	16	49.3	
	26/31			Placebo		2.5	
Agras et al. 1992[a]	12		24	Combination	70	89.2	Advantage of 24-week combined treatment; CBT prevented relapse after desipramine
	23			CBT	55	71.3	
	12	168 (mean)		Desipramine	42	44.1	
Leitenberg et al. 1994	5/7		20	Combination	57		High dropout rate with desipramine; no advantage of combined treatment over CBT alone
	6/7	—[b]		CBT	71.4		
	3/7			Desipramine	0		
Goldbloom et al. 1997	12/29		16	Combination	25	87	No advantage for combined treatment over CBT alone; high dropout rate
	14/24			CBT	43	80	
	12/23	60		Fluoxetine	17	70	

Table 7–2.   Comparison of trials of medication and psychotherapy alone and in combination *(continued)*

Author	N	Maximum dosage (mg/day)	Duration (weeks)	Treatment	% Abstinence	Out-come	Comment
Walsh et al. 1997	23	Desipramine 300; followed by fluoxetine 60	16	Combination	52	87	CBT sign > supportive therapy
	25			CBT	24	64.5	Medication sign > placebo
	28			Desipramine/ fluoxetine	29	68.8	Medication improves outcome of
	22			Supportive + placebo	18	46.3	CBT
	22			Supportive + medication	18	55	
Jacobi et al. 2002	12/18	60	16	Combination	16.7	50	No advantage for combined
	11/19			CBT	26.3	42	treatment over CBT alone;
	12/16			Fluoxetine	12.5	46	high dropout rate

[a]Only 24-week data displayed.
[b]Desipramine serum level = 150–275 ng/mL.

Sequential-Treatment Studies

Response rates to subsequent therapies for patients who have not responded to initial treatment have been variable. One controlled sequential-treatment trial (Walsh et al. 1997) demonstrating modest benefits involved initial treatment with desipramine for 8 weeks. Those subjects who did not experience a 75% reduction in binge frequency were switched to a second treatment, fluoxetine 60 mg/day for 8 weeks. Pharmacological treatment occurred in combination with CBT or supportive psychotherapy, or alone. Overall, 74% of eligible patients required the switch to the second pharmacological treatment. Cessation of binge behavior was found in 29% of the medication-only subjects by the end of the second treatment period. Subjects who did not respond to CBT or IPT were given fluoxetine or placebo in another trial by Walsh and colleagues (2000). The active drug was found to be superior to placebo in improving symptoms. In another study of patients in whom CBT had not produced remission, patients were subsequently randomly assigned to IPT or pharmacotherapy. The rate of response to IPT was 16%, and the rate of response to pharmacotherapy (fluoxetine or desipramine) was 10% (Mitchell et al. 2002). The authors of this trial concluded that sequencing of treatment was of little clinical utility. Thus, the data are mixed regarding the benefit of subsequent treatments after the first therapy fails.

Maintenance Studies

Two maintenance studies have been published. Fichter et al. (1996) conducted a 15-week trial involving patients who had received intensive inpatient psychotherapy. At the end of the inpatient phase, the patients were randomly assigned to fluvoxamine or placebo for 15 weeks. A significant effect was found for fluvoxamine over placebo in delaying recurrence of symptoms. However, the dropout rate for the drug group was 51.4%, compared with 14.3% for the placebo group. The largest maintenance trial was reported by Romano et al. (2002). Subjects were initially treated in a single-blind acute treatment phase, and those who met the response criteria (i.e., achieved a minimum of 50% reduction of baseline frequency of vomiting during one of the final 2 weeks of a single-blind entry phase) were then randomly assigned to fluoxetine 60 mg/ day or placebo. In total, 150 patients were randomly assigned to active drug or placebo for a period of 1 year. However, of the 150 patients who entered the double-blind phase, only 19 completed the trial. The total number of patients who relapsed did not differ between groups. Fluoxetine did prolong the time to relapse. Thus, the weight of the evidence suggests that single-agent pharmacological treatment does not provide a robust maintenance therapy for bulimia nervosa.

Monitoring and Follow-Up

It is widely recognized that even patients who do very well with cognitive therapy and achieve remission are at risk for relapse, particularly in the first 6 months after treatment. Therefore, it is very reasonable for patients to be regularly scheduled for brief visits to assess how they are doing and, if necessary, to undertake refresher sessions.

Although firm guidelines have not been established, it is generally suggested that patients who have had a good response to medication should maintain the same medication at the dose at which response was achieved for an absolute minimum of 6 months and often for a year, during which time they should continue to have scheduled medication-monitoring visits. The most commonly encountered laboratory abnormalities are fluid and electrolyte problems. These abnormalities should be ruled out at baseline, and if patients remain symptomatic, values should be rechecked periodically.

References

Agras WS, Dorian B, Kirkley BG, et al: Imipramine in the treatment of bulimia: a double-blind controlled study. Int J Eat Disord 6:29–38, 1987

Agras WS, Schneider JA, Arnow B, et al: Cognitive-behavioral and response-prevention treatments for bulimia nervosa: a controlled comparison. Am J Psychiatry 149:82–87, 1989

Agras W, Rossiter E, Arnow B, et al: Pharmacologic and cognitive-behavioral treatment for bulimia nervosa: a controlled comparison. Am J Psychiatry 149:82–87, 1992

Agras WS, Walsh T, Fairburn CB, et al: A multicenter comparison of cognitive-behavioral therapy and interpersonal psychotherapy for bulimia nervosa. Arch Gen Psychiatry 57:459–466, 2000

Alger SA, Schwalberg MD, Bigaoutte JM, et al: Effect of a tricyclic antidepressant and opiate antagonist on binge-eating behavior in normoweight bulimic and obese, binge-eating subjects. Am J Clin Nutr 53:865–871, 1991

Bacaltchuk J, Hay P: Antidepressants versus placebo for people with bulimia nervosa. Cochrane Database Syst Rev (4):CD003391

Barbee JG: Topiramate in the treatment of severe bulimia nervosa with comorbid mood disorders: a case series. Int J Eat Disord 33:468–472, 2003

Barlow J, Bloudin J, Bloudin A, et al: Treatment of bulimia with desipramine: a double-blind crossover study. Can J Psychiatry 33:129–133, 1988

Blouin AG, Blouin JH, Perez EL, et al: Treatment of bulimia with fenfluramine and desipramine. J Clin Psychopharmacol 8:261–269, 1988

Bulik CM, Sullivan PF, Carter FA, et al: The role of exposure with response prevention in the cognitive-behavioural therapy for bulimia nervosa. Psychol Med 28:611–623, 1998

Carruba MD, Cuzzolaro M, Riva L, et al: Efficacy and tolerability of moclobemide in bulimia nervosa: a placebo-controlled trial. Int Clin Psychopharmacol 16:27–32, 2001

Chen E, Touyz SW, Beumont PJ, et al: Comparison of group and individual cognitive-behavioral therapy for patients with bulimia nervosa. Int J Eat Disord 33:241–254, 2003

Cotrufo P, Monteleone P, d'Istria M, et al: Aggressive behavioral characteristics and endogenous hormones in women with bulimia nervosa. Neuropsychobiology 42:58–61, 2000

Dumoulin SC, de Glisezinski I, Saint-Martin F, et al: Hormonal changes related to eating behaviour in oligomenorrheic women. J Endocrinol 135:328–334, 1996

El-Giamal N, de Zwaan M, Bailer U, et al: Reboxetine in the treatment of bulimia nervosa: a report of seven cases. Int Clin Psychopharmacol 15:351–356, 2000

El-Giamal N, de Zwaan M, Bailer U, et al: Milnacipran in the treatment of bulimia nervosa: a report of 15 cases. Eur Neuropsychopharmacol 13:73–79, 2002

Fahy TA, Eisler I, Russell FM: A placebo-controlled trial of D-fenfluramine in bulimia nervosa. Br J Psychiatry 162:597–603, 1993

Fairburn CG: A cognitive behavioral treatment for bulimia, in Psychotherapy for Anorexia Nervosa and Bulimia. Edited by Garner DM, Garfinkel PE. New York, Guilford, 1981, pp 160–192

Faris PL, Kim SW, Meller WH, et al: Effect of decreasing afferent vagal activity with ondansetron on symptoms of bulimia nervosa: a randomised, double-blind trial. Lancet 355:792–797, 2000

Fassino S, Daga GA, Boggio S, et al: Use of reboxetine in bulimia nervosa: a pilot study. J Psychopharmacol 18:423–428, 2004

Fichter MM, Kruger R, Rief W, et al: Fluvoxamine in prevention of relapse in bulimia nervosa: effects on eating-specific psychopathology. J Clin Psychopharmacol 16:9–18, 1996

Fluoxetine in the treatment of bulimia nervosa: a multi-center, placebo-controlled, double-blind trial. Fluoxetine Bulimia Nervosa Collaborative Study Group. Arch Gen Psychiatry 49:139–147, 1992

Garner DM, Rockert W, Davis R, et al: Comparison of cognitive-behavioral and supportive-expressive therapy for bulimia nervosa. Am J Psychiatry 150:37–46, 1993

Goldbloom DS, Olmsted M, Davis R, et al: A randomized controlled trial of fluoxetine and cognitive behavioral therapy for bulimia nervosa: short-term outcome. Behav Res Ther 35:803–811, 1997

Goldstein DJ, Wilson MG, Thompson VL, et al, and Fluoxetine Bulimia Nervosa Research Group: Long-term fluoxetine treatment of bulimia nervosa. Br J Psychiatry 166:660–666, 1995

Goldstein DJ, Wilson MG, Ascroft RC, et al: Effectiveness of fluoxetine therapy in bulimia nervosa regardless of comorbid depression. Int J Eat Disord 25:19–27, 1999

Hartman BK, Faris PL, Kim SW, et al: Treatment of bulimia nervosa with ondansetron. Arch Gen Psychiatry 54:969–970, 1997

Hay PJ, Bacaltchuk J, Stefano S: Psychotherapy for bulimia nervosa and binging. Cochrane Database Syst Rev CD000562; 2004

Hedges DW, Reimherr FW, Hoopes SP, et al: Treatment of bulimia nervosa with topiramate in a randomized, double-blind, placebo-controlled trial, Part 2: improvement in psychiatric measures. J Clin Psychiatry 64:1449–1454, 2003

Hoopes SP, Reimherr FW, Hedges DW, et al: Treatment of bulimia nervosa with topiramate in a randomized, double-blind, placebo-controlled trial, Part 1: improvement in binge and purge measures. J Clin Psychiatry 64:1335–1341, 2003

Horne RL, Ferguson JM, Pope HG Jr, et al: Treatment of bulimia with bupropion: a multicenter controlled trial. J Clin Psychiatry 49:262–266, 1988

Hsu LK, Clement L, Santhouse R, et al: Treatment of bulimia nervosa with lithium carbonate: a controlled study. J Nerv Ment Dis 179:351–355, 1999

Hughes PL, Wells LA, Cunningham CJ, et al: Treating bulimia with desipramine. Arch Gen Psychiatry 43:182–186, 1986

Ingoin-Apfelbaum L, Apfelbaum M: Naltrexone and bulimic symptoms. Lancet 2:1087–1088, 1987

Jacobi C, Dahme B, Dittmann RW: Cognitive-behavioral, fluoxetine and combined treatment for bulimia nervosa: short-term and long-term results. European Eating Disorders Review 10:179–198, 2002

Kennedy SH, Piran N, Warsh JJ, et al: A trial of isocarboxazid in the treatment of bulimia nervosa. J Psychopharmacol 8:391–396, 1988

Management of Bulimia Nervosa   191

Kennedy SH, Goldbloom DS, Ralevski E: Is there a role for selective monoamine oxidase inhibitor therapy in bulimia nervosa? A placebo-controlled trial of brofaromine. J Clin Psychopharmacol 13:415–422, 1993

le Grange D, Lock J, Dymek M: Family-based therapy for adolescents with bulimia nervosa. Am J Psychother 57:237–251, 2003

Leitenberg H, Rosen JC, Gross J, et al: Exposure plus response-prevention treatment of bulimia nervosa. J Consult Clin Psychol 56:535–541, 1988

Leitenberg H, Rosen J, Vara L, et al: Comparison of cognitive-behavior therapy and desipramine in the treatment of bulimia nervosa. Behav Res Ther 32:37–45, 1994

Marrazzi MA, Bacon JP, Kinzie J, et al: Naltrexone use in the treatment of anorexia nervosa and bulimia nervosa. Int J Clin Psychopharmacol 10:163–172, 1995

Mitchell JE, Groat R: A placebo-controlled double-blind trial of amitriptyline in bulimia. J Clin Psychopharmacol 4:186–193, 1984

Mitchell JE, Christenson G, Jennings J, et al: A placebo-controlled, double-blind crossover study of naltrexone hydrochloride in outpatients with normal weight bulimia. J Clin Psychopharmacol 9:94–97, 1989

Mitchell JE, Pyle RL, Eckert ED, et al: A comparison study of antidepressants and structured group therapy in the treatment of bulimia nervosa. Arch Gen Psychiatry 47:149–157, 1990

Mitchell JE, Pyle RL, Pomeroy C, et al: Cognitive-behavioral group psychotherapy of bulimia nervosa: importance of logistical variables. Int J Eat Disord 14:277–287, 1993

Mitchell JE, Peterson CB, Myers T, et al: Combining pharmacotherapy and psycho therapy in the treatment of patients with eating disorders. Psychiatr Clin North Am 24:315–323, 2001

Mitchell JE, Halmi K, Wilson GT, et al: A randomized secondary treatment study of women with bulimia nervosa who fail to respond to CBT. Int J Eat Disord 32:271–281, 2002

Morgan JF, McCluskey SE, Brunton JN, et al: Polycystic ovarian morphology and bulimia nervosa: a 9-year follow-up study. Fertil Steril 77:928–931, 2002

Nickel C, Tritt K, Muehlbacher M, et al: Topiramate treatment in bulimia nervosa patients: a randomized, double-blind, placebo-controlled trial. Int J Eat Disord 38:295–300, 2005

Pope HG Jr, Hudson JL, Jonas JM, et al: Bulimia treated with imipramine: a placebo-controlled, double-blind study. Am J Psychiatry 140:554–558, 1983

Pope HG Jr, Keck PE Jr, McElroy SL, et al: A placebo-controlled study of trazodone in bulimia nervosa. J Clin Psychopharmacol 9:254–259, 1989

Romano SJ, Halmi KA, Sarkar NP, et al: A placebo-controlled study of fluoxetine in continued treatment of bulimia nervosa after successful acute fluoxetine treatment. Am J Psychiatry 159:96–102, 2002

Rothschild R, Quitkin HM, Quitkin FM, et al: A double-blind placebo-controlled comparison of phenelzine and imipramine in the treatment of bulimia in atypical depressives. Int J Eat Disord 15:1–9, 1994

Russell GF, Checkley SA, Feldman J, et al: A controlled trial of D-fenfluramine in bulimia nervosa. Clin Neuropharmacol 11 (suppl 1):S146–S159, 1988

Sabine EJ, Yonace A, Farrington AJ, et al: Bulimia nervosa: a placebo-controlled double-blind therapeutic trial of mianserin. Br J Clin Pharmacol 15 (suppl 2):195S–202S, 1983

Safer DL, Telch CG, Agras WS: Dialectical behavior therapy for bulimia nervosa. Am J Psychiatry 158:632–634, 2001

Schwartz RC, Barrett MJ, Saba G: Family Therapy for Bulimia. New York, Guilford, 1985

Sokol MS, Gray NS, Goldstein A, et al: Methylphenidate treatment for bulimia nervosa associated with a cluster B personality disorder. Int J Eat Disord 25:233–237, 1999

Sundblad C, Bergman L, Eriksson E: High levels of free testosterone in women with bulimia nervosa. Acta Psychiatr Scand 90:397–398, 1994

Sundblad C, Landen M, Eriksson T, et al: Effects of the androgen antagonist flutamide and the serotonin reuptake inhibitor citalopram in bulimia nervosa. J Clin Psychopharmacol 25:85–88, 2005

Walsh BT, Devlin MJ: Psychopharmacology of anorexia nervosa, bulimia nervosa, and binge eating, in Psychopharmacology: The Fourth Generation of Progress. Nashville, TN, American College of Neuropsychopharmacology, 2000. Available at: http://www.acnp.org/g4/GN401000153/CH149.html. Accessed December 28, 2006.

Walsh BT, Stewart JW, Roose SP, et al: A double-blind trial of phenelzine in bulimia. J Psychiatry Res 19:485–489, 1985

Walsh BT, Gladis M, Roose SP, et al: Phenelzine vs placebo in 50 patients with bulimia. Arch Gen Psychiatry 45:471–475, 1988

Walsh BT, Hadigan CM, Devlin MJ, et al: Long-term outcome of antidepressant treatment for bulimia nervosa. Am J Psychiatry 148:1206–1212, 1991

Walsh BT, Wilson T, Loeb K, et al: Medication and psychotherapy in the treatment of bulimia nervosa. Am J Psychiatry 154:523–531, 1997

Walsh BT, Agras WS, Devlin MJ, et al: Fluoxetine for bulimia nervosa following poor response to psychotherapy. Am J Psychiatry 157:1332–1334, 2000

Wermuth BM, Davis KL, Hollister LE, et al: Phenytoin treatment of the binge-eating syndrome. Am J Psychiatry 134:1249–1253, 1977

Wilson GT, Fairburn CC, Agras WS, et al: Cognitive-behavioral therapy for bulimia nervosa: time course and mechanisms of change. J Consult Clin Psychol 70:267–274, 2002

Yager J, Landsverg J, Edelstein CK: Help seeking and satisfaction with care in 651 women with eating disorders, I: patterns of utilization, attributed change, and perceived efficacy of treatment. J Nerv Ment Dis 177:632–637, 1989

8

Management of Eating Disorders Not Otherwise Specified

Michael J. Devlin, M.D.

Kelly C. Allison, Ph.D.

Juli A. Goldfein, Ph.D.

Alexia Spanos

The DSM-IV-TR diagnostic category of eating disorder not otherwise specified (EDNOS) (American Psychiatric Association 2000) is both the least studied and the most prevalent eating disorder diagnosis (Fairburn and Bohn 2005). Several disparate groups of conditions are included under the rubric of EDNOS, including anorexia nervosa–like or bulimia nervosa–like syndromes; binge-eating disorder (BED); night-eating syndrome (NES) or other nocturnal eating syndromes (in obese and nonobese individuals); and other serious disorders of eating that do not fit easily into any of the above groups. To qualify for a diagnosis of EDNOS, the affected individual's symptoms must be of clinical severity. Thus, it is imperative that a classification of "not otherwise specified" not be regarded by clinicians, providers, or insurers as indicating a subthreshold or marginally significant eating disorder. Rather, individuals with EDNOS should be seen as equally deserving of treatment as those with anorexia nervosa and bulimia nervosa, and systematic study of the characteristics and treatment of these disorders should be viewed as of equal importance to that of the classic eating disorders.

At present, there is still a great deal to be learned about the optimal classification of diagnostic clusters presently labeled EDNOS. While BED, currently included in Appendix B of DSM-IV, has received a significant amount of attention in the past decade and has considerable face validity, there remain significant questions regarding the validity of the current diagnostic concept (Devlin et al. 2003). Similarly, although a disorder centered on night eating has been recognized since the 1950s (Stunkard et al. 1955), there is still no real consensus regarding the best criteria for this disorder. Both binge eating in the absence of compensatory behavior and night eating are known to occur in individuals of normal weight as well as overweight and obese individuals. However, most individuals who present for treatment for BED and NES are in fact overweight (i.e., body mass index [BMI] = 25–29.9) or obese (i.e., BMI = 30 or greater). Whether or how obesity should be included in the categorization of these disorders is another as yet unanswered question.

What we do know at this point is that there are several treatment approaches that are useful for some patients with EDNOS. While nosologists and epidemiologists study the prevalence, course, and optimal categorization of individuals with EDNOS, clinicians must provide the best available treatments to relieve the suffering and promote the well-being of those who present for evaluation and treatment. In this chapter, we describe the currently available treatments for EDNOS, focusing on BED and NES. For treatment of individuals with anorexia nervosa–like and bulimia nervosa–like syndromes, readers are referred to the chapters in this volume describing treatment for anorexia nervosa and bulimia nervosa, as systematic studies of the modification of standard treatment for individuals with variants of these disorders have, for the most part, not yet been carried out.

Binge-Eating Disorder

Fran is a 38-year-old, single, African American personnel manager with a BMI of 39.7. She tends to feel out of control of her eating and snacks on three or four candy bars throughout the day, in addition to eating a normal breakfast and lunch. Fran binges nearly every evening, starting either on her way home from work then continuing when she is alone at home, or after a normal dinner. A typical binge episode consists of two pieces of chicken, a small bowl of salad, two servings of mashed potatoes, a hamburger, a large serving of French fries, a fast food apple pie, a large chocolate shake, a large bag of potato chips, and 15–20 small cookies, all eaten within a 2-hour period. During her binge episodes Fran eats much more rapidly than usual until she feels uncomfortably full, eats large amounts of food when she does not feel physically hungry, eats alone because she is embarrassed by how much she is eating, and feels disgusted with herself and very guilty after eating. She is also extremely distressed about her weight and readily admits that her weight and shape are the most important factors that affect how she feels about herself.

From childhood, Fran remembers being singled out by her family as "the only one who wasn't very athletic and very thin." She was teased by her family about her weight and was the only one who did not have to clean her plate at meals. However, when she looked back at pictures of herself as an adolescent, she was surprised and confused to see that she did not look overweight. "Everybody thought I was fatter than I ever really was." Fran began binge eating in secret at age 11 after her family enrolled her in a weight-loss program and she was restricted to snacking on celery and carrots while her siblings ate potato chips. Fran's intense concerns about her appearance and history of extreme weight fluctuations also date from the time she began dieting. Over the years she went on and off numerous diets, and each time she lost and then regained 25–90 pounds through binge eating and overeating large amounts of fast food. Fran avoided wearing shorts, pants, and swimsuits at all costs, even if it meant depriving herself of opportunities to swim, which was one of her favorite activities.

Target Symptoms and Treatment Goals

Individuals like Fran who present with BED often have more than one target symptom. By definition, uncontrolled eating binges occur regularly and are associated with significant distress, so the cessation of binge eating and the institution of healthy eating patterns are virtually always important goals. Like Fran, most individuals with BED seen in clinical settings are overweight or obese. Obesity has several associated medical risks, including diabetes mellitus, hypertension, osteoarthritis, and certain forms of cancer, and as we now know, a weight loss of as little as 5%–10%, if maintained, can yield significant medical benefits. For both medical and psychological reasons, most patients with BED desire weight loss. Finally, weight stabilization and enhanced self-acceptance at a higher-than-average weight for height may be important goals for many patients. Even patients who are successful in losing significant amounts of weight often do not lose sufficient weight to fall within a normal weight range, and therefore, as is true for patients with anorexia nervosa and bulimia nervosa, self-acceptance is often of vital importance to the patient's overall health.

A striking feature of patients with BED is the frequent occurrence of co-morbid psychopathology. It is beyond the scope of this chapter to review in detail the many studies that have documented increased levels of general psychopathology in individuals with BED compared with normal-weight or obese control groups, including higher levels of depression, anxiety, anger, and impulsivity, and comorbid psychiatric diagnoses, most notably current and lifetime major depression. Although many of the available studies of comorbidity in BED have been conducted in clinical samples, population-based studies have also borne out the relationship between binge eating or BED and risk for lifetime major depression (Bulik et al. 2002; Telch and Stice 1998). While the evidence is mixed regarding rates of comorbid psychiatric diagnoses in individuals with BED versus those with bulimia nervosa, several studies have reported comparable rates of comorbid affective disorders in the two patient groups, and one large epidemiological study found that rates of comorbidity did not differ among samples of patients with purging bulimia nervosa, nonpurging bulimia nervosa, or BED (Striegel-Moore et al. 2001).

The first generation of treatments for BED tended to develop along two lines: those emphasizing dieting and those emphasizing nondieting approaches. The former type of program, often including obese patients with BED along with their obese non-binge-eating counterparts, placed the emphasis on weight loss, with binge cessation being viewed mainly as a means toward that end. The latter type of program placed a greater emphasis on psychological well-being and self-acceptance, with flexibility in eating seen as more desirable than rigid restraint. The most recent generation of studies has attempted to combine the goals of dieting and nondieting programs, promoting a balanced emphasis on healthy lifestyle, medical well-being, and satisfaction with body image. In fact, self-acceptance and healthy change may be seen not as competing goals but rather as mutually reinforcing goals (Wilson 1996).

In any case, the initial step in treating patients with BED should be a discussion of the several possible goals of treatment, the advantages and disadvantages of attempting to change along each of the above dimensions, the patient's priorities, and the available options for treatment, with clinician and patient working collaboratively to select the treatment approach that is best suited to the patient's priorities. When other resources are not available, various forms of self-help conducted by patients alone or with therapist guidance may prove beneficial (Perkins et al. 2006).

Nutritional Issues

Many overweight or obese individuals with BED present, first and foremost, for weight-loss treatment. For these individuals, the most important question is whether standard treatment programs for obesity—that is, behavioral weight control programs such as the LEARN program (Brownell 2004), accompanied by low-calorie diet (LCD) or very low-calorie diet (VLCD)/liquid fast— have beneficial effects in obese individuals with BED that are comparable to those seen in nonbingeing individuals. Behavioral weight control programs are typically offered in either an individual or a group format and consist of a combination of nutritional advice, lifestyle counseling, implementation of both structured exercise and increased daily activity, and problem solving regarding family-related and psychological barriers to healthy lifestyles.

A theoretical concern is that the dietary restriction imposed by such programs might promote binge eating either in the short or in the long term. However, the evidence on this point is limited and does not clearly suggest a need for a distinct treatment approach. For instance, in programs using VLCD in individuals who binge eat, whereas some patients experience a reemergence of binge eating during the transition from liquid diet to regular foods, many patients appear to do as well as individuals without BED (Yanovski et al. 1994). Similarly, while the response to LCD programs is variable and tends to deteriorate over time, it is not clear that individuals who binge eat fare markedly worse than nonbingeing individuals in such programs (Gladis et al. 1998). One recent study has demonstrated that among nonbingeing individuals, LCD does not promote the de novo emergence of binge eating (Wadden et al. 2004).

In the absence of evidence that patients with BED do not do well in VLCD or LCD programs, clinicians should seriously consider these approaches in patients whose primary goal is weight loss. There is some evidence that structured exercise may facilitate weight loss when superimposed on treatments, such as cognitive-behavioral therapy (CBT), that in and of themselves typically do not yield significant weight loss (Pendleton et al. 2002), although this approach is less well studied than VLCD or LCD programs. Given the relatively frequent occurrence of comorbid psychiatric conditions such as depression in these patients (Yanovski et al. 1993), and the marked distress related to eating, body image dissatisfaction, and weight fluctuation that is characteristic of these patients (Dingemans et al. 2002), clinicians should carefully monitor these patients and perhaps consider the use of supplemental psychosocial and/ or medication treatments in selected cases.

A question that has emerged more recently is whether the presence of binge eating or of full-syndrome BED adversely affects outcome in patients receiving bariatric surgery, such as Roux-en-Y gastric bypass or laparoscopic adjustable band placement. While clinical practice in this regard is quite variable (Devlin et al. 2004), most studies suggest that, at least in the short term, binge eating tends to resolve following such procedures (de Zwaan 2005). However, given the absence of definitive long-term data demonstrating that patients with eating disorders are not at risk for resurgence of eating disorder symptoms, careful postoperative follow-up of BED patients who undergo bariatric surgery would nonetheless seem prudent. In addition, reports have appeared of patients who have developed significant eating disorders following bariatric surgery (Segal et al. 2004), further underscoring the utility of postoperative monitoring for symptoms of emergent eating disorders. A more complete discussion of these issues is presented in Chapter 9 ("Psychiatric Aspects of Bariatric Surgery") in this volume.

Although most obese or overweight patients with BED would welcome some amount of weight loss, some patients present with binge cessation and a healthy lifestyle as their primary goals. Unfortunately, a definitive study comparing weight outcomes following treatment with nutritionally based approaches versus psychological approaches, such as CBT, in patients who present primarily for treatment of binge eating has yet to be reported. However, even for obese or overweight patients for whom weight loss is not the initial goal of treatment, it is important to consider obesity-related comorbidity, implement healthy lifestyle changes, and ensure adequate medical care for any obesity-related comorbid conditions.

Psychosocial Approaches

CBT, the most widely studied form of psychotherapy for BED, is a time-limited, structured treatment that directly targets eating disorder symptoms of binge eating, strict dieting, extreme concerns about shape and weight, and low self-esteem, as well as subthreshold compensatory behaviors such as vomiting and laxative abuse (Fairburn et al. 1993; Marcus 1997). A course of CBT for BED typically consists of 20 weekly 45-minute sessions and may be delivered either in an individual or in a group format. A course of CBT for BED is outlined in Table 8–1.

The initial stage (sessions 1–8) focuses primarily on psychoeducational and behavioral strategies. The foundation of CBT is daily self-monitoring to increase awareness of high-risk situations that trigger binge eating and associated behaviors, thoughts, and feelings. Patients are encouraged to work toward a moderate, realistic, and flexible level of dietary restraint to facilitate healthy eating and eliminate binge eating. A regular pattern of eating is prescribed—typically three meals plus two to three snacks per day, incorporating a wide variety of foods, including favorite foods served in moderate portions. Other behavioral strategies emphasized early in treatment include using stimulus control techniques (e.g., slowing eating by putting the fork down between bites, serving and eating one portion at a time) and practicing pleasurable alternatives to binge eating (e.g., playing a musical instrument, taking a bubble bath, calling a friend). Subjects are also given information about the complex causes of obesity and binge eating, including the degree to which obesity is genetically and environmentally influenced.

Stage 2 (sessions 9–16) emphasizes cognitive interventions and problem-solving strategies targeting problematic eating and concerns about body weight and shape. Patients are taught to use automatic thought records and cognitive restructuring to identify and modify maladaptive rules, beliefs, and assumptions, such as dichotomous thinking (e.g., foods are either good or bad), imperatives (e.g., "I should never eat more than 1,200 calories a day"), and jump-

Table 8–1.   Cognitive-behavioral therapy (CBT) for binge-eating disorder

Phase 1 (Sessions 1–8)

Psychoeducation

    Relationship between binge eating and obesity, complex causes of obesity

    Elimination of binge eating will not necessarily lead to weight loss

    Benefits of weekly weighing, focus on long-term trends

    Nutritional guidance (e.g., benefits of fruits and vegetables, complex carbohydrates)

    Emphasis on overall moderation and flexible restraint (e.g., enjoyable foods in controlled portions)

    Benefits of exercise

Behavioral techniques

    Self-monitoring of food, circumstances, thoughts, feelings

    Regular pattern of meals and snacks, planning

    Stimulus-control strategies (e.g., putting fork down between bites)

    Alternative activities (e.g., calling a friend, taking a bubble bath)

    Systematic delay (wait 15 minutes)

Phase 2 (Sessions 9–16)

Problem-solving skills

    Systematic problem solving, seven steps

    Decisional analysis to enhance motivation, reduce ambivalence

Cognitive techniques

    Identification and modification of dysfunctional thoughts and beliefs about eating, food, weight

    Promotion of acceptance of larger-than-average body size

    Reduction in body image disparagement and shame

Phase 3 (Sessions 17–20)

Psychoeducation

    Lapse versus relapse, recovery from slips possible

    Inevitability of setbacks: importance of planning ahead, being proactive

Problem-solving skills

    Comprehensive maintenance plan/list of CBT strategies

    Current and anticipated high-risk situations plus specific coping strategies

    Decisional analysis about weight-loss treatment

ing to conclusions (e.g., "I'll never have a boyfriend because no man could ever be attracted to me at this weight"). CBT for overweight or obese patients with BED differs from CBT for bulimia nervosa in that patients are, in fact, undesirably heavy by cultural standards and are challenged to work toward acceptance of a larger than average body size. Problem-solving strategies include a seven-step approach detailed by Fairburn, Marcus, and Wilson (1993) and decisional analysis. The latter technique consists of identifying the short- and long-term costs and benefits of big-picture decisions such as whether to stop or to continue to binge eat, as well as decisions about more specific behaviors such as whether or not to self-monitor food intake.

Stage 3 (sessions 17–20) focuses on the maintenance of improvement and on relapse prevention. Patients develop a comprehensive relapse prevention plan listing CBT strategies to be used on an ongoing basis, as well as strategies to resume as needed. For example, it is not uncommon for patients to decide to discontinue self-monitoring unless their eating habits begin to deteriorate, when they may resume food records on a short-term basis. It can be useful to identify a list of current and anticipated high-risk situations to help patients plan for potential problems. Patients are also encouraged to be proactive in implementing CBT strategies as soon as possible to prevent the progression of eating slips from occasional lapses to full-blown relapse. In addition, patients who have been successful in controlling their binge eating but have not lost a significant amount of weight may wish to consider undertaking a form of treatment that is more specifically directed toward weight loss.

Interpersonal therapy (IPT) is a short-term, semistructured approach that addresses interpersonal problems that contribute to the onset and maintenance of the eating disorder, focusing primarily on current, rather than historical, social functioning (Wilfley et al. 2000). A primary goal is to enhance interpersonal functioning and communication skills, rather than directly addressing the symptoms of the eating disorder (Tantleff-Dunn et al. 2004). IPT typically consists of 4–6 months of weekly sessions, conducted in either an individual or group modality. Phase 1 (4–5 sessions) is focused on diagnostic evaluation and obtaining a history of interpersonal relationships. One or two potential problem areas are then targeted from four types of interpersonal challenges: grief, role transitions, role disputes, and interpersonal deficits. Phase 2 (8–10 sessions) is focused on the present, and various options are explored for changes in each of the target problem areas. The therapist is active but nondirective in identifying themes and inconsistencies. In Phase 3 (4–5 sessions), progress is summarized, termination with the therapist is processed, and relapse prevention strategies focusing on the identification of symptoms that require active attention are discussed.

Dialectical behavior therapy (DBT) was originally developed for treatment of patients with borderline personality disorder (Linehan 1993a, 1993b) and has more recently been adapted for treatment of severe eating disorders, including BED (as reviewed in Kotler et al. 2003). DBT is based on cognitive-behavioral techniques but also incorporates Zen Buddhism and other acceptance-based philosophies and approaches. Because DBT is a longer-term, time- and labor-intensive approach, it is generally recommended for treatment-refractory patients for whom other treatments have failed. DBT typically consists of four treatment modalities: weekly individual psychotherapy, weekly DBT skills training groups, telephone consultations, and case consultations for therapists. In the model of DBT for BED described by Blocher and colleagues (2004), treatment is conducted in four sequential stages. The pretreatment stage focuses on preparation and commitment to therapy. Stage 1 identifies behavioral targets, with the goal of reducing problematic eating disorder symptoms by means of adaptive coping strategies and behavioral skills. This stage requires a 1-year commitment from the patient, with the option of extending treatment beyond this time frame. Once there is substantial improvement in target behaviors, treatment moves to stage 2, which is focused on decreasing posttraumatic stress. After patients are relatively stable behaviorally and emotionally, treatment shifts to stage 3, in which issues related to personal goals, self-respect, and dependency issues are addressed.

Medication Treatment

Studies using medication to treat overweight or obese patients with BED typically have focused on reduction in binge eating and weight loss as desired outcomes (Table 8–2). A variety of selective serotonin reuptake inhibitor (SSRI) antidepressant medications, prescribed at dosages toward the high end of the recommended range (e.g., fluoxetine up to 60–80 mg/day, sertraline up to 200 mg/day, citalopram up to 60 mg/day, escitalopram up to 30 mg/day, fluvoxamine up to 300 mg/day), have been found to be helpful in reducing binge eating. In most cases treatment with SSRIs yields a significant reduction in binge-eating episodes that exceeds that seen with placebo treatment (Appoli-

nario and McElroy 2004). However, it is important to note that 1) most studies to date have been short-term, and little is known about how patients might
fare in the longer term, either with continuation treatment or after medication
discontinuation; and 2) placebo response rates in several studies have been
strikingly high (as shown in Table 8–2), suggesting that short-term binge reduction may in many cases be at least in part attributable to the nonspecific effect of being in treatment or taking a medication as opposed to the specific
effect of that medication. These medications are generally well tolerated, with
few patients discontinuing treatment due to side effects.

More recently, investigators have used medications indicated for obesity
treatment and anticonvulsant medications in an attempt to help patients both
to stop binge eating and to lose weight. Studies using the appetite suppressant
sibutramine, which is typically associated with weight losses of about 10% of
starting weight (Appolinario et al. 2003), have reported both binge reduction
and weight loss that are comparable to those seen in obese nonbingeing individuals. Although most patients do not have clinically significant elevations in
heart rate or blood pressure, these should be monitored in patients treated with
sibutramine. Treatment with orlistat, a weight-management agent that promotes weight loss by inhibiting fat absorption, also has been found to yield
weight loss in binge-eating individuals that is comparable to that seen in nonbingeing individuals, and is associated with improvement in eating disorder
symptoms that is modestly greater than that seen in a placebo group (Golay et
al. 2005). The anticonvulsants topiramate (McElroy et al. 2003) and, more recently, zonisamide (McElroy et al. 2004a) have been found to have utility both
for binge suppression and for weight loss. Significantly, topiramate has been
studied over a 1-year period and has been found to yield continued binge suppression and ongoing weight loss during that period in patients who tolerate the
medication. However, side effects such as cognitive problems, paresthesias,
and somnolence preclude long-term medication maintenance treatment in a
substantial minority of patients (McElroy et al. 2004b).

The paucity of studies of combined psychotherapy and pharmacotherapy
does not allow for firm recommendations. However, it appears that when offered in combination with expertly delivered psychosocial interventions for
BED, medication confers little additional benefit in terms of binge suppression or remission but may enhance outcome in terms of weight loss (Agras et
al. 1994) or improvement in depressive symptoms (Devlin et al. 2005).

Table 8–2. Medications for binge-eating disorder

Medication	Maximum dosage studied (mg/day)	Effect on binge reduction	Effect on weight loss	Comments
SSRI antidepressants				
Fluoxetine	80	+++	+	
Sertraline	200	+++	++	
Fluvoxamine	300	+++	+	
Citalopram	60	+++	+	
Other antidepressants				
Desipramine	200	+++	–	
Imipramine	200	+++	–	
Appetite suppressants				
Dexfenfluramine	30	+++	–	Removed from market
Sibutramine	15	+++	+++	Monitoring of heart rate and blood pressure necessary
Anticonvulsants				
Topiramate	400	+++	+++	Cognitive effects sometimes problematic
Other agents				
Naltrexone	150	+++	–	
Orlistat	120	++	+++	
Placebo	NA	++	–	

Note. NA=not applicable; SSRI=selective serotonin reuptake inhibitor.

It is worth noting that dexfenfluramine, which was reported to reduce binge eating in patients with BED (Stunkard et al. 1996), was removed from the market because of the increased risk of primary pulmonary hypertension and heart valve abnormalities found with the drug. Patients who report having used fenfluramine or dexfenfluramine either alone or in combination with other agents (e.g., phentermine/fenfluramine) should be evaluated for potential complications.

Monitoring and Follow-Up

While short-term remission of binge eating in patients with BED is common, longer-term follow-up studies of both community and clinical samples suggest that the course of BED over time is rather unstable, with at least a substantial minority of patients still symptomatic 5–6 years after initial evaluation (Fairburn et al. 2000; Fichter et al. 1998). The degree to which treatment impacts the long-term course of BED is still uncertain.

One association that has been supported by several studies is the association between binge eating and weight gain over time. A large community study of young women with BED reported that the prevalence of obesity in those with binge eating nearly doubled over the 5-year follow-up period. Several studies have suggested that remission of binge eating is associated with weight stabilization, whereas continued binge eating tends to give rise to weight gain over time (Agras et al. 1997; Raymond et al. 2002; Sherwood et al. 1999; Wilfley et al. 2002). On the basis of these findings, clinical prudence dictates that patients with BED who achieve short-term remission be carefully monitored for lapse or relapse. In addition, full and sustained remission of binge eating should be viewed as a worthwhile treatment goal with implications for medical as well as psychological health.

Night-Eating and Nocturnal Eating Syndromes

Bob is a 57-year-old physician with a BMI of 38. He describes himself as a "model eater" until evening. He eats a breakfast at 8 A.M., not because he is hungry but because he thinks he should. He sometimes feels nauseated in the morning because he has eaten during the night. During the day, Bob passes up snacks at the office and eats lunch at 12:30 P.M. At home he eats dinner between 7 and 9 P.M. After dinner he may doze off, but he will usually have two or three snacks before bedtime, which is typically at midnight. He wakes two to four times each night and eats whatever is available—donuts, peanut butter and jelly sandwiches, leftovers from dinner, or chips. He drinks regular soda at night, although he does not drink it during the day. Bob describes having no control over his eating during this time. He reports that his best sleep occurs between 4 and 6 A.M.

Bob's night eating began soon after he got married in his mid-20s, when he was still normal weight. For a couple of years, he was up late some nights as a resident, and his wife usually had home-cooked food readily available for him. He also remembers waking and eating cold soup and beans out of a can in the middle of the night. Currently, there is no difference in his night eating from weekdays to weekends, and he makes sure he has a minibar or room service available to him if he is traveling. There are only two nights per year that he does not eat: before getting blood work done for his yearly physical and on Yom Kippur. He is unable to sleep on those nights. Three years ago he had surgery and was unable to get out of bed to eat for 2 weeks. His wife left him healthy snacks to eat instead of the "junk food" he usually consumed, and he lost 15 pounds.

Target Symptoms and Treatment Goals

NES is not included in DSM-IV-TR (American Psychiatric Association 2000), and its diagnostic criteria have varied. Its original definition included morning anorexia, evening hyperphagia (i.e., eating 25% of the daily food intake after 6 P.M.), and insomnia, and it was linked to stress (Stunkard et al. 1955). There have been many variations in this definition, most commonly for evening hyperphagia, including at least 50% of the daily food intake after 7 P.M. (Stunkard et al. 1996); excessive evening eating (Rand et al. 1997); and eating on and off throughout the evening without enjoyment (Kuldau and Rand 1986). Notably, Birketvedt et al. (1999) acknowledged the presence of nocturnal ingestions (eating on awakening during the night) in their provisional criteria for NES, which included morning anorexia; evening hyperphagia (i.e., 50% of intake after evening meal); awakenings at least once per night; consumption of snacks during awakenings; and a duration of 3 months, in the absence of bulimia nervosa and BED.

More recently, a group of 46 overweight and obese persons who were recruited for a study of NES using the Birketvedt et al. (1999) criteria were evaluated for 10 days with a food and sleep diary (O'Reardon et al. 2004a). Although the participants reported eating half of their intake after dinner and during the night during a screening interview, their diaries revealed that they consumed 35% (SD = 10%), on average—a proportion still considerably higher than the 10% (SD = 7%) consumed by 43 similar control subjects. Given this reality, it is likely that persons have difficulty estimating their evening intake independent of the evening meal. On the basis of the findings above, two standard deviations above the average evening food intake for "normal eaters" would be 24%, suggesting that consumption of 25% or more of the day's calories after dinner would be an unusually large amount.

In the same study (O'Reardon et al. 2004a), individuals with NES awoke 1.5 (SD = 1.0) times per night and ate on 74% of those occasions, as compared with control subjects, who awoke 0.5 (SD = 0.5) times per night and did not eat. These diary reports of awakenings were confirmed with actigraphy, which also showed that individuals with NES and control subjects maintained similar bedtimes and morning awakening times throughout the study. Overall, these researchers concluded that the main aspect of NES is a delay in the circadian pattern of eating that interferes with the usual sleep pattern. Since that time, this research group has used the following definition for NES: a phase delay in the circadian pattern of eating, manifested by 1) evening hyperphagia (i.e., ≥25% of calories after the evening meal), 2) awakenings accompanied by nocturnal ingestions (at least three times per week), or 3) both (Allison and Stunkard 2005).

More research is needed to validate a definition of NES, including the criteria for evening hyperphagia, the required frequency of nocturnal ingestions, and whether both of these features should be required for a diagnosis of NES (Allison and Stunkard 2005). The presence of morning anorexia also needs more investigation, as it may be a symptom that is neither necessary nor sufficient for the diagnosis of NES (Engel 2005). It is important to note that most individuals with NES do not have BED (there seems to be a 15%–20% rate of comorbidity with BED; see Allison et al. 2004a, 2006; Powers et al. 1999; Stunkard et al. 1996) and that nocturnal ingestions typically consist of about 300 kcal (Birketvedt et al. 1999).

The target of treatment for NES is shifting the delayed eating schedule back to the day by promoting a regular daytime eating schedule and eliminating nocturnal ingestions. Many individuals with NES are distressed that their evening and nocturnal eating episodes contribute to weight gain and/or sabotage their daytime weight-loss efforts. The compulsion to eat is just too overwhelming to overcome, and they feel it is necessary to eat in order to fall back to sleep. Many individuals with NES have no appetite or attempt to restrict their eating the following morning in order to mitigate the effects of their nighttime snacking. Thus, they establish a circular pattern of restriction during the day followed by grazing during the evening and nocturnal ingestions during the night.

A review of thoughts recorded by individuals with NES before and after they ate at night revealed four major themes: experiencing a specific food craving, feeling anxious or agitated, needing to eat to fall back to sleep, and physical hunger or compulsion to eat. Other, less common themes were feeling stressed, depressed, or bored (Allison et al. 2004b). Examples of these thoughts are shown in Table 8–3. These records suggest that individuals with NES experience dysfunctional thoughts that maintain their distressing eating patterns, and that psychotherapeutic treatments may be effective in changing the thoughts and reducing the night-eating behaviors. It also seems plausible that psychopharmacology could help to decrease the compulsion to eat at night and to regulate eating and sleeping schedules. Treatment will be discussed in more detail later in this section.

Two other nocturnal eating disorders have been reported in the sleep literature: nocturnal eating and drinking syndrome (NEDS) and sleep-related eating disorder (SRED). The construct for NEDS emphasizes a sleep disorder with recurrent awakenings often accompanied by eating or drinking (Thorpy 1990), and the construct for SREDs adds to this a reduced level of awareness or recall of nocturnal eating episodes. NEDS is not well differentiated from NES and SRED and has not received much independent attention. Persons with SRED often consume nonfood items and suffer injuries attempting to prepare foods while in a parasomnic state (Schenck et al. 1993). SRED is associated with additional sleep disorders, such as somnambulism associated with noneating behaviors, restless legs syndrome, obstructive sleep apnea, and periodic leg movements (Schenck et al. 1991). SRED has also been linked to the presence of daytime anorexia nervosa and bulimia nervosa (Gupta 1991; Winkelman 1998; Winkelman et al. 1999). The nocturnal eating may provide the opportunity to eat when control and awareness of food consumption are low for those who are undernourished during the day (de Zwaan et al. 2003).

For persons with SRED, the goal of treatment is to stop their parasomnic episodes of eating. Since they have little to no awareness of these episodes, traditional psychotherapies may be difficult to employ. Medication, which will be discussed later in this section, may be the more fruitful approach in treating this disorder.

Table 8–3. Examples of four common themes of thoughts recorded before and after night-eating episodes

Theme	Thoughts before eating	Thoughts after eating
Compelled evening hyperphagia	I'm very relaxed. I really am not hungry, but I feel an overwhelming compulsion to eat.	I'm disgusted that I ate just before going to bed and by my lack of control and willpower.
Anxious/agitated	I was very tired and just wanted to go to sleep. I was anxious and upset because we are going away on vacation Saturday and my husband has yet to pack. So we had a little argument before bed.	When I got up and found the chocolate, I knew I was in trouble. I started to eat it very fast and my heart was pounding. It is very hard for me to stop once I start, but I only ate a little and then went back to bed.
Craving	I woke up at 2 A.M. I had purchased pastry cakes earlier in the day. I knew they were there and wanted them. I knew if I didn't go downstairs and eat a pack I wouldn't get back to sleep.	Good. Now I can go right back to sleep as soon as I go up to my bed.
Need to eat to sleep	Very tired, can't sleep. If I just eat something, I will be able to sleep. My stomach bugs me—if I don't eat, I will just keep getting up.	Hope I can sleep through to morning. Very tired. Just want to sleep all the way through. Don't want to get up again.

Nutritional Issues

Limited information is known about the impact of NES and SRED on traditional weight loss efforts or weight gain over time. Stunkard et al. (1955) reported that persons with NES were much less successful at losing excess weight and were more likely to have adverse reactions to weight-loss programs than non-night-eating individuals. Gluck et al. (2001) reported that the dropout rate between individuals with NES and those without night eating in a behavioral weight-loss group did not differ. After BMI was controlled for, the NES group lost less weight (4.4 kg) than the non-NES group (7.3 kg) ($P=0.003$), suggesting that pure weight-loss efforts, in the absence of interventions that address evening and nocturnal eating behaviors, may be difficult for individuals with NES. Conversely, a structured 4-week inpatient cognitive-behavioral weight-loss program produced greater weight loss among patients who reported night eating more than half of the time prior to treatment than for those who reported night-eating behaviors less than half of the time (22.6 pounds vs. 15.6 pounds, $P<0.05$). It is likely that the lack of access to food after 7:00 P.M. in this environment promoted this large weight loss, but it is not clear why the individuals with NES lost more weight than the non-night-eating controls.

In the population-based Danish MONICA study (Andersen et al. 2004), which included 1,051 women and 1,061 men, the presence of nocturnal ingestions was linked with greater weight gain among obese women (5.2 kg vs. 0.9 kg) over a 6-year period. No relationship between nocturnal ingestions and weight gain was found among the men.

Not much is known about the success of persons with SRED in weight-loss programs, although the behavior would not be conducive to success. Reports suggest that about 40% of those with SRED are overweight, and individuals with SRED often complain that the nocturnal eating episodes have contributed to difficulties with weight management (Schenck et al. 1993; Winkelman 1998).

Psychosocial Approaches

Studies of psychosocial approaches to treatment for NES are few. Case studies using behavioral treatment have been reported, indicating mixed success (Coates 1978; Williamson et al. 1989). Pawlow et al. (2003) conducted the only placebo-controlled treatment trial comparing abbreviated progressive muscle relaxation (PMR) with sitting quietly for a 1-week trial. The PMR group had significantly increased levels of morning hunger and reduced evening hunger ratings, and there was a trend for more breakfasts consumed and less nighttime eating in this group. Levels of stress, anxiety, and depression were also significantly reduced in the PMR group. A longer trial is needed to test the extended effect of PMR.

CBT has been tested in a pilot study for treatment of NES, with some success (Allison et al. 2005). This treatment was modified from CBT treatment for BED, with a specific emphasis on regulating eating during the day and attending to thoughts and behaviors associated with after-dinner eating and nocturnal ingestions. Weight loss was included as an objective for overweight and obese participants, because this was a major reason for their seeking treatment. The 10-session treatment occurred weekly for 8 weeks and biweekly for the last 2 sessions (Table 8–4).

Key aspects of CBT treatment for NES include keeping a food and sleep diary every day and completing assessments of hunger, cravings, and emotions before eating at night. Participants are encouraged to pick a "kitchen is closed" time, and behavioral techniques are used to provide obstacles and discouragement to eating after this time. Raising awareness about food choices during the night and establishing a consistent daytime eating schedule are promoted, and caloric restriction is introduced at the third session for those with a weight loss goal. Other topics addressed include sleep hygiene, stress reduction through deep breathing and muscle relaxation, and exercise.

Sixteen participants enrolled in the pilot study, and nine completed the study (Allison et al. 2005). Last-observation-carried-forward analyses revealed significant reductions in the four major outcome measures at treatment end, including the Night Eating Symptom Scale (NESS; O'Reardon et al. 2004a), proportion of caloric intake consumed after dinner, number of awakenings, and number of nocturnal ingestions (Figure 8–1). Completers showed more dramatic improvements, decreasing their nocturnal ingestions from 6.4 to 0.3 per week ($P<0.01$) and reducing the percentage of calories consumed after dinner from 33.7% to 18.7% ($P<0.05$). Completers also lost a significant amount of weight (84.4 ± 23.5 kg at baseline to 81.5 ± 22.0 kg at session 10, $P<0.01$). A controlled trial of CBT for NES, with longer-term follow-up, is needed to investigate its efficacy further.

Table 8–4.   Cognitive-behavioral therapy (CBT) for night-eating syndrome (NES)

Session number	CBT session themes
1	Introduce the CBT model. Review symptoms and history of NES. Assign food and sleep diary and Night Eating Assessment (NEA)[a] to be completed at nocturnal ingestions. Begin to establish regular meal and snack times and sleeping times.
2	Review diary and NEAs for past week and identify the most common feelings associated with night-eating episodes. Identify a particular night-eating situation. Review automatic thoughts, themes, and decisions, and begin a behavior chain for night eating episodes. Discuss strategies for decreasing amounts eaten during night through stimulus-control techniques and portion control. Assign food and sleep diary and NEAs.
3	Review diary and NEAs for past week. Apply behavior chain to specific eating episodes. Introduce a calorie counting system, and start to identify how many calories can be alloted at night, with idea of trying to shift energy intake to earlier in the day. Assign food and sleep diary and NEAs.
4	Review diary for past week and recordings of calories. Assess total calories per day, and aim for a specified calorie range, as appropriate for body mass index status. Introduce dysfunctional thought records (DTRs). Work through an example and identify typical cognitive distortions and alternative responses. Assign food and sleep diary and DTRs.
5	Review diary, including caloric intake, and DTRs for past week. Discuss alternatives to eating at night. Introduce deep breathing exercises and brief progressive muscle relaxation (PMR) exercises to be used when resisting night eating episodes. Assign food and sleep diary and DTRs.
6	Review diary, including calorie goals, and DTRs for past week. Review breathing and PMR exercises and the times they were used during the week. Discuss particular themes and triggers for night-eating episodes and precipitants that may occur during the day. Assign food and sleep diary and DTRs.
7	Review diary, including calorie goals, and DTRs for past week. Examine sleep hygiene behaviors and obstacles for achieving a regular sleep schedule. Discuss the role of physical activity in relation to eating, any weight-loss goals, and sleeping. Assign food and sleep diary and DTRs.

Table 8–4.   Cognitive-behavioral therapy (CBT) for night-eating syndrome (NES) *(continued)*

Session number	CBT session themes
8	Review diary, including calorie goals, and DTRs for past week. Discuss progress in reducing night eating. Assess what areas remain most problematic. Review skills learned specific to those areas. Assign food, sleep, and thought diary.
9	Review diary, including calorie goals, and DTRs for past week. Identify any problems or regression to past behaviors that have occurred. Review skills learned specific to those areas. Discuss how to anticipate setbacks and how to bolster self-efficacy. Assign food and sleep diary and DTRs. Next session in 2 weeks.
10	Review diary, including calorie goals, and DTRs for past 2 weeks. Discuss reactions to the CBT treatment, and emphasize again how to troubleshoot for future setbacks, with review of skills learned in program.

[a]Night Eating Assessment consists of visual analog scales to identify to what degree the individual with NES is hungry, sad, craving a food, anxious, agitated, compelled to eat, and bored. The patient is encouraged to complete this before each night-eating episode.

Medication Treatment

As with psychosocial approaches to NES treatment, medication trials are also in their early stages. Case reports of success with D-fenfluramine (O'Reardon et al. 2004b; Spaggiari et al. 1994) suggested that treatment with SSRIs may be beneficial. A case series using paroxetine yielded success with four patients (Miyaoka et al. 2003). Additionally, an open-label 12-week trial of sertraline with 17 individuals with NES yielded significant reductions in NESS score, number of nocturnal awakenings and ingestions, percentage of caloric intake after dinner, and weight (−4.8 kg) (O'Reardon et al. 2004b).

A double-blind, placebo-controlled 8-week trial was recently reported comparing sertraline ($n=17$) with placebo ($n=17$) (O'Reardon et al. 2006). One participant from each group was unblinded early because of no response; there were no other dropouts. The results were similar to those of the open-label trial, with significant reductions for the sertraline group versus the placebo group in NESS score and number of nocturnal awakenings and ingestions. Percentage of caloric intake after the evening meal was reduced by 68% in the sertraline group versus 29% in the placebo group, but this difference

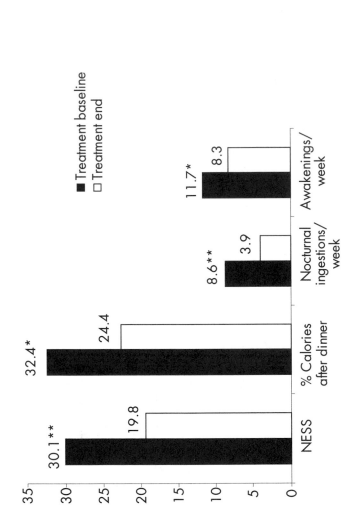

Figure 8–1. Cognitive-behavioral therapy treatment for night-eating syndrome: last-observation-carried-forward analyses for the major outcome measures.

NESS=Night Eating Symptom Scale. *$P < 0.05$; **$P < 0.01$.

was not significant after Bonferroni correction. Seventy-one percent of the individuals taking sertraline were classified as "responders" according to the Clinical Global Impression of Improvement Scale (CGI-I<2), and 41% were classified as "remitters" (CGI-I=1). Only 18% of the placebo group reached responder status. Individuals with a BMI>25 lost a significant amount of weight while taking sertraline (−2.9±3.8 kg) as compared to receiving placebo (−0.3 ±2.7 kg, $P<0.01$).

Case reports of topiramate have also shown some promise in treating NES. Winkelman (2003) reported success in two patients with NES and two patients with SRED, with accompanying significant weight loss. In an additional case series of six nonresponders to sertraline, there were significant reductions in NESS score, percentage of calories consumed after dinner, and weight (−4.6 kg over 12 weeks, $P<0.05$), with nonsignificant drops in nocturnal awakenings and ingestions (Allison 2005). One participant withdrew because of cognitive side effects. Controlled trials of topiramate for NES and possibly for SRED seem warranted.

Finally, pharmacotherapy treatments reported to be helpful in SRED are carbidopa/L-dopa, bromocriptine, codeine, and clonazepam (Schenck and Mahowald 2000; Schenck et al. 1993). SREDs including somnambulism have reportedly been induced by risperidone, olanzapine, bupropion, and zolpidem, among other medications (Khazaal et al. 2003; Lu and Shen 2004; Paquet et al. 2002; Schenck et al. 2005).

Monitoring and Follow-Up

The available information on the long-term course of NES is limited to one recent report of open-label maintenance treatment with sertraline (O'Reardon et al. 2005). In this study, 15 patients were followed for 6 months, with 10 of these patients completing 12 months of treatment. At 6 months, 11 of 13 patients who responded to acute treatment with sertraline had maintained their responder status (CGI-I<2), and 2 patients with only minimal improvement after the first 8 weeks had converted to responder status, which in turn corresponded to a remission rate (CGI-I=1) of 67% for the sample. All 10 patients who completed the 12-month follow-up were responders, including 1 patient who had relapsed at month 6. The mean dosage at week 8 was 96.7± 44.2 mg/day. At 6 months and 12 months, the average total daily dose increased to 123.3±45.8 mg and 150±47.1 mg, respectively. Treatment-related improvements were maintained at 6 and 12 months, and weight loss appeared to continue during the maintenance phase (−4.4 kg at week 8, −6.4 kg at month 6, and −8 kg at month 12). Studies of the natural course of NES and other nocturnal eating disorders and follow-up studies of patients who have received treatment, including both psychosocial and pharmacological approaches, are greatly needed.

Other EDNOS Syndromes

Patients who present with EDNOS comprise, in addition to those with binge-eating disorder and night-eating syndrome described earlier, mostly patients with subthreshold or variant forms of anorexia nervosa or bulimia nervosa. These patients may include

1. Individuals with the behavioral and psychological features of anorexia nervosa who are not below 85% of ideal body weight (e.g., those who were overweight or obese and lost a great deal of weight) or those who meet criteria for anorexia nervosa but have not been amenorrheic for at least 3 months.
2. Individuals who binge eat and purge less than twice per week.
3. Normal-weight individuals who purge but do not binge eat (e.g., individuals with subjective bulimic episodes and purging).
4. Individuals who chew and spit out food but do not swallow in order to avoid weight gain.
5. Individuals who, following bariatric surgery, manifest psychological and behavioral features similar to those seen in anorexia nervosa and bulimia nervosa (Segal et al. 2004).

In the absence of systematic studies of the treatment of patients with these and other conditions currently classified as EDNOS, treatment should follow a plan based on symptoms that most closely resemble the full-fledged disorder. In tailoring the treatment plan to the individual, it is useful to consider the various dimensions of the patient's presentation, including nutritional status (obese, overweight, normal weight, underweight), behavior (restrained eating, binge eating, compensatory behaviors, checking or avoidance behaviors), psychological factors (body image dissatisfaction, comorbid psychopathology), and motivation for change (ego-syntonicity vs. ego-dystonicity of symptoms). A consideration of these dimensions of functioning may assist the clinician in structuring an individually tailored treatment that applies various aspects of treatment programs for anorexia nervosa, bulimia nervosa, binge-eating disorder, or night-eating syndrome based on the patient's particular symptom profile and goals.

References

Agras WS, Telch CF, Arnow B, et al: Weight loss, cognitive-behavioral, and desipramine treatments in binge eating disorder: an additive design. Behav Ther 25:225–238, 1994

Agras WS, Telch CF, Arnow B, et al: One-year follow-up of cognitive-behavioral therapy for obese individuals with binge eating disorder. J Consult Clin Psychol 65:343–347, 1997

Allison K: Treatment of the night eating syndrome. Presentation at the annual meeting of the Eating Disorders Research Society, Toronto, ON, September 2005

Allison KC, Stunkard AJ: Obesity and eating disorders. Psychiatr Clin North Am 28:55–67, 2005

Allison K, Crow S, Stunkard A, and Eating Disorders Look AHEAD Study Group: The prevalence of binge eating disorder and night eating syndrome in adults with type 2 diabetes mellitus (abstract). Obes Res 12:A89, 2004a

Allison KC, Stunkard AJ, Thier SL: Overcoming Night Eating Syndrome: A Step-by-Step Guide to Breaking the Cycle. Oakland, CA, New Harbinger, 2004b

Allison K, Martino N, O'Reardon J, et al: CBT treatment for night eating syndrome: a pilot study (abstract). Obes Res 13:A83, 2005

Allison KC, Wadden TA, Sarwer DB, et al: Night eating syndrome and binge eating disorder among persons seeking bariatric surgery: prevalence and related features. Surg Obes Relat Dis 2:153–158, 2006

American Psychiatric Association: Diagnostic and Statistical Manual of Mental Disorders, 4th Edition, Text Revision. Washington, DC, American Psychiatric Association, 2000

Anderson GS, Stunkard AJ, Sorensen TIA, et al: Night eating and weight change in middle-aged men and women. Int J Obes Relat Metab Disord 28:1338–1343, 2004

Appolinario JC, McElroy SL: Pharmacological approaches in the treatment of binge eating disorder. Curr Drug Targets 5:301–307, 2004

Appolinario JC, Bacaltchuk J, Sichieri R, et al: A randomized, double-blind, placebo-controlled study of sibutramine in the treatment of binge-eating disorder. Arch Gen Psychiatry 60:1109–1116, 2003

Birketvedt G, Florholmen J, Sundsfjord J, et al: Behavioral and neuroendocrine characteristics of the night-eating syndrome. JAMA 282:657–663, 1999

Blocher McCabe E, LaVia MC, Marcus MD: Dialectical behavior therapy for eating disorders, in Handbook of Eating Disorders and Obesity. Edited by Thompson JK. New York, Wiley, 2004, pp 232–244

Brownell KD: The LEARN Program for Weight Management, 10th Edition. Dallas, TX, American Health Publishing Company, 2004

Bulik CM, Sullivan PF, Kendler KS: Medical and psychiatric morbidity in obese women with and without binge eating. Int J Eat Disord 32:72–78, 2002

Coates TJ: Successive self-management strategies towards coping with night eating. J Behav Ther Exp Psychiatry 9:181–183, 1978

Devlin MJ, Goldfein JA, Dobrow IJ: What is this thing called BED? Update on binge eating disorder nosology. Int J Eat Disord 34:1–17, 2003

Devlin MJ, Goldfein JA, Flancbaum L, et al: Surgical management of obese patients with eating disorders: a survey of current practice. Obes Surg 14:1252–1257, 2004

Devlin MJ, Goldfein JA, Petkova E, et al: Cognitive behavioral therapy and fluoxetine as adjuncts to group behavioral therapy for binge eating disorder. Obes Res 13:1077–1088, 2005

de Zwaan M: Weight and eating changes after bariatric surgery, in Bariatric Surgery: A Guide for Mental Health Professionals. Edited by Mitchell JE, de Zwaan M. New York, Routledge, 2005, pp 77–99

de Zwaan M, Burgard MA, Schenck CH, et al: Night time eating: a review of the literature. European Eating Disorders Review 11:7–24, 2003

Dingemans AE, Bruna MJ, van Furth EF: Binge eating disorder: a review. Int J Obes Relat Metab Disord 26:299–307, 2002

Engel S: Item response theory of the night eating syndrome. Presentation at the annual meeting of the Eating Disorders Research Society, Toronto, Canada, ON, September 2005

Fairburn CG, Bohn K: Eating disorder NOS (EDNOS): an example of the troublesome "not otherwise specified" (NOS) category in DSM-IV. Behav Res Ther 43:691–701, 2005

Fairburn CG, Marcus MD, Wilson GT: Cognitive-behavioral therapy for binge eating and bulimia nervosa: a comprehensive treatment manual, in Binge Eating: Nature, Assessment, and Treatment. Edited by Fairburn CG, Wilson GT. New York, Guilford, 1993, pp 361–404

Fairburn CG, Cooper Z, Doll HA, et al: The natural course of bulimia nervosa and binge eating disorder in young women. Arch Gen Psychiatry 57:659–665, 2000

Fichter MM, Quadflieg N, Gnutzmann A: Binge eating disorder: treatment outcome over a 6-year course. J Psychosom Res 44:385–405, 1998

Gladis MM, Wadden TA, Vogt R, et al: Behavioral treatment of obese binge eaters: do they need different care? J Psychosom Res 44:375–384, 1998

Gluck ME, Geliebter A, Satov T: Night eating syndrome is associated with depression, low self-esteem, reduced daytime hunger, and less weight loss in obese outpatients. Obes Res 9:264–267, 2001

Golay A, Laurent-Jaccard A, Habicht F, et al: Effect of orlistat in obese patients with binge eating disorder. Obes Res 13:1701–1708, 2005

Gupta MA: Sleep related eating in bulimia nervosa: an underreported parasomnia disorder (abstract). Sleep Research 20:182, 1991

Khazaal Y, Krenz S, Zullino DF: Bupropion-induced somnambulism. Addict Biol 8:359–362, 2003

Kotler LA, Boudreau GS, Devlin MJ: Emerging psychotherapies for eating disorders. J Psychiatr Pract 9:431–441, 2003

Kuldau JM, Rand CSW: The night eating syndrome and bulimia in the morbidly obese. Int J Eat Disord 5:143–148, 1986

Linehan MM: Cognitive-Behavioral Treatment of Borderline Personality Disorder. New York, Guilford, 1993a

Linehan MM: Skills Training for Treating Borderline Personality Disorder. New York, Guilford, 1993b

Lu ML, Shen WW: Sleep-related eating disorder induced by risperidone. J Clin Psychiatry 65:273–274, 2004

Marcus MD: Adapting treatment for patients with binge-eating disorder, in Handbook of Treatment for Eating Disorders, 2nd Edition. Edited by Garner DM, Garfinkel PE. New York, Guilford, 1997, pp 484–493

McElroy SL, Arnold LM, Shapira NA, et al: Topiramate in the treatment of binge eating disorder associated with obesity: a randomized, placebo-controlled trial. Am J Psychiatry 160:255–261, 2003

McElroy SL, Kotwal R, Hudson JI, et al: Zonisamide in the treatment of binge-eating disorder: an open-label, prospective trial. J Clin Psychiatry 65:50–56, 2004a

McElroy SL, Shapira NA, Arnold LM, et al: Topiramate in the long-term treatment of binge-eating disorder associated with obesity. J Clin Psychiatry 65:1463–1469, 2004b

Miyaoka T, Yasukawa R, Tsubouchi K, et al: Successful treatment of nocturnal eating/drinking syndrome with selective serotonin reuptake inhibitors. Int Clin Psychopharmacol 18:175–177, 2003

O'Reardon JP, Ringel BL, Dinges DF, et al: Circadian eating and sleeping patterns in the night eating syndrome. Obes Res 12:1789–1796, 2004a

O'Reardon JP, Stunkard AJ, Allison KC: A clinical trial of sertraline in the treatment of the night eating syndrome. Int J Eat Disord 35:16–26, 2004b

O'Reardon J, Allison K, Martino N, et al: Maintenance treatment of the night eating syndrome with sertraline, a selective serotonin reuptake inhibitor (abstract). Obes Res 13:A193, 2005

O'Reardon JO, Allison KC, Martino NS, et al: A randomized placebo-controlled trial of sertraline in the treatment of the night eating syndrome. Am J Psychiatry 163:893–898, 2006

Paquet V, Strul J, Servais L, et al: Sleep-related eating disorder induced by olanzapine (letter). J Clin Psychiatry 63:597, 2002

Pawlow LA, O'Neil PM, Malcolm RJ: Night eating syndrome: effects of brief relaxation training on stress, mood, hunger, and eating patterns. Int J Obes Relat Metab Disord 27:970–978, 2003

Pendleton VR, Goodrick GK, Poston SC, et al: Exercise augments the effects of cognitive-behavioral therapy in the treatment of binge eating. Int J Eat Disord 31:172–184, 2002

Perkins SJ, Murphy R, Schmidt U, et al: Self-help and guided self-help for eating disorders. Cochrane Database Syst Rev (3):CD004191, 2006

Powers PS, Perez A, Boyd F, et al: Eating pathology before and after bariatric surgery: a prospective study. Int J Eat Disord 25:293–300, 1999

Rand CSW, Macgregor MD, Stunkard AJ: The night eating syndrome in the general population and among postoperative obesity surgery patients. Int J Eat Disord 22:65–69, 1997

Raymond NC, de Zwaan M, Mitchell JE, et al: Effect of a very low calorie diet on the diagnostic category of individuals with binge eating disorder. Int J Eat Disord 31:49–56, 2002

Schenck CH, Mahowald MW: Combined bupropion-levodopa-trazodone therapy of sleep-related eating and sleep disruption in two adults with chemical dependency. Sleep 23:587–588, 2000

Schenck CH, Hurwitz TD, Bundlie SR, et al: Sleep-related eating disorders: polysomnographic correlates of a heterogeneous syndrome distinct from daytime eating disorders. Sleep 14:419–431, 1991

Schenck CH, Hurwitz T, O'Connor KA, et al: Additional categories of sleep-related eating disorders and the current status of treatment. Sleep 16:457–466, 1993

Schenck CH, Connoy DA, Castellanos M, et al: Zolpidem-induced sleep-related eating disorder (SRED) in 19 patients (abstract). Sleep 28(suppl):A259, 2005

Segal A, Kinoshita KD, Larino MA: Postsurgical refusal to eat: anorexia nervosa, bulimia nervosa or a new eating disorder? A case series. Obes Surg 14:353–360, 2004

Sherwood NE, Jeffery RW, Wing RR: Binge status as a predictor of weight loss treatment outcome. Int J Obes Relat Metab Disord 23:485–493, 1999

Spaggiari MC, Granella F, Parrino L, et al: Nocturnal eating syndrome in adults. Sleep 17:339–344, 1994

Striegel-Moore RH, Cachelin FM, Dohm FA, et al: Comparison of binge eating disorder and bulimia nervosa in a community sample. Int J Eat Disord 29:157–165, 2001

Stunkard AJ, Grace WJ, Wolff HG: The night-eating syndrome: a pattern of food intake among certain obese patients. Am J Med 19:78–86, 1955

Stunkard AJ, Berkowitz R, Wadden T, et al: Binge eating disorder and the night eating syndrome. Int J Obes Relat Metab Disord 20:1–6, 1996

Tantleff-Dunn S, Gokee-LaRose J, Peterson RD: Interpersonal psychotherapy for the treatment of anorexia nervosa, bulimia nervosa, and binge eating disorder, in Handbook of Eating Disorders and Obesity. Edited by Thompson JK. New York, Wiley, 2004, pp 163–185

Telch CF, Stice E: Psychiatric comorbidity in women with binge eating disorder: prevalence rates from a non-treatment-seeking sample. J Consult Clin Psychol 66:768–776, 1998

Thorpy MJ (ed): International Classification of Sleep Disorders: Diagnostic and Coding Manual. American Sleep Disorders Association, Diagnostic Classification Steering Committee. Lawrence, KS, Allen Press, 1990

Wadden TA, Foster GD, Sarwer DB, et al: Dieting and the development of eating disorders in obese women: results of a randomized controlled trial. Am J Clin Nutr 80:560–568, 2004

Wilfley DE, MacKenzie KR, Robinson Welch R, et al: Interpersonal Psychotherapy for Group. New York, Basic Books, 2000

Wilfley DE, Welch RR, Stein RI, et al: A randomized comparison of group cognitive behavioral therapy and group interpersonal therapy for the treatment of overweight individuals with binge-eating disorder. Arch Gen Psychiatry 59:713–721, 2002

Williamson DA, Lawson OD, Bennett SM, et al: Behavioral treatment of night bingeing and rumination in an adult case of bulimia nervosa. J Behav Ther Exp Psychiatry 20:73–77, 1989

Wilson GT: Acceptance and change in the treatment of eating disorders and obesity. Behav Ther 27:417–439, 1996

Winkelman JW: Clinical and polysomnographic features of sleep-related eating disorder. J Clin Psychiatry 59:14–19, 1998

Winkelman JW: Treatment of nocturnal eating syndrome and sleep-related eating disorder with topiramate. Sleep Med 4:243–246, 2003

Winkelman JW, Herzog DB, Fava M: The prevalence of sleep-related eating disorder in psychiatric and non-psychiatric populations. Psychol Med 29:1461–1466, 1999

Yanovski SZ, Nelson JE, Dubbert BK, et al: Association of binge eating disorder and psychiatric comorbidity in obese subjects. Am J Psychiatry 150:1472–1479, 1993

Yanovski SZ, Gormally JF, Leser MS, et al: Binge eating disorder affects outcome of comprehensive very-low calorie diet treatment. Obes Res 2:205–212, 1994

9

Psychiatric Aspects of Bariatric Surgery

James E. Mitchell, M.D.

Lorraine Swan-Kremeier, Ph.D.

Tricia Myers, Ph.D.

It is now widely appreciated that the majority of adult Americans are over-weight or obese and that the rate of obesity has markedly accelerated over the last two decades (Ogden et al. 2003). Severe obesity has been associated with a plethora of medical complications, including diabetes mellitus, hypertension, dyslipidemia, urinary incontinence, cardiovascular disease, respiratory problems (including obstructive sleep apnea), osteoarthritis, and a variety of cancers (including cancer of the breast, uterus, prostate, and colon) (Kushner and Roth 2003). Paralleling this increase in obesity has been the increasing use of bariatric surgery procedures as a means of treating individuals with severe obesity, in particular those with a body mass index (BMI) greater than 40 or a

BMI greater than 35 in patients with certain comorbid conditions such as hypertension, type 2 diabetes, and dyslipidemia.

Our purpose in this chapter is to provide an overview of the current state of knowledge concerning bariatric surgery, including the history of the procedures, procedures currently being used, and complications resulting from these procedures. We then discuss the psychological assessment of patients who are candidates for bariatric surgery, relationships between psychopathology and bariatric surgery, psychosocial outcomes of patients who undergo bariatric surgery, and the psychological management of these patients pre- and postoperatively.

Overview of Bariatric Surgery Procedures

The first widely used procedure, known as the *jejunoileal bypass,* or JIB (Balsiger et al. 2000), involved an intestinal bypass in which the proximal duodenum was bypassed to the distal ileum (Figure 9–2). (For purposes of comparison, normal gastrointestinal anatomy is shown in Figure 9–1.) This procedure resulted in profound malabsorption associated with a variety of untoward effects, including diarrhea, protein-calorie malnutrition, and various vitamin and mineral deficiencies, as well as kidney stones, gallstones, and the risk of liver failure from cirrhosis (Latifi et al. 2002). Because of these complications, jejunoileal bypass is no longer a recommended procedure.

Following the introduction of surgical stapling devices during World War II, researchers developed a number of gastric restriction procedures, including *horizontal gastroplasty* and *vertical-banded gastroplasty.* In the former a pouch was created in the upper stomach by introducing a horizontal suture line (Figure 9–3), but, unfortunately, the stomach enlarged with time, resulting in limited weight loss. In vertical-banded gastroplasty (Figure 9–4), a vertical staple line was placed, with a proximal pouch draining into the distal pouch. While this method also had the advantage of lack of metabolic complications, the consumption of high-calorie liquids was not restricted, and consequently weight gain following surgery was not uncommon. Because of such limitations, these purely restrictive procedures have now been abandoned as well.

Gastric bypass was originally introduced in 1969. This procedure involved the creation of a pouch in the upper stomach with bypass of the larger gastric volume and connection of the gastric pouch to a proximal intestine loop. This

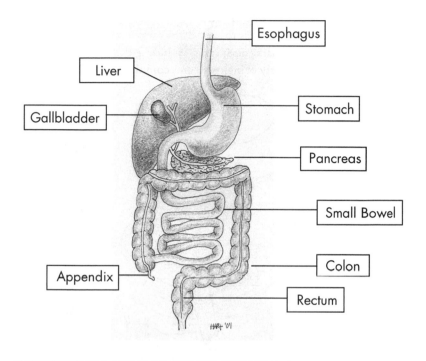

Figure 9–1. Normal gastrointestinal anatomy.

procedure was modified to include a Roux-en-Y technique for drainage of the pouch to prevent bile reflux. The size of the pouch was subsequently reduced to approximately 15–20 mL. In addition, the staple line was transectioned to prevent staple line failures. This operation is now considered the preferred procedure in bariatric surgery in the United States and is now performed laparoscopically at many centers (Figure 9–5).

A brief clinical vignette may illustrate the outcome of this procedure:

> N.C. was a 42-year-old white woman who had had trouble with obesity since adolescence. When she graduated from high school, she was 5 feet, 6 inches tall and weighed about 160 pounds, which meant she was about 30 pounds overweight. Throughout her adulthood she battled obesity. She tried many commercial weight-loss diets and bought literally dozens of diet books. During

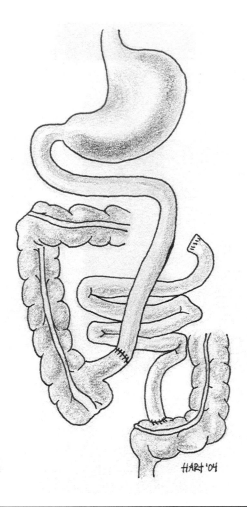

Figure 9–2.   Jejunoileal bypass, which involves intestinal bypass in which the proximal duodenum is bypassed to the distal ileum.

This procedure resulted in profound malabsorption associated with a variety of untoward effects, including diarrhea, protein-calorie malnutrition, and various vitamin and mineral deficiencies, as well as kidney stones, gallstones, and the risk of liver failure from cirrhosis (Latifi et al. 2002). Because of these complications, jejunoileal bypass is no longer a recommended procedure.

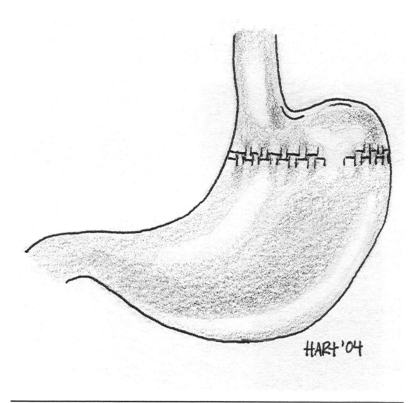

Figure 9–3.   Horizontal gastroplasty, in which a pouch is created in the upper stomach by introducing a horizontal suture line.
The stomach enlarged with time, resulting in limited weight loss. Because of this limitation, this purely restrictive procedure has been abandoned.

some of these attempts at weight loss she would lose significant amounts of weight, at times as much as 30 pounds, but she would always return to her prior weight and then gain beyond it. This was a source of continued concern and frustration for her. By the time she finally began seriously considering bariatric surgery at age 40, she weighed 260 pounds. She was beginning to experience medical complications of obesity, including dyslipidemia, hypertension, and frequent pain in her knees and ankles. Socially she suffered as well. She had two daughters, now grown, but during most of their youth, she had felt very uncomfortable about her weight and many times would not go to school activities in support of her children because of embarrassment.

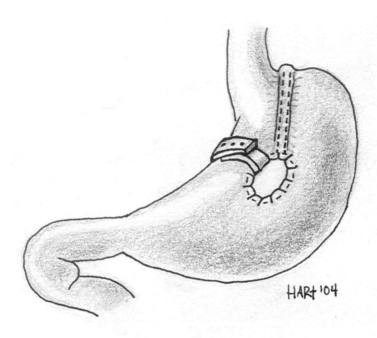

Figure 9–4.   Vertical-banded gastroplasty, in which a vertical staple line is placed, with a proximal pouch draining into the distal pouch.

While this method also had the advantage of lack of metabolic complications, the consumption of high-calorie liquids was not restricted, and consequently weight gain following surgery was not uncommon. Because of such limitations, this purely restrictive procedure has been abandoned.

She was working regularly and was married, but her social network was limited to a few friends who were also overweight. She avoided going to places like the shopping mall or other public places. Her relationship with her husband was strained at best. He was modestly overweight but could not understand why she continued to gain weight at such a rapid rate. They rarely did things together socially and had not been sexually active for several years.

She underwent Roux-en-Y gastric bypass. She was dedicated to achieving the best results possible, was compliant with the dietary information she received, went to her follow-up visits, and lost weight rapidly. Within a period of about 4 months, she lost 50 pounds, and continued losing at this rate for another 6 months. At that point, her weight loss began to level off, which was

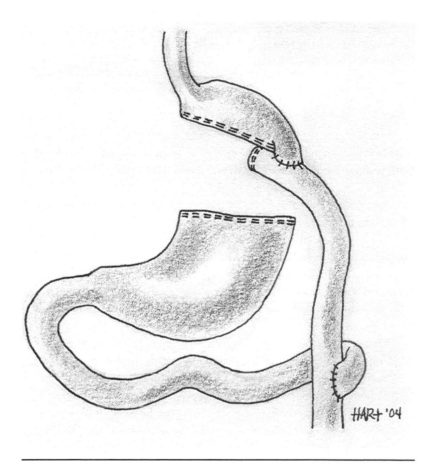

Figure 9–5. Gastric bypass, which involves the creation of a pouch in the upper stomach with bypass of the larger gastric volume and connection of the gastric pouch to a proximal intestine loop.

This procedure was modified to include a Roux-en-Y technique for drainage of the pouch to prevent bile reflux. The size of the pouch was subsequently reduced to approximately 15–20 mL. In addition, the staple line was transectioned to prevent staple line failures. This operation is now considered the preferred procedure in bariatric surgery in the United States and is now performed laparoscopically at many centers.

a source of great concern for her, and she returned to the doctor who had performed the procedure. She was referred for counseling with a dietitian. At that point she decided that she needed more lifestyle modification and began being very careful about her dietary intake, in particular avoiding foods high in fats, and began a regular program of exercise. With this new lifestyle pattern, she was able to stabilize her weight and at least in the short term prevent further weight regain.

Gastric banding was introduced in 1983, with an adjustable form of the band being introduced in 1992. Adjustable gastric banding (Figure 9–6) has become quite popular in many parts of the world. It has only been available in the United States since 2000.

Generally patients lose 60%–80% of their excess weight during the first 18 months following Roux-en-Y gastric bypass. Weight loss is more modest with banding procedures. Most recently, *biliopancreatic diversion,* with and without the duodenal switch, has been introduced for "super obese" patients (see Scopinaro et al. 2002) (Figure 9–7). These procedures result in fairly profound malabsorption and a significantly greater complication rate than is seen with other procedures, and they are reserved for patients with very extreme obesity at certain centers.

Bariatric surgery procedures can be associated with serious, sometimes fatal, complications. Problems that develop during the surgery proper include trauma to organs such as the spleen, bleeding, and the complications of anesthesia. Short-term perioperative complications include bowel obstruction, lung collapse, and distension of the bypassed portion of the stomach (Byrne 2001). Postoperative leaking is also a very serious complication and may require surgical reintervention. Wound infections can also occur. Long-term complications include bowel obstruction, gallbladder disease, and various nutritional deficiencies, including deficiencies of vitamin B_{12}, magnesium, and calcium (Byrne 2001; Elliot 2003). In a recent report concerning insurance claims for 2,522 bariatric surgeries in nonelderly patients, although the complication rate was 21.9% during the initial surgical stay, the rate increased to 39.6% over the 180 days after discharge. A total of 10.8% of the patients without 30-day complications developed a complication between 30 days and 180 days. Overall, 18.2% of the patients had some type of postoperative visit to the hospital with a complication (through readmission, outpatient hospital visit, or emergency room visit) within 180 days (Encinosa et al. 2006).

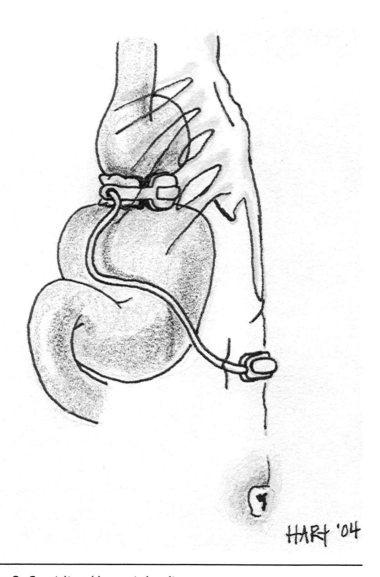

Figure 9–6. Adjustable gastric banding.

Gastric banding was introduced in 1983, with an adjustable form of the band being introduced in 1992. Adjustable gastric banding has become quite popular in many parts of the world. It has only been available in the United States since 2000.

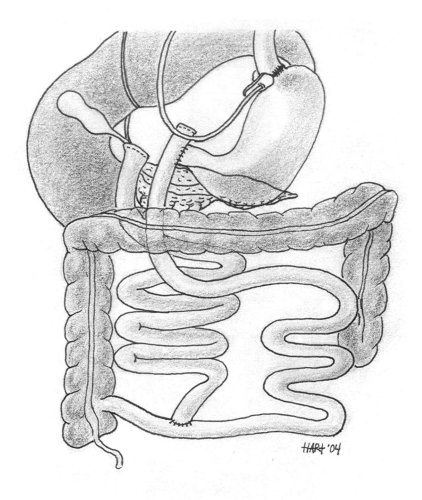

Figure 9–7.   Biliopancreatic diversion.

This method, with and without the duodenal switch, has been introduced for "super obese" patients (Scopinaro et al. 2002). These procedures result in fairly profound malabsorption and a significantly greater complication rate than is seen with other procedures, and they are reserved for patients with very extreme obesity at certain centers.

Psychiatric Issues in Bariatric Surgery Candidates and Patients

Psychiatric Comorbidity

The potential benefits of weight loss on obesity-related medical conditions most often serve as the primary impetus for pursuing bariatric surgery. However, psychosocial consequences of obesity often influence the patient's motivation and ultimate decision to undergo surgical intervention. Consequently, clinicians should be acquainted with what is known about the psychological and psychosocial experiences of bariatric surgery candidates.

Psychiatric conditions are not uncommon in obese individuals pursuing bariatric surgery, and, accordingly, careful assessment of psychopathology is a critical component of presurgical evaluation. A history of Axis I diagnoses has been reported in 27%–42% of bariatric surgery patients (Gentry et al. 1984; Gertler and Ramsey-Stewart 1986), most commonly adjustment disorders, affective disorders, anxiety disorders, and eating disorders. An investigation of psychiatric diagnoses and treatment history in bariatric surgery candidates conducted by Sarwer and colleagues (2004) highlighted the prevalence of psychiatric comorbidity in these patients. Of the 90 patients interviewed, 56 met criteria for a lifetime Axis I diagnosis, and half of these individuals met criteria for multiple diagnoses. Major depressive disorder, followed by binge-eating disorder (BED) and substance use disorders, was among the most common. Approximately 40% of subjects had reportedly received treatment for these conditions, primarily in the form of psychiatric medications. Interestingly, the majority of patients (71.9%) had been prescribed psychiatric medications by their primary physician versus a mental health professional.

Previous studies demonstrate similar findings. Larsen (1990) reported lifetime histories of adjustment disorders (15%), anxiety disorders (14%), and affective disorders (8%) in a sample of bariatric surgery candidates. In a study conducted by Powers et al. (1992), 62 Axis I disorders were represented among bariatric surgery patients, with affective disorders (34%), anxiety disorders (9%), and substance use disorders (8%) among the most common diagnoses. These prevalence rates, which are likely based on subjects meeting full criteria for Axis I diagnoses, may actually underestimate psychiatric comorbidity in bariatric surgery populations. If subthreshold diagnoses were considered, it is likely that the presence of depression, anxiety, substance abuse, and other psychopathology would be even more prevalent.

Although personality disorders have been less commonly studied in bariatric surgery patients, increased rates of these disorders have also been found. A presurgical history of Axis II diagnoses was found in 22% of bariatric surgery patients in Larsen's (1990) study. Powers et al. (1992) reported similar findings. Glinski et al. (2001) reported even higher prevalence rates, with 36% of their sample meeting criteria for an Axis II diagnosis. A review of the literature suggests that a "mixed" personality disorder profile, usually reflecting dependent and avoidant features, is most common (Glinski et al. 2001; Larsen 1990; Powers et al. 1992).

Although available research suggests that psychiatric and personality pathology are common among bariatric surgery patients, these results must be interpreted cautiously in light of several limitations in these studies. Variations in demographics, methods, and assessment measures across studies make it difficult to arrive at definitive conclusions. Few studies have included a control group of nonsurgical obese patients or comparison with nonobese norms. Furthermore, it is important to consider the context in which obese individuals pursue bariatric surgery. In a society that espouses an ideal of thinness while stigmatizing and discriminating against obese persons, it is not surprising that obese individuals who do not match societal ideals and are subjected to social, occupational, and personal mistreatment often experience psychological distress and adopt appropriately defensive personality styles. These perspectives may help health professionals more fully understand the multifaceted experiences of patients pursuing bariatric surgery and guide them in anticipating their patients' postsurgical needs.

Eating-Specific Psychopathology

As noted above, there is a relatively high rate of eating disorders, primarily BED, in bariatric surgery patients. (A full account of BED is presented in Chapter 8, "Management of Eating Disorders Not Otherwise Specified," in this volume.)

Investigations into the prevalence of eating pathology in bariatric surgery patients highlight the pervasiveness of binge eating, BED, and other aberrant eating behavior in these patients. Studies have reported prevalence rates of binge eating of 50% or more in patients seeking bariatric surgery (Hsu et al. 1996,

1997; Powers et al. 1999). In a study conducted by Mitchell and colleagues (2001), nearly half of patients interviewed 13–15 years following gastric bypass surgery admitted to symptoms and behaviors presurgically that would have met full criteria for BED. Similar rates were reported by Powers et al. (1999) and Hsu et al. (1996).

Other aberrant eating behaviors in bariatric surgery patients have been the topic of investigation. Although less common than binge eating, night-eating syndrome (NES) and "grazing" have been found to occur in bariatric surgery patients. NES, a variant of eating disorder not otherwise specified (more fully described in Chapter 8), is currently not included in DSM-IV-TR (American Psychiatric Association 2000). This syndrome constitutes a form of eating pathology characterized by lack of hunger in the morning, overeating in the evening, and initial and intermittent insomnia (Stunkard et al. 1955). In one review, prevalence ratings of NES in obese populations ranged from 8% to 64% (Ceru'-Bjork et al. 2001). Prevalence ratings for NES in bariatric surgery patients vary from 10% to 42% (Hsu et al. 1996; Powers et al. 1999). Continuous eating over extended periods of time, oftentimes referred to as "grazing," "picking," or "nibbling," has also been found to be a significant problem for patients pursuing bariatric surgery (Saunders et al. 1998). The consequences of NES and grazing are primarily related to excessive weight gain, obesity, and obesity-related medical conditions.

Psychosocial Issues

To fully understand the experience of bariatric surgery patients, it is necessary to consider the impact of obesity on self-esteem, body image, interpersonal and occupational functioning, and overall quality of life. Research in the area of psychosocial functioning in bariatric surgery patients is highly variable with regard to sample demographics, surgical procedures, study design, and measures of assessment and outcome. Despite these limitations, there is a consensus among the research reports that the psychosocial functioning of obese patients is significantly impaired.

For some, the negative impact of severe obesity on self-evaluation results in levels of impairment comparable to those attributed to the medical sequelae of obesity. Embarrassment, shame, and dissatisfaction with one's appearance frequently become the primary influence affecting one's self-evaluation. Consequently, the belief that weight loss will enhance self-esteem is often a driving hope for bariatric surgery patients. Fantasies of improving self-image, self-confidence, and social ease frequently become strong motivators for pursuing surgery. Libeton et al. (2004) reported that dissatisfaction and embarrassment regarding appearance, weight, and shape was the primary motivation (second only to medical concerns) for pursuing bariatric surgery in 32% of their sample.

Social, sexual, and occupational functioning are also impaired in bariatric surgery patients, yet these issues are rarely the specific focus of research investigation. Much of what is known about these areas is based on clinical anecdotes. As noted in the previous subsection on psychiatric comorbidity, avoidant and dependent personality characteristics are not uncommon. Many patients report significant avoidance of social activities and/or activities that involve eating, physical activity, and bodily exposure, fearing embarrassment and ridicule because of their weight and shape. Similarly, sexual intimacy is often avoided due to shame, embarrassment, and physical limitations. At times, obesity-related medical conditions such as sleep apnea, heart disease, and/or osteoarthritis impact patients' abilities to perform occupational responsibilities and affect attendance patterns and employment leave. For some, employment may be impossible. Impairment in these crucial aspects of psychosocial functioning is virtually always significant for bariatric surgery candidates, is often at the forefront of reasons for pursuing surgery, and always requires investigation.

The impact of obesity on medical status is well documented. Less is known regarding the impact of obesity on *quality of life*, the individual's experience of happiness and satisfaction related to physical, psychological, emotional, social, and spiritual aspects of life (Livingston and Fink 2003). Health-related quality of life (HRQOL) measures, such as the Impact of Weight on Quality of Life—Lite (IWQOL-Lite), are commonly used to assess quality of life in bariatric surgery patients. Although the available studies on this issue have been variable in methodology and measures, the results consistently point to significant impairment in several areas of quality of life for bariatric surgery candidates (Wadden et al. 2001).

Psychosocial Outcomes of Bariatric Surgery

Systematic reviews of the psychosocial outcomes of bariatric surgery (Herpertz et al. 2003) have attempted to ascertain how bariatric surgery impacts psychological and psychosocial functioning as well as how psychosocial functioning impacts bariatric surgery outcome, most often measured by percentage of excess weight lost (%EWL).

Bariatric surgery appears to have an overall positive impact on psychiatric symptomatology. Several investigations reported improvement in depressive symptoms following bariatric surgery (Gentry et al. 1984; Gertler and Ramsey-Stewart 1986; Larsen 1990; Powers et al. 1997). Improvements in anxiety symptoms have also been reported (Hafner et al. 1990; Larsen 1990). In general, although bariatric surgery appears to have an overall positive impact on psychopathology, longer-term follow-up studies suggest that improvements in some areas may erode over time. Mitchell and colleagues (2001) conducted a 13- to 15-year follow-up study of 86 gastric bypass surgery patients. At some point following surgery, 29% of patients had experienced a major depressive episode, and 24.4% struggled with symptoms of specific phobia; 2 patients died of complications of psychiatric conditions (suicide and gastrointestinal bleeding associated with chronic alcoholism).

Research also suggests that some personality pathology may decrease following surgery, although the reductions are not as striking as for Axis I disorders. Larsen and Torgersen (1989) reported reductions in self-doubt, insecurity, sensitivity, dependence, overcompliance, and emotional instability. Another study (Chandarana et al. 1990) found reductions in schizoid, avoidant, and passive-aggressive traits .

How psychopathology impacts bariatric surgery outcome has also been of interest. Most research in this area has used weight loss as a primary outcome measure. Although methods have varied widely, research has not shown that psychiatric comorbidity negatively impacts weight loss in bariatric surgery patients. However, some evidence suggests that more severe psychopathology and particular types of psychopathology, such as emotional lability, self-injurious behaviors, impairment in interpersonal functioning, suspiciousness, and self-defeating behaviors, might place patients at risk for poorer weight loss (Barrash et al. 1987). Presurgical psychiatric comorbidity has also been implicated as a risk for increased medical complications (Clark et al. 2003; Powers et al. 1988; Saltzstein and Gutmann 1980) and decreased satisfaction with surgical outcome (Valley and Grace 1987).

Since binge eating and BED are the most common preexisting eating pathologies seen in bariatric surgery patients, how surgery impacts these conditions is of considerable interest. If a strict definition of binge eating as involving the consumption of an objectively large amount of food in a discrete period of time is used (American Psychiatric Association 2000), bariatric surgery may very well offer a cure for binge eating—given anatomical restriction. However, critical aspects of binge eating, including loss of control while eating and significant distress, may persist or reemerge following surgery. Kalarchian and colleagues (2002) reported postsurgical loss of control during eating in 46% of gastric bypass patients. Hsu et al. (1996, 1997) also cited the presence of loss of control with postsurgical eating. In fact in their studies, 25.9% of vertical-banded gastroplasty patients met the full criteria for BED (not requiring consumption of an objectively large amount of food).

Whether or not a presurgical history of aberrant eating behaviors (including binge eating, NES, and grazing) negatively impacts bariatric surgery outcome has been the subject of controversy. Some have argued that presurgical binge eating or night eating is not negatively associated with weight trajectory following surgery (Powers et al. 1999). Others have argued that presurgical eating pathology does in fact result in less weight loss and/or greater weight gain at long-term follow-up. Although presurgical BED did not impact weight loss in the first postsurgical year in a study conducted by Pekkarinen et al. (1994), presurgical BED was associated with greater weight regain at 2-year follow-up. More recent studies confirm that presurgical binge eating places a patient at risk for a reemergence of overeating and loss of control postsurgically, which in turn is associated with less weight loss and greater weight regain (Kalarchian et al. 2002; Mitchell et al. 2001).

Less controversial is the positive impact of bariatric surgery on psychosocial variables of self-esteem, body image, and social, sexual, and occupational functioning. Similarly, little question exists regarding whether weight loss secondary to bariatric surgery improves quality of life. What is perhaps most interesting is that significant improvements in quality of life are found relatively early, before maximal weight is lost. In a cross-sectional investigation of HRQOL in gastric bypass patients prior to surgery, shortly after surgery, and at 6 and 12 months postsurgically, Dymek and colleagues (2002) found significant differences in HRQOL in the early weeks following surgery. Despite recovering from a major surgical procedure, patients who were 2–4 weeks postsurgery reported significant improvements in their appraisal of general health, self-esteem, vitality, and physical functioning. HRQOL was similar to that of normal control subjects at 6-month follow-up. Furthermore, a linear relationship was found between amount of weight lost and improvements in HRQOL (Dymek et al. 2001). Even patients who may have experienced post-surgical complications (i.e., vomiting, plugging, and dumping) reported these improvements in quality of life (Arcila et al. 2002).

To summarize, the literature highlights the high prevalence of psychiatric comorbidity and impaired psychosocial functioning of bariatric surgery patients. Although it appears that presurgical psychological and eating-specific pathology do impact bariatric surgery outcome, particularly related to medical complications, weight loss, and weight maintenance, considerable methodological variability clouds the field. Consequently, it is imperative that efforts be made to standardize the presurgical psychological assessment of bariatric surgery candidates and that research continue to explore psychiatric and psychosocial variables in examining bariatric surgery outcome. These efforts will be necessary to guide development in patient selection and preparation, as well as development of appropriate interventions for patients at risk of poor outcome.

Psychological Assessment for Bariatric Surgery

A comprehensive behavioral assessment of current and past psychological status must include an evaluation of any psychological indicators that may negatively impact the outcome of bariatric surgery. Such an assessment is of paramount importance in light of the potential for untoward physical complications as well as the drastic and long-term behavioral changes necessitated by the surgery. Typically, this assessment includes a review of self-report inventories as well as a face-to-face interview with the patient. Ideally, the assessment should be conducted by a behavioral specialist who is closely connected to the surgical team.

Self-Report Databases

Self-report databases can be used to obtain a detailed history about the patient's weight, eating patterns, previous weight loss attempts, and concerns about shape and weight. These databases can be especially helpful when completed by the patient in advance of the face-to-face interview, providing the clinical interviewer with pertinent information that can be used to streamline and target the assessment. Several databases with good reliability and validity have previously been developed for this purpose—for example, the Eating Disorders Questionnaire (EDQ [Version 9.0]; Mitchell et al. 1985 (included as an appendix to Chapter 2, "Assessment and Determination of Initial Treatment Approaches for Patients With Eating Disorders," in this volume) and the Weight and Lifestyle Inventory (WALI; Wadden and Phelan 2002).

One of these databases can be mailed to patients prior to the scheduled appointment, with instructions to complete and return it either in the mail or in person at the time of the clinic visit. This method is advantageous in that patients will be able to access information, such as dates and medication names and dosages, that they may not be able to recall at the time of their face-to-face evaluation. Alternatively, the clinician may request that patients arrive 45 minutes early for their appointment to complete a self-report database on-site. Either way, the clinical interviewer should have ample time to review the contents of the inventories in preparation for the in-person interview.

Self-report measures such as these appear to be well accepted by clinicians and patients alike. They allow patients to provide detailed information about their individual circumstances while enabling clinicians to ask appropriate follow-up questions and still wisely manage their time by relying on these instruments to provide valuable background information. Some of these databases are formatted such that they can be scanned to yield a narrative text about the patient for the medical record. At present, such databases require appropriate software to interpret reports and are used predominately for research; however, Internet-based databases on the horizon should allow for more widespread application of these useful tools in clinical settings.

Regardless of which self-report inventories are used, it is important to assess several key topics, including success at prior weight-loss attempts, mood, disordered eating behaviors and beliefs, and quality of life. It is also useful to include several blank food logs when the assessment packet is mailed out, in order to obtain a clearer picture of current eating habits. Table 9–1 offers some suggestions for self-report measures that may be used when the clinician is assessing the suitability of weight-loss surgery for a particular patient.

The Clinical Interview

Increasingly, insurance companies and surgical teams are requesting that patients have psychological evaluations prior to undergoing bariatric surgery.

Table 9–1. Available self-report questionnaires

Questionnaire	Comments
Eating Disorders Questionnaire (EDQ; Mitchell et al. 1985), Version 8.4	Yields demographic information and an in-depth history of eating and weight and previous treatment. A recently updated version (9.0) can be obtained from the Neuropsychiatric Research Institute (also see appendix to Chapter 2, this volume) and will be available online in the near future.
Three-Factor Eating Questionnaire (TFEQ; Stunkard and Messick 1985)	A 51-item inventory that consists of three subscales: restraint, disinhibition, and hunger. Good reliability and validity.
Questionnaire on Eating and Weight Patterns—Revised (QEWP-R; Spitzer et al. 1992)	A 28-item questionnaire that assesses binge eating and binge-eating disorder.
Social Function–36 (SF-36; Ware et al. 1994)	A widely used health-related quality-of-life instrument with available norms for several patient groups. Eight areas of social functioning are assessed: physical function, role physical, bodily pain, general health, vitality, social function, role emotional, and mental health.
Impact of Weight on Quality of Life—Lite (IWQOL-Lite; Kolotikin et al. 2001)	Assesses quality of life specific to obesity. Yields scores on five domains: physical function, self-esteem, sexual life, public distress, and work. Also provides a total score.
Beck Depression Inventory (BDI; Beck et al. 1961)	A 21-item measure used widely to assess level of depression. Very good reliability and validity.

Unfortunately, at present there is no standardized approach to assessment. The lack of agreement regarding what ought to be included in such assessments is further complicated by a paucity of information about which factors are likely to improve or impede successful surgical outcomes. In fact, at the present time, overall, very few psychological factors are thought to preclude bariatric surgery a priori. Currently, even such conditions as psychosis, mental retardation, active substance dependence, excessive impulsivity, and severe hypochondriasis are not considered to be firm contraindications. Even in the face of such obstacles, case-by-case decisions that allow the surgery are presently made by surgical teams.

In an effort to provide a standardized approach to the bariatric psychological assessment procedure, the Boston Interview for Gastric Bypass (Sogg and Mori 2004) was recently developed. This semistructured interview assesses several key topics, on the basis of empirical studies as well as the authors' clinical impressions, and focuses on data that can readily be used to make behavioral recommendations likely to improve outcome. Since it appears to offer a "state of the art" approach at this time, the recommendations that follow are consistent with that protocol.

Weight, Diet, and Nutrition History

A weight history should be obtained to enable the clinician to better understand environmental and physiological contributions to the patient's obesity as well as the effect that the patient's obesity has had on his or her life. Both medically supervised and commercial program-based weight-loss attempts should be identified, as should self-help groups and prescription and nonprescription medications. The patient should be directly asked about the use of any of the herbal preparations that are increasingly marketed for weight reduction and should be encouraged to discuss his or her successes. The clinician should follow through with each of these methods in an attempt to identify potential issues related to adherence that could negatively impact surgical outcome.

Current Eating Behaviors

The clinical interviewer should gain a clear picture of the patient's eating patterns, including any problematic behaviors that could hinder surgical outcome. This line of inquiry should include an assessment for BED and excessive consumption of high-calorie beverages, both of which are thought to limit weight loss or encourage weight regain postsurgery. The food logs included with the self-report questionnaires can be quite helpful when reviewing this information; however, it is important to note that obese patients are likely to underreport what and how much they have eaten, and patients' responses on these questionnaires should be reviewed with this in mind.

Medical History

Aside from gathering a detailed medical history, which is ultimately the responsibility of the surgical team, it is also important to assess patients' understandings of their medical status, how well they adhere to general medical recommendations, and the extent of their usual compliance with prescribed medications.

Knowledge of Surgical Procedures and Risks and
Recommended Postsurgery Regimen

Patients should be asked about their knowledge of the planned surgical procedure and inherent risks, recovery procedures, and the recommended dietary regimen once the surgery is performed. This line of questioning is intended to assess whether or not the patient is making an informed decision about the surgery and allows the clinician to provide additional education about these issues should the need arise. In particular, this assessment can help the clinician detect the presence of any cognitive or motivational deficits that might require additional intervention prior to the surgery or even preclude approval for surgery.

Motivation and Expectations of Surgical Outcome

The clinician should also confirm that the patient's expectations are reasonable by asking the patient to identify reasons for seeking bariatric surgery and expectations of physical and psychosocial outcomes. Many patients have unrealistic expectations about the amount of weight they will lose and may need to be reminded that although they can expect to lose about 60%–70% of extra weight, they may continue to be overweight when weight loss plateaus. Others may seek the surgery for superficial reasons or expect weight loss to improve major deficits in other areas such as interpersonal relationships. In this case, additional education will also be necessary. Further, the authors of the Boston Interview for Gastric Bypass (Sogg and Mori 2004) point out the importance of determining the patient's level of preparedness for the stringent changes in

eating required postsurgery. An inability to demonstrate appropriate problem-solving skills in this regard may trigger referral to a behavior change professional prior to surgery.

Support System and Relationships

Typically, it is very beneficial for patients to have an identified support per-
son(s) who can provide help immediately postsurgery and who is alert and at-
tentive to changes in the home that would likely increase compliance. It is also
important to note that the dramatic changes in weight following surgery can
have a potentially negative impact on existing relationships. For example, members of the person's support system can feel threatened and/or might hinder
weight loss, consciously or not. Therefore, patients should be asked to predict
how current relationships might be influenced by the surgery. In some instances,
referrals for couples or family counseling may be necessary.

Psychiatric Functioning

The Boston Interview for Gastric Bypass contains a mini-mental status examination to identify cognitive factors that may interfere with successful participation in treatment recommendations or competence to make educated decisions. It also gathers information on psychiatric factors, such as psychosis or
mood instability, that may negatively impact the ability of patients to take care
of themselves following surgery..

Psychological Management

As noted in the previous section, a subset of bariatric patients will experience
mood, relationship, or eating problems following surgery. Most will be non-
compliant in at least one area of postsurgical recommendations, typically those
about exercise and/or snacking. We also know that those who struggled with
BED prior to surgery are particularly vulnerable to recurrences of difficulties toward the end of the second year after surgery. Unfortunately, limited information is available regarding how to manage these symptoms postsurgery; only a
handful of anecdotal reports and research studies are found in the literature.

In the single published controlled trial, bariatric patients were randomly assigned to either a minimal ($n=15$) or behavioral ($n=17$) intervention (Tucker et

al. 1991). Both groups received education presurgery about recommended dietary changes. Those in the behavioral intervention group also received, via the mail, 12 educational packets about eating and lifestyle changes, and they had six monthly consultations following the surgery. Although both groups failed to eat as recommended, those in the behavioral intervention group ate less dietary fat and reported greater physical activity and better family satisfaction than did the minimal intervention group. However, the minimal intervention group consumed more protein. No statistical differences resulted with regard to weight loss or ratings of daily caloric intake, frequency of vomiting, stomach pain, or emotional health.

Although results have been somewhat inconsistent and several of the studies have lacked statistical rigor, available data suggest that surgical outcome can be enhanced with ongoing therapist contact and/or regular attendance at support groups postsurgery. They also suggest that a supportive and solution-focused presurgical intervention can benefit those individuals with identified risk factors such as BED. However, those in clinical practice can attest to the fact that this subset of patients is rarely seen for psychological intervention in a timely manner, if at all.

Presurgical and Postsurgical Interventions

Bariatric patients progress through three phases, and, therefore, interventions should match their unique needs at these various points in time. The first, the *preoperative phase,* is when patients are actively preparing for surgery by gathering information and working through the assessment process. Most are excited about the possibility of dramatic weight loss; however, for some, apprehension and uncertainty are prominent. In addition to conducting an appropriate assessment, the clinician can also help the patient explore these and other key issues before the decision to proceed with surgery. One approach to this exploration is the nonjudgmental stance taken in motivational interviewing (Miller and Rollnick 1991). Originally developed for use with substance users, motivational interviewing can also help guide bariatric patients through self-discovery. Furthermore, the presurgical recommendations may also prompt individual treatment for comorbidities such as substance abuse or dependence, significant depressive disorders, and/or unchecked anxiety disorders that, depending on severity, could lead to complications postsurgery.

In addition, because BED can reemerge approximately 2 years postsurgery, it may be helpful to provide psychoeducation and, possibly, intervention prior to surgery, in an effort to prevent difficulties from occurring. Finally, clinicians, especially those with a background in behavioral and cognitive-behavioral therapies, can also provide nonsurgical interventions for weight loss either as an alternative to bariatric surgery or as a way to help prepare those patients whose BMI is too high to safely undergo anesthesia or laparoscopic procedures.

In the months immediately following surgery, a majority of bariatric patients will experience rapid weight loss and improvements in emotional functioning. During this second, early postoperative phase, some will struggle with making the behavioral adjustments required for optimum outcome. The clinician can work to increase compliance with recommendations to eat more slowly, avoid high-calorie beverages, chew thoroughly, and recognize and respond to sensations of fullness (Kalarchian and Marcus 2003). When difficulties do occur, the clinician can problem-solve with the surgical team to reinforce appropriate changes.

One area with which most bariatric patients struggle is compliance with exercise recommendations. Clinicians should consider the patient's current level of physical conditioning and set appropriate goals based on that information. When goals are set too high, patients often experience frustration and may give up prematurely; therefore, exercise goals should initially be short in duration and at an appropriate frequency. Patients can also benefit from self-monitoring, scheduling a regular exercise time, and finding someone to exercise with in order to increase accountability.

In contrast to the first 6 months, when physical adjustment is paramount, the next 12–18 months can, for some patients, bring about a decline in psychological functioning or social relationships. During this third, later postoperative phase, premorbid conditions may reemerge or new difficulties may surface that should be addressed with individual counseling to minimize impact on outcome. It may be advantageous for the clinician to maintain intermittent contact during this time with those patients who have a history of psychiatric disorders so that intervention, if necessary, can be instituted in a timely manner. Psychoeducation and supportive therapy can also be offered during monthly check-in sessions. If a patient is noted to experience increased difficulty, sessions can be scheduled more frequently, or the patient can be referred for specialized treatment. Psychotropic medication may also be appropriate.

Marital discord can also surface during these months, especially in those relationships that were already troubled prior to surgery. Couples counseling would be prudent in these cases. The patient should continue to meet with his or her individual counselor to track postsurgical adjustment, and at the same time, the couple may be referred to another clinician to address relationship issues, so that in instances where this might present a problem, questions of the clinician's potential allegiance to one member of the couple over the other are minimized. On the other hand, in some cases bringing a significant other into one or a few individual sessions as a collateral source of information and/or to provide education and perspective to the other person may prove beneficial.

As mentioned previously, approximately 2 years postsurgery a subset of bariatric patients experience weight regain as well as increased psychological difficulties. In these patients it is imperative to continue to reinforce the need for physical activity and healthy eating behaviors to maximize weight loss. Because of associated weight gain, it is also important to provide cognitive-behavioral treatment for BED in those patients in whom this emerges (Peterson et al. 1998; Telch et al. 1990; Wilfley et al. 1993). Even though the stomach pouch is substantially altered, some patients nevertheless begin to experience a loss of control over eating or begin to engage in unproductive eating habits, such as constant grazing, that can significantly impact outcome.

Treatment for BED can be provided in a group or individual format. Patients self-monitor types and quantities of food and liquid consumed and also report thoughts and feelings that they experience as triggering, during, and subsequent to binge eating. Because underreporting by patients is typical, and since the importance of this self-monitoring intervention needs to be stressed, careful review of the food logs is necessary. Obese individuals often avoid eating during the first portion of the day, so a regular pattern of three meals and two snacks is advised. Setting reasonable goals for increased exercise and other physical activity is also a focus of treatment. Patients are also urged to engage in distracting activities or behaviors during vulnerable times that are incompatible with eating. Cognitive restructuring, a specialized technique used to challenge the accuracy of problematic and self-sabotaging thoughts, is used to help patients explore the evidence that supports such thoughts and the evidence that does not support the troublesome thoughts, and to reach a more reasoned conclusion based on this evidence, rather than simply accepting the thoughts and feelings distorted by the eating disorder. Other associated difficulties may also be the focus of treatment. For example, body image distortions, ineffective coping strategies, poor problem solving, and lack of assertiveness may all be targeted with appropriate interventions. Finally, relapse prevention techniques should be incorporated in all treatment plans to address ongoing maintenance of change.

References

American Psychiatric Association: Diagnostic and Statistical Manual of Mental Disorders, 4th Edition, Text Revision. Washington, DC, American Psychiatric Association, 2000

Arcila D, Velazquez D, Gamino R, et al: Quality of life in bariatric surgery. Obes Surg 12:661–665, 2002

Balsiger BM, Murr MM, Poggio JL, et al: Surgery for weight control in patients with morbid obesity. Med Clin North Am 84:477–489, 2000

Barrash J, Rodriguez E, Scott DH, et al: The utility of MMPI subtypes for the prediction of weight loss after bariatric surgery. Int J Obes 11:115–128, 1987

Beck AT, Ward CH, Medelson M, et al: An inventory for measuring depression. Arch Gen Psychiatry 4:561–571, 1961

Byrne TK: Complications of surgery for obesity. Surg Clin North Am 81:1181–1193, vii–viii, 2001

Ceru'-Bjork C, Andersson I, Rossner S: Night eating and nocturnal eating—two different or similar syndromes among obese patients? Int J Obes Relat Metab Disord 25:365–372, 2001

Chandarana PC, Conlon P, Holliday RL, et al: A prospective study of psychosocial aspects of gastric stapling surgery. Psychiatr J Univ Ott 15:32–35, 1990

Clark MM, Balsiger BM, Sletten CD, et al: Psychosocial factors and 2-year outcome following bariatric surgery for weight loss. Obes Surg 13:739–745, 2003

Dymek MP, le Grange D, Neven K, et al: Quality of life and psychosocial adjustment in patients after Roux-en-Y gastric bypass: a brief report. Obes Surg 11:32–39, 2001

Dymek MP, le Grange D, Neven K, et al: Quality of life after gastric bypass surgery: a cross-sectional study. Obes Res 10:1135–1142, 2002

Elliot K: Nutritional considerations after bariatric surgery. Crit Care Nurs Q 26:133–138, 2003

Encinosa WE, Bernard DM, Chen CC, et al: Healthcare utilization and outcomes after bariatric surgery. Med Care 44:706–712, 2006

Gentry K, Halverson JD, Heisler S: Psychologic assessment of morbidly obese patients undergoing gastric bypass: a comparison of preoperative and postoperative adjustment. Surgery 95:215–220, 1984

Gertler R, Ramsey-Stewart G: Pre-operative psychiatric assessment of patients presenting for gastric bariatric surgery (surgical control of morbid obesity). Aust N Z J Surg 56:157–161, 1986

Glinski J, Wetzler S, Goodman E: The psychology of gastric bypass surgery. Obes Surg 11:581–588, 2001

Hafner RJ, Rogers J, Watts JM: Psychological status before and after gastric restriction as predictors of weight loss in the morbidly obese. J Psychosom Res 34:295–302, 1990

Herpertz A, Kielmann R, Wolf AM, et al: Does obesity surgery improve psychosocial functioning? A systematic review. Int J Obes Relat Metab Disord 27:1300–1314, 2003

Hsu LKG, Betancourt S, Sullivan SP: Eating disturbances before and after vertical banded gastroplasty: a pilot study. Int J Eat Disord 19:23–34, 1996

Hsu LKG, Sullivan SP, Benotti PN: Eating disturbances and outcome of gastric bypass surgery: a pilot study. Int J Eat Disord 21:385–390, 1997

Kalarchian MA, Marcus MD: Management of the bariatric surgery patient: is there a role for the cognitive behavior therapist? Cogn Behav Pract 10:112–119, 2003

Kalarchian MA, Marcus MD, Wilson GT, et al: Binge eating among gastric bypass patients at long-term follow-up. Obes Surg 12:270–275, 2002

Kolotikin RL, Crosby RD, Kosloski KD, et al: Development of a brief measure to assess quality of life in obesity. Obes Res 9:102–111, 2001

Kushner RF, Roth JL: Assessment of the obese patient. Endocrinol Metab Clin North Am 32:915–933, 2003

Larsen F: Psychosocial function before and after gastric banding surgery for morbid obesity: a prospective psychiatric study. Acta Psychiatr Scand Suppl 359:1–57, 1990

Larsen F, Torgersen S: Personality changes after gastric banding surgery for morbid obesity: a prospective study. J Psychosom Res 33:323–334, 1989

Latifi R, Kellum JM, De Maria EJ, et al: Surgical treatment of obesity, in Handbook of Obesity Treatment. Edited by Wadden TA, Stunkard AJ. New York, Guilford, 2002, pp 339–356

Libeton M, Dixon JB, Laurie C, et al: Patient motivation for bariatric surgery: characteristics and impact on outcomes. Obes Surg 14:392–398, 2004

Livingston EH, Fink AS: Quality of life: cost and future of bariatric surgery. Arch Surg 138:383–387, 2003

Miller WR, Rollnick S: Motivational Interviewing: Preparing People to Change Addictive Behavior. New York, Guilford, 1991

Mitchell JE, Hatsukami D, Eckert ED, et al: Eating Disorders Questionnaire. Psychopharmacol Bull 21:1025–1042, 1985

Mitchell JE, Lancaster KL, Burgard MA, et al: Long-term follow-up of patients' status after gastric bypass. Obes Surg 11:464–468, 2001

Ogden CL, Carroll MD, Flegal KM: Epidemiologic trends in overweight and obesity. Endocrinol Metab Clin North Am 32:741–760, 2003

Pekkarinen T, Koskela K, Hulkuri K, et al: Long-term results of gastroplasty for morbid obesity: binge-eating as a predictor of poor outcome. Obes Surg 4:248–255, 1994

Peterson CB, Mitchell JE, Engbloom S, et al: Binge eating disorder with and without a history of purging symptoms. Int J Eat Disord 24:251–257, 1998

Powers PS, Rosemurgy AS, Coovert DL, et al: Psychosocial sequelae of bariatric surgery: a pilot study. Psychosomatics 29:283–288, 1988

Powers PS, Boyd F, Blair CR, et al: Psychiatric issues in bariatric surgery. Obes Surg 2:315–325, 1992

Powers PS, Rosemurgy A, Boyd F, et al: Outcome of gastric restriction procedures: weight, psychiatric diagnoses and satisfaction. Obes Surg 7:471–477, 1997

Powers PS, Perez A, Boyd F, et al: Eating pathology before and after bariatric surgery: a prospective study. Int J Eat Disord 25:293–300, 1999

Saltzstein EC, Gutmann MC: Gastric bypass for morbid obesity: preoperative and postoperative psychological evaluation of patients. Arch Surg 115:21–28, 1980

Sarwer DB, Cohn NI, Gibbons LM, et al: Psychiatric diagnoses and psychiatric treatment among bariatric surgery candidates. Obes Surg 14:1148–1156, 2004

Saunders R, Johnson L, Teschner J: Prevalence of eating disorders among bariatric surgery patients. Int J Eat Disord 6:309–317, 1998

Scopinaro N, Marinari BM, Camerini G: Laparoscopic standard biliopancreatic diversion: technique and preliminary results. Obes Surg 12:241–244, 2002

Sogg S, Mori DL: The Boston Interview for Gastric Bypass: determining the psychological suitability of surgical candidates. Obes Surg 14:370–380, 2004

Spitzer RL, Devlin M, Walsh TB, et al: Binge eating disorder: a multi-site field trial of the diagnostic criteria. Int J Eat Disord 11:191–203, 1992

Stunkard AJ, Messick S: The Three-Factor Eating Questionnaire to measure dietary restraint, disinhibition, and hunger. J Psychosom Res 29:71–83, 1985

Stunkard AJ, Grace WJ, Wolff HG: The night-eating syndrome: a pattern of food intake among certain obese patients. Am J Med 19:78–86, 1955

Telch CF, Agras WS, Rossiter EM, et al: Group cognitive-behavioral treatment for the non-purging bulimic: an initial evaluation. J Consult Clin Psychol 58:629–635, 1990

Tucker JA, Samo JA, Rand CSW, et al: Behavioral interventions to promote adaptive eating behavior and lifestyle changes following surgery for obesity: results of a two-year outcome evaluation. Int J Eat Disord 10:689–698, 1991

Valley V, Grace DM: Psychosocial risk factors in gastric surgery for obesity: identifying guidelines for screening. Int J Obes 11:105–113, 1987

Wadden TA, Phelan S: Behavioral assessment of the obese patient, in Handbook of Obesity Treatment. Edited by Wadden TA, Stunkard AJ. New York, Guilford, 2002, pp 186–226

Wadden TA, Sarwer DB, Womble LG, et al: Psychosocial aspects of obesity and obesity surgery. Obes Surg 81:1001–1024, 2001

Ware JE, Kosinski M, Keller SD: SF-36 Physical and Mental Summary Scales: A User's Manual. Boston, MA, The Health Institute, 1994

Wilfley DE, Agras WS, Telch CF, et al: Group cognitive-behavioral therapy and group interpersonal psychotherapy for the non-purging bulimic individual: a controlled comparison. J Consult Clin Psychol 61:296–305, 1993

10

Medication-Related Weight Changes

Impact on Treatment of Eating Disorder Patients

Pauline S. Powers, M.D.

Nancy L. Cloak, M.D.

Links between psychotropic medications and weight changes have been recognized for decades, but interest in these connections has increased dramatically in recent years. This heightened awareness has paralleled the increasing prevalence of obesity and growing recognition of its complications, especially type 2 diabetes mellitus. Other contributing factors likely include the growing number of psychotropic medications on the market, increasing awareness of medication adverse effects, and expanding use of atypical antipsychotics and mood stabilizers for indications other than schizophrenia and classic mania.

As evidenced by the 2004 publication of guidelines for preventing and managing antipsychotic-induced obesity and diabetes (American Diabetes Association et al. 2004), the impact of psychotropic medications on weight, glucose, and lipid levels is rapidly becoming a key consideration in treatment planning.

Less visible, but equally important, are the potential effects of weight-altering medications on patients with eating disorders. In 2004 more than 25 million prescriptions were written for atypical antipsychotics alone (NDC Health Pharmaceutical Audit Suite 2004). Inevitably, some of these would have been given to patients with eating disorders or who were at risk for developing eating disorders. Because psychiatric comorbidities are common among eating disorder patients (see Table 10–1), psychotropic medications are of particular concern, but any agent that affects weight could impact the development or course of an eating disorder. As clinicians who prescribe these medications for eating disorder patients can attest, significant clinical issues often arise around medication nonadherence and/or worsening of eating disorder symptoms.

The role of weight-altering medications in precipitating or exacerbating eating disorders has not been widely addressed in the literature. Likewise, the impact of eating disorder pathology on adherence to medications has not been systematically examined. In this chapter, we review medications known to affect weight and discuss case examples and reports illustrating the relationship of eating disorders to weight-altering medications. We then offer some preliminary recommendations for managing these important problems.

Physiology of Weight Regulation

The concept of homeostatic energy regulation provides the foundation for understanding the effects of medications on weight. Through a series of complicated systems, the body maintains *energy balance:* the food eaten (called "energy in") minus the calories expended ("energy out") results in an individual's increasing, decreasing, or maintaining the same weight. Although measuring the amount of food consumed is relatively easy, assessing energy expenditure accurately is more difficult. Energy expenditure is determined by three important factors: *obligate energy expenditure* (basal metabolic rate or the closely associated resting metabolic rate), which accounts for the majority of energy

Table 10–1.   Psychiatric comorbidity in eating disorder patients: approximate lifetime prevalences (%)

Comorbid disorder	Eating disorder		
	Anorexia nervosa	Bulimia nervosa	BED
Depressive disorders	50–70	50–70	50
Anxiety disorders	23–66	25–75	9–46
Social phobia	24–55	17–59	
OCD	10–66	3–4	
PTSD		37	22
Bipolar disorders	0–8	0–19	0–10
Substance use disorders		22–28	8–33
Personality disorders			
Obsessive-compulsive	35–60	5	4
Borderline		35–40	

Note.   BED = binge-eating disorder; OCD = obsessive-compulsive disorder; PTSD = posttraumatic stress disorder.
Source.   McElroy et al. 2005; O'Brien and Vincent 2003; Rachelle and Lilenfeld 2004.

used by most people; *physical activity;* and *nonexercise adaptive thermogenesis,* which includes the calories used to digest and process food as well as nonpurposeful motoric activities such as fidgeting. Figure 10–1 illustrates the components of energy expenditure.

Among other factors, basal metabolic rate is influenced by age and sex. With aging, there is a decrease in basal metabolic rate (and often physical activity). Because basal metabolic rate increases with muscle mass, males tend to have a metabolic rate about 10% greater than females (Donahoo et al. 2004).

Thus, in considering the effect of medications on weight, the clinician must take into account multiple factors. Medications may cause weight change by altering energy intake, basal metabolic rate, physical activity, nonexercise adaptive thermogenesis, or some combination of these components via their impacts on a myriad of cellular processes involving the brain, neuroendocrine functions, and numerous other organ systems. Research into the causes of medication-associated weight change is just beginning, and in most cases, the precise mechanisms are unknown.

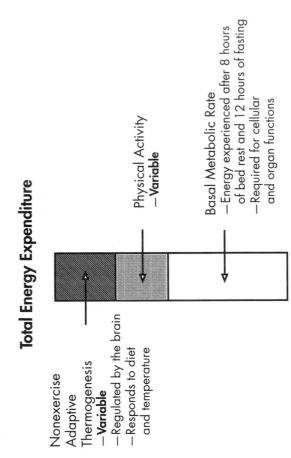

Figure 10–1.   Components of energy expenditure.

Energy expenditure is determined by three important factors: *obligate energy expenditure* (basal metabolic rate or the closely associated resting metabolic rate), which accounts for the majority of energy used by most people; *physical activity*; and *nonexercise adaptive thermogenesis*, which includes the calories used to digest and process food.

Medications That Affect Weight

Most medications that affect weight cause weight gain rather than weight loss. This feature may reflect a biological propensity in which any perturbation in the system is more likely to result in energy storage because of its survival advantage. While the majority of medications that cause weight gain are used for psychiatric or neurological conditions, corticosteroids and some antidiabetic, antihypertensive, and hormonal agents that also affect weight are widely prescribed.

Medications That Cause Weight Gain

Psychotropic Agents

Antipsychotic agents.   Both older neuroleptics and atypical antipsychotics are associated with weight gain, though the prevalence and degree vary among different medications and individual patients. In a widely cited meta-analysis of 81 studies, average weight gain over 10 weeks at standard doses of antipsychotics ranged from 0.28 kg with ziprasidone to 5.67 kg with clozapine (Allison et al. 1999). Figure 10–2 illustrates these differences. Weight gain may be even greater among children and adolescents with the atypical antipsychotics, especially olanzapine (E. Hollander et al. 2006) and risperidone (Aman et al. 2005), which have been studied. Less is known about the newer agent aripiprazole. Two industry-sponsored trials found average weight losses with aripiprazole of 1.26 kg (Pigott et al. 2003) and 1.37 kg (McQuade et al. 2004) after 26 weeks.

The mechanism or mechanisms for antipsychotic-induced weight gain are unclear. One small study found evidence for increased caloric intake in patients taking olanzapine (Gothelf et al. 2002). Weight gain has also been correlated with histamine$_1$ (H$_1$) receptor affinity (Kroeze et al. 2003), presence of the -759C allele for the serotonin$_{2C}$ (5-HT$_{2C}$) receptor (Correll and Malhotra 2004), and activation of orexin neurons in the lateral hypothalamic/perifornical area (Fadel et al. 2002). Given the complexity of weight regulation, multiple mechanisms are likely involved.

Mood stabilizers.   Lithium is associated with a mean weight gain of 10 kg over 6–10 years (Garland et al. 1988). Two large, long-term (up to 17 years) naturalistic studies indicated that about 20% of patients taking lithium will experience weight gain >10 kg (Vestergaard et al. 1980, 1988). Proposed mech-

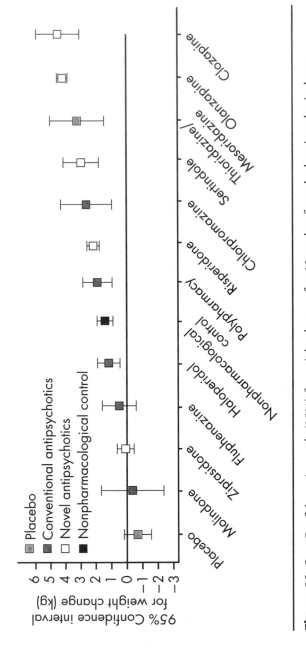

Figure 10–2.   Confidence intervals (95%) for weight change after 10 weeks of standard antipsychotic doses.

Source.   Estimated from a random effects model on page 1690 in Allison et al. 1999.

anisms for lithium-induced weight gain include its insulin-like activity in some patients, possible direct appetite-stimulating effects in the hypothalamus, use of high-calorie beverages to relieve thirst, and fluid retention.

Weight gain has been reported in up to 71% of patients prescribed valproate for epilepsy or mood stabilization (Jallon and Picard 2001). In a 1-year randomized, placebo-controlled trial ($N=187$), 21% of subjects taking valproate for bipolar disorder gained more than 5% of baseline weight, compared with 7% of those taking placebo (Bowden et al. 2000). A 32-week prospective study revealed an average weight gain of 5.8 kg in patients with epilepsy who took valproate (Biton et al. 2001). Mechanisms are unclear but may include stimulation of insulin release and/or increased availability of long-chain fatty acids due to competitive valproate binding.

While carbamazepine is generally regarded as a second-line mood stabilizer because of its toxicities and drug interactions, it appears to cause less weight gain than lithium or valproate. Information about weight gain with carbamazepine in psychiatric patients is limited, although one small controlled study reported an average weight gain of 2 kg versus 0 kg with placebo at 14 weeks (Joffe et al. 1986). In epilepsy trials, rates of weight gain exceeding 7% of baseline were found in 2%–14% of those patients receiving carbamazepine (Jallon and Picard 2001). Proposed mechanisms for this finding include appetite stimulation and fluid retention.

Lamotrigine is a newer anticonvulsant approved by the U.S. Food and Drug Administration (FDA) for treatment of bipolar depression and maintenance therapy in bipolar disorder. It appears to cause minimal weight change. One 6-month randomized controlled trial involving 182 bipolar patients showed a weight gain of 1.1 kg compared with a weight loss of 0.3 kg with placebo (Calabrese et al. 2000). A retrospective review of data from 463 epilepsy patients treated with lamotrigine revealed a mean weight gain of 0.5 kg over an average duration of nearly 1 year (Devinsky et al. 2000).

Antidepressant medications. Antidepressants are probably the most widely prescribed agents for eating disorder patients. The magnitude of weight change with these agents is usually less than for antipsychotics or mood stabilizers. Fortunately, many appear to be weight-neutral. Some, particularly tricyclic antidepressants (TCAs) and mirtazapine, often cause weight gain, and bupropion can cause weight loss.

Weight gain is a well-known side effect of TCAs. For example, 13.3% of 128 subjects in one study of imipramine gained more than 10% of baseline after 33 weeks (Frank et al. 1990). Secondary amines, such as desipramine and nortriptyline, may cause less weight gain than tertiary amines (Fernstrom and Kupfer 1988). Proposed mechanisms include histamine receptor antagonism leading to inhibition of satiety, and alterations in the tumor necrosis factor system, which is known to participate in weight regulation (Hinze-Selch et al. 2000).

Selective serotonin reuptake inhibitors (SSRIs) can cause a decrease in appetite, especially early in treatment, when gastrointestinal side effects are also common. Observations of short-term weight loss with fluoxetine prompted a large-scale controlled trial in obese patients that demonstrated initial weight loss but no treatment difference at 1 year (Michelson et al. 1999). After publication of case reports describing weight gain in patients treated long-term with SSRIs, this effect was investigated further in several large-scale trials. Two of these trials suggested that differences in weight gain liability may exist among individual medications.

One study pooled data from six randomized trials that were originally designed to compare efficacy of various SSRIs with nefazodone ($n=513$). Among the SSRI-treated patients, 4.3% had lost more than 7% of baseline weight at any point in the first 16 weeks. However, during the next 46 weeks, 17.9% had gained more than 7% of baseline weight (Sussman et al. 2001). In a randomized trial comparing fluoxetine, sertraline, and paroxetine in 284 patients with major depressive disorder over a 26- to 32-week period, the percentage of patients whose weight increased more than 7% over baseline was significantly greater for paroxetine-treated (25.5%) than for either fluoxetine-treated (6.8%) or sertraline-treated (4.2%) patients. Extreme weight gain in the paroxetine-treated patients was more common in women (Fava et al. 2000). A 2-year open-label prospective follow-up study comparing several antidepressants in patients with obsessive-compulsive disorder found the percentages of patients gaining more than 7% of baseline weight to be 34.8% for clomipramine, 14.3% for citalopram and paroxetine, 10.7% for fluvoxamine, 8.7% for fluoxetine, and 4.5% for sertaline (Maina et al. 2004). A limitation of these three studies is the lack of placebo control. However, a placebo-controlled trial comparing fluoxetine with placebo over 26 weeks showed that among 388 patients who entered treatment for depression, 4.8% of patients taking fluoxetine and 6.3% of those receiving placebo had a weight increase more than 7%

of baseline, a nonsignificant difference (Michelson et al. 1999). In all of the foregoing studies, weight changes varied greatly between individual patients, including those taking placebo.

Taken together, these findings indicate that weight changes over time in patients taking either SSRIs or placebo vary greatly among individuals. With SSRIs, weight loss is more common acutely, but in the longer term, weight tends to return to baseline. On average, weight gain with most SSRIs is probably equivalent to that with placebo, although individual patients may experience large weight changes. Paroxetine may be more likely to cause weight gain, especially in women.

Mechanisms for weight change due to SSRIs are unknown, although differences in the propensity for causing weight gain among different SSRIs have been related to their unique properties apart from serotonin reuptake inhibition. For example, the H_1 affinity of citalopram and the dopamine reuptake blockade of sertraline are thought to account for the appetite-enhancing and anorectic properties of these agents, respectively (Harvey and Bouwer 2000). The variability of weight change that may occur with the SSRIs is illustrated by the following case example.

> Marie was a 17-year-old girl who presented with classic bulimia nervosa, purging type. Fluoxetine 60 mg/day was started. Her binge eating and purging completely ceased, and then she began restricting her intake to 800 calories per day. Starting initially at 120 pounds at 5 feet, 5 inches in height (body mass index [BMI] = 20), Marie lost weight to 100 pounds (BMI = 16.6) and was brought by her mother to participate in a research medication study for anorexia nervosa. During the screening period the fluoxetine was discontinued, and during this time she gained 10 pounds (BMI = 18.3) and no longer met the criteria for the study. The risk of reemergent bulimia nervosa was considered, and Marie was started in a formal cognitive-behavioral program. Her weight stabilized without recurrence of binge eating or purging.

Among the other antidepressants, venlafaxine and nefazodone appear to be weight-neutral, while bupropion is associated with weight loss more often than weight gain (Sussman and Ginsberg 2000). In contrast, a meta-analysis of the placebo-controlled studies performed during the licensing process for mirtazapine showed that 10% taking medication versus 1% receiving placebo gained more than 7% of baseline weight (Burrows and Kremer 1997). Observations of the effects of trazodone on weight have been mixed, with some studies reporting small weight losses and others noting slight weight gain (Trivedi and Rush 1992). Among the monoamine oxidase inhibitors, phenelzine, and to a lesser extent isocarboxazid, are associated with weight gain, while tranylcypromine appears to be weight-neutral (Cantu and Korek 1988).

Other agents.   While buspirone, hydroxyzine, and benzodiazepines do not generally influence body weight, gabapentin, which is sometimes used off-label for insomnia and anxiety disorders, has been associated with weight gain. One uncontrolled study revealed a weight increase of 5% or more in 35 of 44 patients taking gabapentin as monotherapy or adjunctive therapy for epilepsy (DeToledo et al. 1997). Cyproheptadine, an antihistamine sometimes prescribed for nightmares, is known to cause increased appetite and weight, perhaps because of its anti-serotonergic properties. It is somewhat effective in promoting weight gain in restricting anorexia nervosa patients, but not in those who binge and purge (Halmi et al. 1986).

The newer anticonvulsants are increasingly used off-label in psychiatry for anxiety and mood disorders, and some may be approved for these indications in the future. It can be assumed, on the basis of experience with older agents, that many of them may affect body weight. Significant weight gain has been observed in randomized controlled trials of pregabalin (Arroyo et al. 2004) and vigabatrin (Chadwick 1999), while tiagabine and levetiracetam have not been associated with weight change (Gidal et al. 2003; Loiseau 1999).

Nonpsychotropic Agents

Corticosteroids are well known to cause weight gain by increasing appetite. Systematic evaluation of this effect has been limited, although one 12-month study of renal transplant patients found average weight gains to be 5.3 kg greater in patients receiving steroids compared with patients receiving other immunosuppressive agents (Rogers et al. 2005). Use of inhaled corticosteroids does not seem to be associated with weight gain (Hedberg and Rossner 2000).

Similarly, insulin commonly causes weight gain in patients with diabetes mellitus, with greater increases seen in patients using intensive insulin therapy rather than conventional regimens (Carlson and Campbell 1993). Proposed mechanisms include the anabolic effects of insulin, reduction of glycosuria, and increased food intake related to hypoglycemic episodes. The composition of the weight gain seems to vary among individual patients, with young patients with type 1 diabetes gaining mostly lean mass, and older patients with type 2 diabetes gaining mostly fat (Rigalleau et al. 1999). It has been postulated that the standard treatment of type 1 diabetes mellitus may precipitate an eating disorder in vulnerable individuals (Lawson et al. 1994). This effect may be in part due to the weight gain that ensues with insulin injections (or inhaled insulin).

Oral antidiabetic agents are frequently prescribed for overweight binge-eating disorder (BED) patients with comorbid type 2 diabetes. The sulfonylureas, which stimulate insulin secretion, are associated with average weight gains of 1–4 kg over 6 months (Krentz and Bailey 2005). Thiazolidinediones also cause weight gain, probably by facilitating insulin-stimulated lipid storage in adipose tissue and enhancing fluid retention, especially when combined with other antidiabetic agents. In one randomized trial, patients treated with pioglitazone gained an average of 3.9 kg at 6 months, compared with a weight loss of 0.8 kg in patients receiving placebo, although resting metabolic rate and perceived hunger did not change (Smith et al. 2005). Repaglinide and nateglinide appear to be weight-neutral (Moses 2000; Rosenstock et al. 2004), whereas metformin (Belcher et al. 2005), pramlintide (Hollander et al. 2004), and exenatide (Mikhail 2006) have been associated with weight loss.

Hormonal contraceptives are commonly believed to cause weight gain, and this concern often results in early discontinuation. However, a 2004 systematic review of 42 randomized controlled trials of combination estrogen-progestin contraceptives found no evidence of a causal relationship between these agents and weight change (Gallo et al. 2004). While one study revealed a weight gain of 4.3 kg over 5 years in depot medroxyprogesterone acetate users, compared with 1.8 kg in women using intrauterine devices (Bahamondes et al. 2001), most studies of progestational agents have failed to find evidence for weight gain (Mainwaring et al. 1995; Moore et al. 1995). Similarly, while tamoxifen has been thought to cause weight gain, a 3- to 5-year prospective observational study found no evidence for weight change in patients taking tamoxifen as adjuvant therapy for breast cancer (Kumar et al. 1997).

In addition to being extensively used to treat comorbid hypertension in overweight BED patients, antihypertensive medications are sometimes prescribed off-label in psychiatry for anxiety and medication-induced movement disorders. A systematic review of eight randomized controlled studies of 6 months' duration or greater revealed a median weight gain of 1.2 kg in hypertensive patients treated with β-adrenergic antagonists as compared with placebo (Sharma et al. 2001). Weight gain may result from several effects of these agents, including reductions in basal metabolic rate; exercise intolerance; and adrenergic-agonist–mediated lipolysis. Significant weight gain has not been reported with other antihypertensive agents.

Many gastrointestinal medications are available over the counter, and many are frequently prescribed for patients with eating disorders. For example, metoclopramide has been used to treat symptoms of delayed gastric emptying in anorexia nervosa patients. While theoretically capable of causing weight gain because of its antagonism of dopaminergic (D_2) and serotonergic (5-HT_3) receptors, significant weight change has been described in only one case. In that case, a 19-year-old patient with restricting anorexia experienced a weight gain of nearly 8 kg over 2 months after the dosage was increased from 5 mg qid to 10 mg qid. No changes in eating behavior or physical activity could account for the rapid weight increase, which stopped after the medication was discontinued. Long-term impact on her eating disorder was not described (Sansone and Sansone 2003). Histamine$_2$ (H_2) receptor blockers have been associated with weight loss in some studies, whereas stool softeners, anti-emetics and proton pump inhibitors do not seem to cause weight change.

Medications That Cause Weight Loss

Psychotropic Agents

Apart from medications approved for treatment of obesity, a number of agents are associated with weight loss. (FDA-approved antiobesity medications include sibutramine, orlistat, phentermine, diethylpropion, mazindol, phendimetrazine, and benzphetamine.) Stimulant medications, including amphetamine compounds and methylphenidate, are well known to cause decreased appetite and weight loss. Modafinil, a non-amphetamine wakefulness-promoting agent approved for treatment of sleep disorders, is sometimes used off-label in psychiatry to treat sedating adverse effects of other medications. In this application, it has demonstrated potential for causing substantial weight loss, as illustrated by one case report in which a patient given modafinil for clozapine-associated sedation lost 40 pounds over 1 year (Henderson et al. 2005). However, in a long-term controlled trial with narcolepsy patients, modafinil was not found to differ from placebo in its effects on weight (Moldofsky et al. 2000).

Antipsychotic agents. Molindone is the only medication in this class that consistently has been associated with weight loss. Molindone is a rarely used older antipsychotic that has pharmacological characteristics similar to those of atypical antipsychotics, although its adverse-effect profile does not differ from that of typical agents. Mechanisms may include its lack of histamine receptor antagonism and its ability to selectively inhibit dopamine autoreceptors.

Antidepressants. In one randomized controlled trial, fluoxetine was associated with a small weight decrease during the first month of treatment but an overall weight increase after 1 year, equivalent to that seen with placebo (Michelson et al. 1999). Acute decreases in weight might also be expected with the other SSRIs, given the fact that endogenous hypothalamic serotonin induces satiety. In most studies, bupropion has been associated with modest weight loss of 1–2 pounds, perhaps because of its capacity to inhibit reuptake of norepinephrine and dopamine (Harto-Truax et al. 1983). In one study of 423 patients with major depression, those taking bupropion for 52 weeks achieved weight losses ranging from 0.1 kg to 2.4 kg, with the greatest losses occurring in patients with higher baseline weights (Croft et al. 2002). However, because of its increased potential to cause seizures, bupropion is contraindicated in patients with anorexia nervosa or bulimia nervosa, or a history of those disorders.

Anticonvulsants. Several newer anticonvulsants that cause weight loss are being studied for patients with eating disorders. Topiramate is approved for both adjunctive treatment of seizure disorders and migraine prophylaxis. Observations of an average weight loss of 5.9 kg per year in patients with epilepsy have led to successful applications in the treatment of obesity (Bray et al. 2003), BED (McElroy et al. 2002), bulimia nervosa (Hoopes et al. 2003), and weight gain related to atypical antipsychotic medications (Ko et al. 2005). Weight loss seems to be dose-dependent, as are adverse effects such as impaired cognition and paresthesias. Reports of decreased appetite and weight loss in patients participating in trials of zonisamide for epilepsy prompted a randomized controlled trial in obese adults. In these trials, zonisamide resulted in average weight losses of 5.3 kg greater than those with placebo at 16 weeks (Gadde et al. 2003). Mechanisms for the induction of weight loss by these anticonvulsants are unknown.

Nonpsychotropic Agents

Antidiabetic agents.   Because many patients with BED are overweight or obese, antidiabetic medications are often required, and some of these are associated with weight loss. Metformin is commonly prescribed in treating type 2 diabetes for its insulin-sensitizing effects. It causes weight loss in individuals with type 2 diabetes by reducing food consumption (Lee and Morley 1998). In a large study of nondieting, nondiabetic subjects, metformin-induced weight loss averaging 2 kg over 6 months (Knowler et al. 2002). Efficacy equivalent to that of orlistat in the treatment of obesity has been demonstrated in a randomized trial (Gokcel et al. 2002). Acarbose and miglitol inhibit intestinal alpha-glucosidase enzymes, thereby reducing carbohydrate digestion and absorption. Although acarbose was associated with modest weight loss (about 0.8 kg greater than that seen with placebo) over 1 year in nondieting patients with type 2 diabetes (Wolever et al. 1997), it has been linked to more dramatic weight loss in individual cases (Yoo et al. 1999). Among newer agents for type 2 diabetes are pramlintide and exenatide, analogs of amylin and incretin, respectively—two endogenous peptides that reduce blood glucose. In a 26-week randomized trial, exenatide was associated with dose-dependent weight loss up to an average of 2.8 kg (DeFronzo et al. 2005). A pooled analysis of randomized trials of pramlintide found an average weight loss of 1.8 kg over 26 weeks in patients who were also taking insulin (P. Hollander et al. 2004).

Gastrointestinal medications.   Information about the effect of H_2-receptor blockers on weight is mixed. In randomized controlled trials, these agents have been reported to suppress hunger and enhance weight loss in obese patients on restricted diets (Stoa-Birketvedt 1993) and in nondieting overweight patients with diabetes (Stoa-Birketvedt et al. 1998). Weight loss in the latter trial averaged 3.7 kg greater than placebo after 12 weeks. However, famotidine and nizatidine were not effective in preventing antipsychotic-associated weight gain (Cavazzoni et al. 2003; Poyurovsky et al. 2004), and H_2-receptor blockers have not been reported to be associated with significant weight change when used long term for acid suppression.

Summary of Medications That Affect Weight

As described in the foregoing subsections, numerous medications have been associated with weight changes. The direction of weight change does not seem to be a simple class effect; for example, some anticonvulsants cause weight gain, whereas others are associated with weight loss. In addition, considerable individual variation occurs in the degree of weight change associated with a given agent. It is important for clinicians who work with eating disorder patients to be familiar with the impact of medications on appetite and weight, because the choice of medication may impact both the course of the eating disorder and the patient's willingness to adhere to the regimen. Table 10–2 lists medications associated with weight gain, weight loss, or weight neutrality.

Weight-Altering Medications and Eating Disorders

The association of weight-altering medications and eating disorders is bidirectional. Distorted cognitions related to an eating disorder can result in medication misuse or nonadherence; alternatively, medication-associated weight change can complicate the course of an eating disorder. Clinicians who treat patients with eating disorders should be aware of these reciprocal interactions, which can result in considerable morbidity.

Impact of Eating Disorders on Medication Use

Eating Disorders and Medication Misuse

One facet of the relationship between weight-altering medications and eating disorders is patients' intentional misuse of medications to purge and/or induce weight loss. In fact, misuse of medications is listed among the inappropriate compensatory behaviors meeting criteria for bulimia nervosa (American Psychiatric Association 2000). While excessive or inappropriate use of diuretics, laxatives, and ipecac is commonly assessed in patients with eating disorders, clinicians must also be aware of potential problems with any of the other medications that can affect weight. Even if the patient does not have a medical indication or a prescription, many of these medications are readily available through the Internet or can be obtained from unsuspecting family members or friends.

While misuse of weight-loss-inducing medications among eating disorder patients has not been systematically studied, several case reports and case series attest to its importance. For example, one series of 104 eating disorder consul-

Table 10–2.   Weight effects of some commonly used prescription medications

Medication class	Weight gain	Weight loss	Weight-neutral
Antidepresssants	Mirtazapine Paroxetine Tricyclics Phenelzine Isocarboxazid	Bupropion	Most SSRIs Nefazodone Tranylcypromine Venlafaxine
Mood stabilizers	Valproate Lithium Carbamazepine		Lamotrigine
Anticonvulsants	Valproate Carbamazepine Pregabalin Vigabatrin Gabapentin	Topiramate Zonisamide Felbamate	Tiagabine Lamotrigine
Antipsychotics	Most typical agents Clozapine Olanzapine Risperidone Quetiapine	Molindone	Ziprasidone Aripiprazole
Other psychotropics	Cyproheptadine	Amphetamine Modafinil Methylphenidate	Buspirone Benzodiazepines
Antidiabetics	Insulin Sulfonylureas Thiazolidinediones	Metformin Acarbose Miglitol Pramlintide Exenatide	Repaglinide Nateglinide
Antihypertensives	Beta-blockers		All others
Gastrointestinal	Metoclopramide	H$_2$ blockers[a]	Stool softeners Antiemetics Proton pump inhibitors
Hormonal	Corticosteroids		Contraceptives Tamoxifen

Note.   SSRI = selective serotonin reuptake inhibitors.
[a]Associated with weight loss in some but not all studies.

tations revealed a rate of 6.7% for thyroid hormone abuse (Woodside et al. 1991). Misuse of orlistat as a means of purging in bulimia nervosa has been reported in three patients. Two of the patients obtained the medication through employment in health care (Fernandez-Aranda et al. 2001); the third patient ordered it through the Internet (Malhotra and McElroy 2002). These reports are of particular concern because orlistat was recently approved by the FDA as an over-the-counter medication. Another report describes a patient with bipolar disorder and eating disorder not otherwise specified (NOS) who escalated the dosage of topiramate from 125 to 450 mg/day and lost 6 kg in 15 days while also developing paresthesias and impaired cognition (Colom et al. 2001). When a patient with anorexia nervosa and a history of purging was prescribed fluoxetine for comorbid depression and found that it suppressed her appetite, she increased the dosage from 60 to 120 mg/day and lost 20 pounds over a 2-month period (Wilcox 1987).

Eating Disorders and Medication Nonadherence

Nonadherence to weight-gain-inducing medications in eating disorder patients is best illustrated by the problem of intentional insulin omission in patients with comorbid type 1 diabetes mellitus. If the amount of insulin injected is insufficient, blood glucose rises and exceeds the renal threshold, causing glycosuria, which results in weight loss by excretion of calories and osmotic diuresis. Thus, insulin omission allows patients not only to avoid the weight gain associated with insulin treatment but also to lose weight and/or compensate for eating binges (i.e., purge). Up to one-third of patients with type 1 diabetes report engaging in this behavior at some time (Crow et al. 1998)—a rate that exceeds the prevalence of diagnosable eating disorders in this population. However, insulin omission is more common among patients who do have eating disorders than in those who do not: 44% versus 10% in one study (Bryden et al. 1999) and 54% versus 6% in another (Rodin et al. 1991). Insulin omission almost certainly contributes to the higher rates of impaired metabolic control and diabetes complications found in diabetic individuals with disordered eating (Rydall et al. 1997). The following case example illustrates this problem.

Sharon was a 25-year-old woman when she was first diagnosed with an eating disorder. At age 16, she initially weighed 125 lbs at 5 feet, 6 inches in height

(BMI = 20.2). During the next 4 months, she spontaneously lost 7 pounds and was diagnosed with type 1 diabetes mellitus. At the time of her diabetes diagnosis she weighed 118 pounds (BMI = 19). Insulin was started, and Sharon subsequently gained 12 pounds (BMI = 21). She then tried to compulsively follow the prescribed diabetic diet, but when she did not promptly lose weight she began to binge eat on "forbidden carbohydrates" and gained an additional 10 pounds. Her doctors told her that she had to lose weight or she would die. She began purging by vomiting and by periodically omitting her insulin because she thought it was causing her to gain weight. During the next 9 years she was hospitalized at least four times yearly as a result of ketoacidosis or hypoglycemia. She developed several diabetic complications, including partial blindness and a rising creatinine level. Her weight alternated between 145 and 75 pounds, at which point, at age 25, she was finally evaluated by a psychiatrist and diagnosed with anorexia nervosa.

Now, after 15 years of psychiatric treatment, the comprehensive care of a diabetologist and his team, and two very lengthy inpatient psychiatric hospitalizations, she no longer binge eats, purges, restricts her intake, or omits her insulin. She weighs 145 pounds, is completely blind in one eye, and has multiple other diabetic complications. Although she was clearly predisposed to an eating disorder because of a preexisting obsessive-compulsive disorder, the immediate precipitant to her eating disorder was the weight gain associated with introduction of insulin.

Behaviors similar to insulin omission have also been reported in patients with inflammatory bowel disease. For example, two adolescents with bulimia and inflammatory bowel disease were described as discontinuing their sulfasalazine in order to induce diarrhea as a means of purging (Gryboski 1993). One of these patients subsequently required hospitalization for treatment with intravenous steroids and parenteral hyperalimentation.

Nonadherence to psychotropic medications that cause weight gain is frequently clinically observed in eating disorder patients and has been described in the literature on medication adherence in general psychiatric patients. For example, during a 6-month prospective study of TCAs, 44% of patients taking amitriptyline and 70% of those taking nortriptyline stopped their medications because of weight gain (Berken et al. 1984). In a survey study of 51 psychiatric patients, weight gain was reported as the most distressing of 27 possible medication adverse effects and the most likely to contribute to poor compliance in the future (Gitlin et al. 1989). Another report of 239 National Alliance of the Mentally Ill (now National Alliance on Mental Illness) members concluded that overweight patients who were distressed about weight gain were 2.5 times more likely to report noncompliance (Weiden et al. 2004). Rates of nonadherence among eating disorder patients may well be much higher.

Because medication misuse has the potential for considerable morbidity and even mortality, clinicians who treat patients with eating disorders should carefully monitor their patients' use of medications that affect weight, just as they monitor other behaviors related to the eating disorder. They should also help their colleagues recognize when a patient's treatment refractoriness or unexplained symptoms may be related to medication misuse as part of an eating disorder.

Impact of Medications on Eating Disorders

Externally induced changes in weight or eating habits do seem to precipitate or exacerbate eating disorders in some vulnerable individuals. For example, 9 of 97 patients (9.3%) entering one outpatient eating disorder program reported that their eating problems had worsened after undergoing oral surgery (Maine and Goldberg 2001). One patient's eating disorder symptoms increased rapidly in the context of food restriction during an episode of pancreatitis (Zerbe 1992). Individuals who have surgery for obesity must limit the amount and kinds of foods eaten and may experience vomiting if they overeat. Several cases of anorexia nervosa and bulimia nervosa developing after bariatric surgery have been described in patients who did not have eating disorders prior to their procedures (Guisado et al. 2002). In these examples, eating disorders developed for the first time in a subset of patients whose caloric intake was restricted for medical reasons, just as eating disorders may develop for the first time in a minority of individuals who start to diet.

As with other externally induced changes in weight, medications may have a role in precipitating or exacerbating eating disorders. Because of the significant psychiatric comorbidity with eating disorders, as further described in Chapter 3 ("Eating Disorders and Psychiatric Comorbidity: Prevalence and Treatment Modifications") in this volume, many patients will be exposed to weight-altering psychotropic medications. In addition, some of these medications are prescribed specifically for the eating disorder symptoms. For example, the previously discussed case of Marie illustrates a potential adverse effect of fluoxetine, which is approved for treatment of bulimia nervosa.

In part because atypical antipsychotic agents cause fewer neurological side effects such as extrapyramidal symptoms and tardive dyskinesia, they have been tried in patients with eating disorders, particularly anorexia nervosa. Olanzapine, which is associated with significant weight gain, was reported to be effective for enhancing weight gain in patients with anorexia nervosa in two open-label pilot studies (Barbarich et al. 2004; Powers et al. 2002). However, no large placebo-controlled trials of olanzapine have been reported to date. Quetiapine has also been studied in a pilot open-label study among anorexia nervosa patients. Although some patients gained weight, the mean weight gain was quite small. Modest improvements were noted in symptoms of anxiety and depression (Powers et al. 2007). Other atypical antipsychotic agents, including clozapine, ziprasidone, and aripiprazole, have not been systematically studied. Although olanzapine, risperidone, and quetiapine might be expected to have beneficial effects on weight restoration and perhaps certain other commonly associated symptoms such as anxiety and depression, there are several challenges to using these medications in treating eating disorder patients. The first is that many patients with anorexia nervosa are reluctant to take medications that cause weight gain. The second, and perhaps more important, is that the long-term adverse effects of these drugs in eating disorder patients are not known. The following case example illustrates some of these problems.

Jamie was a 15-year-old girl who was admitted to the hospital with the classic signs and symptoms of restricting anorexia nervosa. Her height was 5 feet, 4 inches, and she weighed 85 pounds (BMI = 14.6); she had been amenorrheic for 6 months and complained that she was fat and needed to lose more weight. She was very resistant to weight gain and heard what she described as an "anorexic male voice" telling her not to eat. After several weeks of trying standard weight restoration treatment methods, her psychiatrist decided to prescribe olanzapine. She was able to become more cooperative and gradually gained to her healthy body weight range of 112–116 pounds.

After discharge, she continued outpatient treatment in another state, where the new treatment team decided to weigh her backward without revealing her weight. After she gained to 120 pounds and discovered on another scale that she exceeded her target weight range, she promptly discontinued the olanzapine and began purging in an attempt to lose weight. Her course over the next 2 years was stormy, and she required rehospitalization before she could be restabilized.

This case illustrates just one of the problems that might be associated with medications that can cause weight gain. For all patients, but particularly for eating disorder patients, it is crucial that the patient be able to maintain trust in her treatment team. Unexpected and unrevealed weight gain is almost certain to erode that trust.

Several published case reports also highlight the role of weight-altering medications in triggering or exacerbating eating disorders. Most involve medications associated with weight gain. For example, among eight young female patients who gained an average of 19 pounds while taking steroids for various medical conditions, two developed anorexia, five were diagnosed with bulimia nervosa, and one with eating disorder NOS (Fornari et al. 2001). While taking risperidone, one patient experienced a weight gain of 20 kg in parallel with preoccupation with weight. She eventually developed bulimia nervosa, which improved when the risperidone was discontinued (Crockford et al. 1997). Clozapine has been associated with worsening of bulimia nervosa (Brewerton and Shannon 1992), and risperidone, olanzapine, and zolpidem have been associated with new onset of sleep-related eating disorders that remitted when the medications were discontinued (Lu and Shen 2004; Morgenthaler and Silber 2002; Paquet et al. 2002). An anorexia nervosa patient who experienced an 8-kg weight gain after taking metoclopramide for gastrointestinal symptoms required an emergency visit with her psychotherapist, although the long-term impact on her eating disorder was not described (Sansone and Sansone 2003). In a group of 74 patients receiving clozapine or olanzapine, 22% of females and 6% of males fulfilled the criteria for BED and 11% of females and 4% of males met the criteria for bulimia nervosa (Theisen et al. 2003). While causality cannot be proven, these percentages are significantly higher than the prevalence of the two disorders in the general population.

Several reports describe how medication reactions associated with weight loss precipitated eating disorders; for example, use of topiramate for epilepsy was associated with relapse of anorexia nervosa in a previously recovered patient (Rosenow et al. 2002), while withdrawal of steroids prescribed for asthma resulted in weight loss and subsequent development of anorexia nervosa in another woman (Morgan and Lacey 1996). Although stimulants prescribed for attention-deficit/hyperactivity disorder (ADHD) might be expected to result in misuse of the medication and aggravation of eating disorder symptoms, several case reports suggest that their use in bulimia nervosa patients actually has a favorable impact in decreasing bingeing and purging, without causing weight loss (Dukarm 2005). However, it should be noted that all of these patients were concurrently receiving specific treatments for their eating disorders.

Clinical Recommendations

Recommendations for clinical management of weight-altering medications in eating disorder patients are summarized in Table 10–3. The goals are twofold: 1) to prevent or minimize adverse effects of weight-altering medications on the eating disorder, and 2) to minimize medication nonadherence or misuse due to eating disorder pathology. Undergirding these recommendations are principles that guide all effective eating disorder treatment: maintaining a positive treatment alliance, monitoring eating disorder symptoms and medical status, working toward specific behavioral goals along with enhanced self-understanding, and communicating frequently among the members of a multidisciplinary treatment team.

A medication's potential impact on weight should be included in risk/benefit assessments before it is prescribed. For patients with anorexia nervosa or bulimia nervosa or histories of these disorders, agents that are weight-neutral are usually preferred to those that cause weight gain or loss, as long as the potential benefit for the primary indication is the same. For example, lamotrigine rather than valproic acid might be recommended for maintenance treatment of bipolar disorder in a bulimia nervosa patient if there are no contraindications for this patient. An exception might be made for the short-term use of olanzapine in anorexia nervosa patients who are involved in eating disorder treatment and who are aware of the medication's potentially positive effects on their weight. If at all possible, medications that cause weight gain should be avoided in patients with BED who are overweight or obese. To these ends, the individual who is treating the eating disorder must communicate with other clinicians who prescribe medications for the patient and, when necessary, educate them about the potential impact of medications on weight and eating disorders.

In many instances, a weight-altering medication may be the best or only choice for the comorbid condition. These circumstances require thorough discussion of the risks and benefits, negotiation of a treatment contract, and on-

Table 10–3.   Recommendations for managing weight-altering medications in eating disorder patients

Include potential weight change in risk/benefit assessments prior to prescribing.

When possible, choose weight-neutral agents in anorexia and bulimia patients.

Communicate with and educate other clinicians who prescribe for the patient.

Initiate discussion of medications' potential impact on weight before prescribing.

Identify and correct patients' misinformation and cognitive distortions related to medications.

Discuss availability of interventions to prevent or treat medication-related weight gain.

Include issues around weight-altering medication adherence and misuse in eating disorder treatment contracts.

Monitor weight and eating disorder symptoms closely after weight-altering medications are initiated or doses are changed.

Monitor medication adherence and symptoms of the comorbid condition.

Follow guidelines for metabolic monitoring of patients taking antipsychotics.

going attention to the quality of the alliance with the patient as well as to his or her weight, eating behaviors, medication adherence, and comorbid conditions. Clinicians should discuss a medication's potential impact on weight before it is prescribed to any psychiatric patient. The patient's concerns should be addressed thoroughly and empathically, with identification and correction of inaccurate information and cognitive distortions. For example, although some medications are commonly associated with weight gain, they still do not cause weight gain in everyone. Patients can also be reassured that strategies for treating medication-induced weight gain—both pharmacological (Malone 2005) and nonpharmacological (Werneke et al. 2003) interventions—are rapidly evolving.

Appropriate use of the medication should be included in the patient's eating disorder treatment contract together with interventions that will be implemented in the event the medication adversely impacts the eating disorder. For example, a patient with a history of anorexia might be prescribed a stimulant for comorbid ADHD with the stipulation that weight loss or evidence of medication misuse would result in discontinuation. A bulimia nervosa patient concerned about weight gain with valproic acid might be encouraged to start an exercise program and be assured that a weight gain of more than

5 pounds would prompt renegotiation regarding this medication. Initiation of a weight-altering medication should also prompt more frequent monitoring of weight and eating behaviors, at least until the impact of the medication on the patient is known. It is also important to monitor adherence to the medication, as well as symptoms of the comorbid disorder for which it is prescribed. While medication adherence can be difficult to measure, a positive response to the question "Have you missed any doses in the past week?" is associated with an adherence rate of less than 60% (Stephenson et al. 1993). Clinicians who prescribe antipsychotic medications should follow established guidelines for metabolic monitoring (American Diabetes Association et al. 2004).

References

Allison DB, Mentore JL, Heo M, et al: Antipsychotic-induced weight gain: a comprehensive research synthesis. Am J Psychiatry 156:1686–1696, 1999

Aman MG, Arnold LE, McDougle CJ, et al: Acute and long-term safety and tolerability of risperidone in children with autism. J Child Adolesc Psychopharmacol 15:869–884, 2005

American Diabetes Association, American Psychiatric Association, American Association of Clinical Endocrinologists, et al: Consensus Development Conference on Antipsychotic Drugs and Obesity and Diabetes. Diabetes Care 27:596–601, 2004

American Psychiatric Association: Diagnostic and Statistical Manual of Mental Disorders, 4th Edition, Text Revision. Washington, DC, American Psychiatric Association, 2000

Arroyo S, Anhut H, Kugler AR, et al: Pregabalin add-on treatment: a randomized, double-blind, placebo-controlled, dose-response study in adults with partial seizures. Epilepsia 45:20–27, 2004

Bahamondes L, Del Castillo S, Tabares G, et al: Comparison of weight increase in users of depot medroxyprogesterone acetate and copper IUD up to 5 years. Contraception 64:223–225, 2001

Barbarich NC, McConaha CW, Gaskill J, et al: An open trial of olanzapine in anorexia nervosa. J Clin Psychiatry 65:1480–1482, 2004

Belcher G, Lambert C, Edwards G, et al: Safety and tolerability of proglitazone, metformin and gliazide in the treatment of type 2 diabetes. Diabetes Res Clin Pract 70:53–62, 2005

Berken GH, Weinstein DO, Stern WC: Weight gain: a side-effect of tricyclic antidepressants. J Affect Disord 7:133–138, 1984

Biton V, Mirza W, Montouris G, et al: Weight change associated with valproate and lamotrigine monotherapy in patients with epilepsy. Neurology 56:172–177, 2001

Bowden CL, Calabrese JR, McElroy SL, et al: A randomized, placebo-controlled 12-month trial of divalproex and lithium in treatment of outpatients with bipolar I disorder. Arch Gen Psychiatry 57:481–489, 2000

Bray GA, Hollander P, Klein S, et al: A 6-month randomized, placebo-controlled, dose-ranging trial of topiramate for weight loss in obesity. Obes Res 11:722–733, 2003

Brewerton TD, Shannon M: Possible clozapine exacerbation of bulimia nervosa (letter). Am J Psychiatry 149:1408, 1992

Bryden KS, Neil A, Mayou RA, et al: Eating habits, body weight, and insulin misuse: a longitudinal study of teenagers and young adults with type 1 diabetes. Diabetes Care 22:1956–1960, 1999

Burrows GD, Kremer CM: Mirtazapine: clinical advantages in the treatment of depression. J Clin Psychopharmacol 17(suppl):34–39, 1997

Calabrese JR, Suppes T, Bowden CL, et al: A double-blind, placebo-controlled, prophylaxis study of lamotrigine in rapid-cycling bipolar disorder. J Clin Psychiatry 61:841–850, 2000

Cantu TG, Korek JS: Monoamine oxidase inhibitors and weight gain. Drug Intell Clin Pharm 22:755–759, 1988

Carlson MG, Campbell PJ: Intensive insulin therapy and weight gain in IDDM. Diabetes 42:1700–1707, 1993

Cavazzoni P, Tanaka Y, Roychowdhury SM, et al: Nizatidine for prevention of weight gain with olanzapine: a double-blind placebo-controlled trial. Eur Neuropsychopharmacol 13:81–85, 2003

Chadwick D: Safety and efficacy of vigabatrin and carbamazepine in newly diagnosed epilepsy: a multicentre randomised double-blind study. Lancet 354:13–19, 1999

Colom F, Vieta E, Benabarre A, et al: Topiramate abuse in a bipolar patient with an eating disorder. J Clin Psychiatry 62:475–476, 2001

Correll CC, Malhotra AK: Pharmacogenetics of antipsychotic-induced weight gain. Psychopharmacology (Berl) 174:477–489, 2004

Crockford DN, Fisher G, Barker P: Risperidone, weight gain, and bulimia nervosa (letter). Can J Psychiatry 42:326–327, 1997

Croft H, Houser TL, Jamerson BD, et al: Effect on body weight of bupropion sustained-release in patients with major depression treated for 52 weeks. Clin Ther 24:662–672, 2002

Crow SJ, Keel PK, Kendall D: Eating disorders and insulin-dependent diabetes mellitus. Psychosomatics 39:233–243, 1998

DeFronzo RA, Ratner RE, Han J, et al: Effects of exenatide (exendin-4) on glycemic control and weight over 30 weeks in metformin-treated patients with type 2 diabetes. Diabetes Care 28:1092–1100, 2005

DeToledo JC, Toledo C, DeCerce J, et al: Changes in body weight with chronic, high-dose gabapentin therapy. Ther Drug Monit 19:394–396, 1997

Devinsky O, Vuong A, Hammer A, et al: Stable weight during lamotrigine therapy: a review of 32 studies. Neurology 54:973–975, 2000

Donahoo WT, Levine JA, Melanson EL: Variability in energy expenditure and its components. Curr Opin Clin Nutr Metab Care 7:599–605, 2004

Dukarm CP: Bulimia nervosa and attention deficit hyperactivity disorder: a possible role for stimulant medication. J Womens Health (Larchmt) 14:345–350, 2005

Fadel J, Bubser M, Deutch AY: Differential activation of orexin neurons by antipsychotic drugs associated with weight gain. J Neurosci 22:6742–6746, 2002

Fava M, Judge R, Hoog SL, et al: Fluoxetine versus sertraline and paroxetine in major depressive disorder: changes in weight with long term treatment. J Clin Psychiatry 61:683–687, 2001

Fernandez-Aranda F, Amor A, Jimenez-Murcia S, et al: Bulimia nervosa and misuse of orlistat: two case reports. Int J Eat Disord 30:458–461, 2001

Fernstrom MH, Kupfer DJ: Antidepressant-induced weight gain: a comparison study of four medications. Psychiatry Res 26:265–271, 1988

Fornari V, Dancyger I La Monaca G, et al: Can steroid use be a precipitant in the development of an eating disorder? Int J Eat Disord 30:118–122, 2001

Frank E, Kupfer DJ, Bulik CM, et al: Imipramine and weight gain during the treatment of recurrent depression. J Affect Disord 30:165–172, 1990

Gadde KM, Franciscy DM, Wagner HR 2nd, et al: Zonisamide for weight loss in obese adults: a randomized controlled trial. JAMA 289:1820–1825, 2003

Gallo MF, Grimes DA, Schulz KF, et al: Combination estrogen-progestin contraceptives and body weight: systematic review of randomized controlled trials. Obstet Gynecol 103:359–373, 2004

Garland EJ, Remick RA, Zis AP: Weight gain: a side effect with antidepressants and lithium. J Clin Psychopharmacol 8:323–330, 1988

Gidal BE, Sheth RD, Magnus L, et al: Levetiracetam does not alter body weight: analysis of randomized, controlled clinical trials. Epilepsy Res 56:121–126, 2003

Gitlin MJ, Cochran SD, Jamison KR: Maintenance lithium treatment: side effects and compliance. J Clin Psychiatry 50:127–131, 1989

Gokcel A, Gumurdulu Y, Karakose H, et al: Evaluation of the safety and efficacy of sibutramine, orlistat and metformin in the treatment of obesity. Diabetes Obes Metab 4:49–55, 2002

Gothelf D, Falk B, Singer P, et al: Weight gain associated with increased food intake and low habitual activity levels in male adolescent schizophrenic inpatients treated with olanzapine. Am J Psychiatry 159:1055–1057, 2002

Gryboski JD: Eating disorders in inflammatory bowel disease. Am J Gastroenterol 88:293–296, 1993

Guisado JA, Vaz FJ, Lopez-Ibor JJ, et al: Gastric surgery and restraint from food as triggering factors of eating disorders in morbid obesity. Int J Eat Disord 31:97–100, 2002

Halmi KA, Eckert E, LaDu TJ, et al: Anorexia nervosa: treatment efficacy of cyproheptadine and amitriptyline. Arch Gen Psychiatry 43:177–181, 1986

Harto-Truax N, Stern WC, Miller LL, et al: Effects of bupropion on body weight. J Clin Psychiatry 44:183–186, 1983

Harvey BH, Bouwer CD: Neuropharmacology of paradoxic weight gain with selective serotonin reuptake inhibitors. Clin Neuropharmacol 23:90–97, 2000

Hedberg A, Rossner S: Body weight characteristics of subjects on asthma medication. Int J Obes Relat Metab Disord 24:1217–1225, 2000

Henderson DC, Louie PM, Koul P, et al: Modafinil-associated weight loss in a clozapine-treated schizoaffective disorder patient. Ann Clin Psychiatry 17:95–97, 2005

Hinze-Selch D, Schuld A, Kraus T, et al: Effects of antidepressants on weight and on the plasma levels of leptin, TNF-alpha, and soluble TNF receptors: a longitudinal study in patients treated with amitriptyline or paroxetine. Neuropsychopharmacology 23:13–19, 2000

Hollander E, Wasserman S, Swanson EN, et al: A double-blind placebo-controlled pilot study of olanzapine in childhood/adolescent pervasive development disorder. J Child Adolesc Psychopharmacol 16:541–548, 2006

Hollander P, Maggs DG, Ruggles JA, et al: Effect of pramlintide on weight in overweight and obese insulin-treated type 2 diabetes patients. Obes Res 12:661–668, 2004

Hoopes SP, Reimherr FW, Hedges DW, et al: Treatment of bulimia nervosa with topiramate in a randomized, double-blind, placebo-controlled trial, Part 1: improvement in binge and purge measures. J Clin Psychiatry 64:1335–1341, 2003

Jallon P, Picard F: Body weight gain and anticonvulsants: a comparative review. Drug Saf 24:969–978, 2001

Joffe RT, Post RM, Uhde TW: Effect of carbamazepine on body weight in affectively ill patients. J Clin Psychiatry 47:313–314, 1986

Knowler WC, Barrett-Connor E, Fowler SE, et al: Reduction in the incidence of type 2 diabetes with lifestyle intervention or metformin. N Engl J Med 346:393–403, 2002

Ko YH, Joe SH, Jung IK, et al: Topiramate as an adjuvant treatment with atypical antipsychotics in schizophrenic patients experiencing weight gain. Clin Neuropharmacol 28:169–175, 2005

Krentz AJ, Bailey CJ: Oral antidiabetic agents: current role in type 2 diabetes mellitus. Drugs 65:385–411, 2005

Kroeze WK, Hufeisen SJ, Popadak BA, et al: H1-histamine receptor affinity predicts short-term weight gain for typical and atypical antipsychotic drugs. Neuropsychopharmacology 28:519–526, 2003

Kumar NB, Allen K, Cantor A, et al: Weight gain associated with adjuvant tamoxifen therapy in stage I and II breast cancer: fact or artifact? Breast Cancer Res Treat 44:135–143, 1997

Lawson ML, Rodin GM, Rydall AC, et al: Eating disorders in young women with IDDM: the need for prevention. Eating Disorders: Journal of Treatment and Prevention 2:261–272, 1994

Lee A, Morley JE: Metformin decreases food consumption and induces weight loss in subjects with obesity with type II non-insulin-dependent diabetes. Obes Res 6:47–53, 1998

Loiseau P: Review of controlled trials of Gabitril (tiagabine): a clinician's viewpoint. Epilepsia 40 (suppl 9):S14–S19, 1999

Lu ML, Shen WW: Sleep-related eating disorder induced by risperidone (letter). J Clin Psychiatry 65:273, 2004

Maina G, Albert U, Salvi V, et al: Weight gain during long term treatment of obsessive-compulsive disorder: a prospective comparison between serotonin reuptake inhibitors. J Clin Psychiatry 65:1365–1371, 2004

Maine M, Goldberg MH: The role of third molar surgery in the exacerbation of eating disorders. J Oral Maxillofac Surg 59:1297–1300, 2001

Mainwaring R, Hales HA, Stevenson K, et al: Metabolic parameter, bleeding, and weight changes in U.S. women using progestin-only contraceptives. Contraception 51:149–153, 1995

Malhotra S, McElroy SL: Orlistat misuse in bulimia nervosa. Am J Psychiatry 159:492–493, 2002

Malone M: Medications associated with weight gain. Ann Pharmacother 39:2046–2055, 2005

McElroy SL, Arnold LM, Shapira NA, et al: Topiramate in the treatment of binge eating disorder associated with obesity: a randomized, placebo-controlled trial. Am J Psychiatry 160:255–261, 2002

McElroy SL, Kotwal R, Keck PE Jr, et al: Comorbidity of bipolar and eating disorders: distinct or related disorders with shared dysregulations. J Affect Disord 86:107–127, 2005

McQuade RD, Stock E, Marcus R, et al: A comparison of weight change during treatment with olanzapine or aripiprazole: results from a randomized, double-blind study. J Clin Psychiatry 65 (suppl 18):47–56, 2004

Michelson D, Amsterdam JD, Quitkin FM, et al: Changes in weight during a 1-year trial of fluoxetine. Am J Psychiatry 156:1170–1176, 1999

Mikhail N: Exanatide: a novel approach for treatment of type 2 diabetes. South Med J 99:1271–1279, 2006

Moldofsky H, Broughton RJ, Hill JD: A randomized trial of the long-term, continued efficacy and safety of modafinil in narcolepsy. Sleep Med 1:109–116, 2000

Moore LL, Valuck R, McDougall C, et al: A comparative study of one-year weight gain among users of medroxyprogesterone acetate, levonorgestrel implants, and oral contraceptives. Contraception 52:215–219, 1995

Morgan J, Lacey JH: Anorexia nervosa and steroid withdrawal. Int J Eat Disord 2:213–215, 1996

Morgenthaler TI, Silber MH: Amnestic sleep-related eating disorder associated with zolpidem. Sleep Med 3:323–327, 2002

Moses R: A review of clinical experience with the prandial glucose regulator, repaglinide, in the treatment of type 2 diabetes. Expert Opin Pharmacother 1:1455–1467, 2000

NDC Health Pharmaceutical Audit Suite: The top 300 prescriptions for 2004. Available at http://www.rxlist.com/top200a.htm. Accessed December 24, 2005.

O'Brien KM, Vincent NK: Psychiatric comorbidity in anorexia and bulimia nervosa: nature, prevalence, and causal relationships. Clin Psychol Rev 23:57–74, 2003

Paquet V, Strul J, Servais L, et al: Sleep related eating disorder induced by olanzapine (letter). J Clin Psychiatry 63:597, 2002

Pigott TA, Carson WH, Saha AR, et al: Aripiprazole for the prevention of relapse in stabilized patients with chronic schizophrenia: a placebo-controlled 26-week study. J Clin Psychiatry 64:1048–1056, 2003

Powers PS, Santana CA, Bannon YS: Olanzapine in the treatment of anorexia nervosa: an open label study. Int J Eat Disord 32:146–154, 2002

Powers PS, Bannon Y, Eubanks R, et al: Quetiapine in anorexia nervosa patients: an open label outpatient pilot study. Int J Eat Disord 40:21–26, 2007

Poyurovsky M, Tal V, Maayan R, et al: The effect of famotidine addition on olanzapine-induced weight gain in first-episode schizophrenia patients: a double-blind placebo-controlled pilot study Eur Neuropsychopharmacol 14:332–336, 2004

Rachelle L, Lilenfeld R: Psychiatric comorbidity associated with anorexia nervosa, bulimia nervosa, and binge eating disorder, in Clinical Handbook of Eating Disorders: An Integrated Approach. Edited by Brewerton TD. New York, Marcel Dekker, 2004, pp 183–207

Rigalleau V, Delafaye C, Baillet L, et al: Composition of insulin-induced body weight gain in diabetic patients: a bio-impedance study. Diabetes Metab 25:321–328, 1999

Rodin G, Craven J, Littlefield C, et al: Eating disorders and intentional insulin under-treatment in adolescent females with diabetes. Psychosomatics 32:171–176, 1991

Rogers CC, Alloway RR, Hanaway M, et al: Body weight alterations under early cor-ticosteroid withdrawal and chronic corticosteroid therapy with modern immuno-suppression. Transplant Proc 37:800–801, 2005

Rosenow F, Knake S, Hebebrand J: Topiramate and anorexia nervosa (letter). Am J Psychi-atry 159:2112–2113, 2002

Rosenstock J, Hassman DR, Madder RD, et al: Repaglinide versus nateglinide mono-therapy: a randomized, multicenter study. Diabetes Care 27:1265–1270, 2004

Rydall AC, Rodin GM, Olmsted MP, et al: Disordered eating behavior and microvas-cular complications in young women with insulin-dependent diabetes mellitus. N Engl J Med 336:1849–1854, 1997

Sansone RA, Sansone LA: Metoclopramide and unintended weight gain. Int J Eat Disord 34:265–268, 2003

Sharma AM, Pischon T, Hardt S, et al: Beta-adrenergic receptor blockers and weight gain: a systematic analysis. Hypertension 37:250–254, 2001

Smith SR, De Jonge L, Volaufova J, et al: Effect of pioglitazone on body composition and energy expenditure: a randomized controlled trial. Metabolism 54:24–32, 2005

Stephenson BJ, Rowe BH, Haynes RB, et al: The rational clinical examination. Is this patient taking the treatment as prescribed? JAMA 269:2779–278, 1993

Stoa-Birketvedt G: Effect of cimetidine suspension on appetite and weight in over-weight subjects. BMJ 306:1091–1093, 1993

Stoa-Birketvedt G, Paus PN, Ganss R, et al: Cimetidine reduces weight and improves metabolic control in overweight patients with type 2 diabetes. Int J Obes Relat Metab Disord 22:1041–1045, 1998

Sussman N, Ginsberg DL: Weight effects of nefazodone, bupropion, mirtazapine, and venlafaxine: a review of the available evidence. Prim Psychiatry 7:33–48, 2000

Sussman N, Ginsberg DL, Bikoff J: Effects of nefazodone on body weight: a pooled analysis of selective serotonin inhibitor– and imipramine-controlled trials. J Clin Psychiatry 62:256–260, 2001

Theisen FM, Linden A, Konig IR, et al: Spectrum of binge eating symptomatology in patients treated with clozapine and olanzapine. J Neural Transm 110:111–121, 2003

Trivedi M, Rush A: A review of randomized controlled medication trials in major depression. Biol Psychiatry 31:188–189, 1992

Vestergaard P, Amdisen A, Schou M: Clinically significant side effects of lithium treat-ment. Acta Psychiatr Scand 62:193–200, 1980

Vestergaard P, Poulstrup I, Schou M: Prospective studies on a lithium cohort, 3: tremor, weight gain, diarrhea, psychological complaints. Acta Psychiatr Scand 78:434–441, 1988

Weiden PJ, Mackell JA, McDonnell DD: Obesity as a risk factor for antipsychotic noncompliance. Schizophr Res 66:51–57, 2004

Werneke U, Taylor D, Sanders TAB, et al: Behavioural management of antipsychotic-induced weight gain: a review. Acta Psychiatr Scand 108:252–259, 2003

Wilcox JA: Abuse of fluoxetine by a patient with anorexia nervosa (letter). Am J Psychiatry 144:1100, 1987

Wolever TM, Chiasson JL, Josse RG, et al: Small weight loss on long-term acarbose therapy with no change in dietary pattern of nutrient intake of individuals with non-insulin-dependent diabetes. Int J Obes Relat Metab Disord 21:756–763, 1997

Woodside DB, Walfish P, Kaplan AS, et al: Graves' disease in a woman with thyroid hormone abuse, bulimia nervosa, and history of anorexia nervosa. Int J Eat Disord 10:111–115, 1991

Yoo W, Park T, Baek H: Marked weight loss in a type 2 diabetic patient treated with acarbose. Diabetes Care 22:645–646, 1999

Zerbe KJ: Recurrent pancreatitis presenting as fever of unknown origin in a recovering bulimic. Int J Eat Disord 12:337–340, 1992

11

Cognitive-Behavioral Therapy for Eating Disorders

Joel Yager, M.D.

The premise that cognitive-behavioral therapy (CBT) is an effective treatment for eating disorders is bolstered by a strong evidence-based literature. In Chapter 7 ("Management of Bulimia Nervosa") and Chapter 8 ("Management of Eating Disorders Not Otherwise Specified"), Mitchell et al. and Devlin et al. review studies supporting the view that CBT is currently the single most effective intervention for bulimia nervosa and binge-eating disorder (BED), respectively. In Chapter 5 ("Management of Anorexia Nervosa in an Ambulatory Setting"), Kaplan and Noble detail that CBT is the only psychotherapeutic treatment demonstrated to be effective for relapse prevention of anorexia nervosa in patients over the age of 18 (Pike et al. 2003), although CBT is certainly no panacea for this difficult-to-treat condition (Walsh et al. 2006). CBT's effectiveness for patients with anorexia nervosa who are acutely ill, seriously underweight, and in a weight restoration phase is even less well supported; many acutely ill anorexia nervosa patients are even less likely than weight-restored patients to engage in CBT and are very prone to drop out of treatment (Halmi et al. 2005).

Given the general support for CBT in bulimia nervosa and BED, this chapter will provide clinicians with some theoretical rationale for CBT in eating disorders; a brief description of commonly employed technical strategies; an overview of resistances and complications and their management; and a guide to additional resources for learning more about administering CBT for patients with eating disorders.

Distorted Cognitions and Maladaptive Behaviors in Eating Disorders

Distorted cognitions about weight and shape constitute core dimensions of the diagnostic criteria for anorexia nervosa, including intense fears of gaining weight and, for both anorexia nervosa and bulimia nervosa, having self-evaluation unduly influenced by shape and weight. Taken together, these cognitions have lent support for a *transdiagnostic* model (Fairburn et al. 2003), in which commonalities of cognitive distortions about weight, shape, and food are linked to self-esteem.

Cognitive theorists describe negative thoughts and beliefs, and dysfunctional attitudes and schemas, as key drivers of negative emotions and behaviors in psychopathology. The individual manifest thoughts and beliefs are often entrenched in far-ranging higher-order cognitive structures that pervasively cover a larger sphere of self-concept. Cognitive therapies not only address the individual beliefs but also attempt to uncover and work with the deeper broad schemes in which they are embedded. Examples of specific forms of distorted cognitions abound in eating disorders and include many types of perverse, maladaptive attitudes and schemes regarding one's own body and body image.

Although there are some perceptual distortions about body size, in which patients perceive their bodies to be larger than they actually are, attitudes about the perceptions seem most pathological. Core higher-order features are often those associated with perfectionism and chronically low self-esteem (Fairburn et al. 2003). Mood and self-esteem are highly overdependent on perceptions regarding shape and weight. Classic examples of cognitive distortions in eating disorders include the following (as summarized by Garner et al. [1997]):

- *Dichotomous "all or none" thinking* that often accompanies perfectionism (e.g.,"If I'm not in complete control, I lose *all* control and everything will become chaotic. If I gain a single ounce, I'll go on to become extremely obese")
- *Magnification* (e.g.,"If I gain a pound, I won't fit into my clothes")
- *Self-referential personalization* (e.g.,"If I gain two pounds, everyone will notice how fat I'm becoming")
- *Catastrophizing* (e.g.,"If I gain a pound, my boyfriend will leave me because I'm becoming a fat pig")
- *Selective abstraction* (e.g., "My dieting makes me morally stronger than all of my friends")
- *Overgeneralization* (e.g., "I gave in to my urge to have that cookie. I'm totally weak willed")
- *Superstitious thinking* (e.g.,"If I give up my strict eating pattern, something bad will happen to my dog").

Other distortions have been described, including *thought-shape fusion,* in which merely thinking about eating a forbidden food increases the person's estimate of his or her shape or weight, elicits a perception of moral wrongdoing, and makes the person feel fat (Shafran et al. 1999).

The cognitive distortions involve not only the content but the processes of thinking, which may be illogical and which may take on the unswerving intensity of zealously held overvalued ideas (McKenna 1984) that approach delusional proportions. The distorted cognitions may be subtly and continuously strengthened by negatively self-reinforcing behaviors such as constant mirror-gazing and body checking experienced through self-derogatory appraisal biases that are selectively biased to find fault (Fairburn 2006). Often, patients discount positive information, feedback, or observations and selectively perceive and appraise and focus on negative interpretations.

Several cognitive models of eating disorders suggest that these distorted cognitions lead to alterations in eating behavior, exercise, and other related behaviors that bring about the physiological impairments of eating disorders. In a complex set of feedback loop interactions in which various elements positively reinforce one another in a downward spiral, low self-esteem may contribute to extreme concerns about shape and weight that in turn produce restrictive eating and strict dieting that may promote binge eating, which then may provoke self-induced vomiting that feeds back to all of the above, particularly low self-esteem (Fairburn et al. 1993). The interacting cognitive subsystems of weight and shape vis-à-vis self-esteem are central to this model (Waller and Kennerley 2003).

It is also conceivable that, for whatever reasons, behavioral abnormalities are initiated through as yet ill-defined biological mechanisms, and that at least some cognitive distortions in thinking subsequently develop as epiphenomena, to help reduce cognitive dissonance. In a vicious negative feedback cycle, poor nutrition affects brain functions, often leading to more primitive thinking, with more intense and stereotypical obsessions, many of which appear to ameliorate "spontaneously" (i.e., without formal psychotherapy) once weight is restored.

Maladaptive behaviors related to eating disorders include those specifically associated with anorectic behavioral patterns such as restrictive, ritualistic eating as well as rituals around eating binges. Compulsive behaviors often surround exercise and laxative misuse and abuse. In addition, far more subtle repetitive behaviors may be in play that surreptitiously reinforce negative thoughts and attitudes toward the self, such as constantly checking weight by frequent weighing on the scale, and checking out body features by feeling parts of the body (e.g., thighs) or constantly mirror-gazing, and reinforcing whatever one sees with negative self-statements (Fairburn 2006).

To summarize, the ubiquitous cognitive distortions concern both the form of thinking and the content of thinking. Although still in some dispute, many theories posit that distorted and maladaptive cognitive schemes drive the abnormal behaviors that in turn yield the physiological impairments that characterize eating disorders. Regardless of how the distorted cognitions and maladaptive behaviors of eating disorders originate, they offer useful grappling points around which patients and clinicians can attempt interventions to reverse the pathological processes of these disorders. The rationale is empirical and straightforward: by pushing back on distorted thinking, patients should experience remissions in their unrelenting self-deprecating stances and be able to act differently with regard to eating, purging, and related behaviors. By identifying other emotional issues and cognitive concerns that eating disorder-related cognitive distortions may be masking, patients may be better able to directly deal with those issues, alleviating some of the tendency to keep generating eating disorder psychopathology. By pushing back on maladaptive eating-related behaviors, patients should be able to interrupt the distorted cognitive patterns that accompany them as never-ceasing themes of background music. The bottom-line premises are that correcting the behaviors and the thinking leads to healthier behaviors and a gradual disappearance of the core features of the eating disorders.

Patient Selection for CBT

Before CBT is prescribed for a given patient, several clinical points should be kept in mind. CBT is unlikely to work and should not be prescribed for patients who are psychotic, severely depressed, or suicidal, or who are actively abusing substances (Wilson et al. 1997). Furthermore, in the presence of certain other complicating conditions, such as ambivalent motivations or complex personality difficulties, particularly those associated with Cluster B diagnoses, CBT is less likely to be effective in the usual brief course and may require modification and extension, although it may still be used. The usual course of CBT is less likely to help patients with severe restrictive eating in anorexia nervosa or to help patients with BED and obesity to lose weight and maintain weight loss. Patients who are more likely to benefit from CBT are those who are best able to access specific cognitions; identify, label, and discriminate among emotional states; understand and accept the cognitive model; accept personal responsibility for working toward change; and form a strong working alliance with their clinicians (Safran and Segal 1990).

The case of Heather illustrates a typical patient selected for CBT:

At age 21 Heather, a senior nursing student, presented with a history of increasing episodes of binge eating and purging since age 16. She recalled being anxious and perfectionistic from early childhood on and prone to get upset if she was not excelling in school and athletics, and had always been normal in weight. In high school a gym teacher had made an offhand comment suggesting that she could do better in her sport if she lost a few pounds, and Heather recalled feeling humiliated and demoralized from that moment on. After attempting to severely restrict her caloric intake, Heather found that she could "have my cake and eat it too" by eating what she wanted when she wanted and purging immediately afterward. However, these "bad habits" started to "run away with me," and she could not control their urgency and frequency. The harder she tried, the worse she felt about herself. Her daily thoughts were riddled with ruminations about needing to be thinner, being a "loser" for not being able to control herself, and being a "fat pig" whenever she "gave in" to her food cravings.

Applying CBT in Treating Patients With Eating Disorders

Several important background issues bear mention. To start, each individual requires an individualized appraisal regarding her particular paramount cognitive and behavioral symptoms and the relative contributions of each to the patient's impairments, and these should be constantly reassessed during treatment, as working hypotheses. Inevitably, good CBT requires clinicians to appraise not only the patient's thoughts, beliefs, and schemas, but also her motivation, temperament, personality structure, and attachment style, as well as other social and interpersonal issues. Clinicians who fall back on pat formulas and generalizations about cognitive distortions and schemes will too often miss the most salient issues and themes and err in treatment. In addition, although close adherence to the CBT manual is most likely to assure success, some flexibility is necessary, and the clinician must always stay attuned to what the dominant clinical issues are at any time with the patient. At times, major life crises and/or other psychiatric problems may surface that should take precedence, and the planned CBT eating disorder agenda may need to be set aside temporarily so that more pressing issues can be addressed. It should be clear that psychiatric medications may be used in conjunction with CBT.

Finally, the importance of so-called nonspecific factors in CBT, as in all forms of psychotherapy, needs to be underscored. No psychotherapy occurs in a sterile vacuum, and no manualized psychotherapy that includes various protocols is (or should be) applied in a robotic manner. A recent study of psychotherapy for adult patients with relatively long-standing anorexia nervosa showed that certain nonspecific supportive factors in clinical management, when applied systematically and diligently in psychotherapy, made as much impact in this patient population as formal CBT (McIntosh et al. 2005). These included such straightforward components of clinician-patient interactions as education, care, support, and the fostering of a therapeutic relationship designed to promote adherence to treatment through the use of praise, reassurance, and advice. The CBT relationship works best in an atmosphere of collaboration, where the clinician is frequently checking in with the patient to make certain that they are attuned to the important issues, strategies, and tactics. When difficulties, resistances, and impasses arise, the clinician should be curious, open to feedback, empathic, flexible, and empirical. On occasion, it might be important to see other family members to enlist their support, for clarification or dispute resolution. The take-home implication for clinicians is that these dimensions of psychotherapy can be very helpful by themselves and should certainly not be ignored when other more specific CBT interventions are implemented.

A very important nonspecific factor of these treatments is the very fact that they are structured and prescriptive, necessarily increasing the diligent and inescapable attention and mindfulness that patients must pay to the fact that they are engaged in a treatment. They are also expected to do something in the nature of homework, requiring effort and commitment. Clearly, patients who are too chaotic and undisciplined to do the work, or who lack sufficient motivation or mental energy to diligently apply themselves to the tasks, show these tendencies quickly and early, between the first and second visit, and may either drop out or show that they require modifications of treatment early on—for example, the application of motivational interviewing techniques (Miller and Rollnick 2002).

Over the past several decades, a number of groups have devised, tested, and iteratively evolved CBT programs focusing on bulimia nervosa, most notably based on the CBT–bulimia nervosa manual of Fairburn et al. (1993). These have been variably modified for BED, obesity, and anorexia nervosa. For bulimia nervosa and BED, most treatments are scheduled for 4–6 months. Patients with anorexia nervosa usually require longer therapy, generally in the order of 1–2 years, at least.

The synthesized overview presented in a somewhat schematized fashion in Table 11–1 is based on several of these programs, to offer a current blend of the best-practice CBT approaches to eating disorders. A parallel program for BED is described in Chapter 8 in this volume.

Most programs are conceptualized as occurring in three to four stages. Typically, the sessions are scheduled more frequently at the start, perhaps twice per

Table 11–1.   Prototypical cognitive-behavioral therapy (CBT) program elements for bulimia nervosa (modifiable for other eating disorders)

Stage 1 (approximately eight sessions)

Aims

Establishing a therapeutic relationship, educating the patient about the condition and the model, establishing weekly weighings if appropriate, and changing behaviors such as restrictive eating, binge eating, and purging.

Techniques

Establishing a trusting relationship, assessing the patient's motivational state, and establishing treatment expectations and parameters, while being constantly attune to patient's concerns and resistances.

  Note: When the patient is ambivalent about treatment, it may be useless to jump into the usual protocols for CBT. Instead, initial periods of time should be devoted to motivational interviewing and motivational enhancement. This may include discussion of the adaptive functions of the eating disorder (including pros and cons of staying with the disorder versus changing).

Self-monitoring:

  Record specific information about meals (which may include calorie estimates of each item consumed) as well as eating binges, purges, and exercise; and the *a*ntecedents, *b*ehaviors, and *c*onsequences of each event ("ABCs") on a monitoring sheet. The patient may be asked to record the time of the event; environmental, cognitive-emotional, and interoceptive triggers; the actual eating and associated behaviors; and what was consumed and what happened after consumption, including associated thoughts, emotions, behaviors. Patients who are reluctant to self-monitor should be empathically but firmly encouraged to apply themselves to completing their diaries.

Weekly weighing (for patients where the specific weight shifts are matters of close attention):

  Weighings should usually be once per week only, to reduce tendency to overfocus attention on weight, stemming from daily (or more frequent) weighings.

Education about weight, eating, and the biological and psychological consequences of undereating, binge eating, and purging, through discussions and assigned readings.

Prescriptive eating in regular, structured, scheduled patterns

  The importance here is to ensure that patients are not skipping meals and that patients who require snacks for adequate intake and/or to avert hunger-induced binges actually consume the snacks.

Table 11–1.   Prototypical cognitive-behavioral therapy (CBT) program elements for bulimia nervosa (modifiable for other eating disorders) *(continued)*

Stage 1 *(continued)*

Self-control strategies, including:

Increasing mindfulness about eating. Self-monitoring techniques offer one approach. Doing nothing else while eating except attending to and sensing the acts of eating are others (e.g., avoiding such distractions to mindful eating such as watching television or driving while eating).

Avoiding body-checking, mirror-gazing, weighing, and looking at fashion magazines, and noting the frequency and intensity of urges to do just those behaviors.

Providing suitable and alternative pleasurable and adaptive activities to replace or distract from binge eating, purging, or excessive exercise (so-called healthy pleasures).

Offering stimulus-control instructions such as environmental manipulations to avoid "poison foods" or "toxic" social situations; assuring portion size control.

Developing delaying tactics to resist giving in to impulsive urges, to stretch out the time between consumption and purging until the urge to purge may either pass or result in much fewer calories being purged because sufficient time has passed to ensure some digestion of what has been ingested (i.e., exposure and response prevention); developing the concept of "healthy days" on the calendar, where "permissible days" to binge eat and purge are gradually pushed further and further apart, and other pleasurable rewards are provided for successes.

Explicitly giving permission for the patient to be kinder to herself with respect to perfectionistic expectations and strivings (e.g., formulating prescribed circumstances around which she can practice being less than perfect).

Stage 2 (approximately seven sessions)

Aims

Developing additional coping skills for reducing dieting and restrictive eating behaviors, and resisting or delaying binge eating and purging behaviors. The emphasis is increasingly on cognitive issues.

Techniques

Generating lists of frightening foods, and beginning to introduce them, sequentially, as meal components starting with the least intimidating, to deal with restrictive eating.

Table 11–1. Prototypical cognitive-behavioral therapy (CBT) program elements for bulimia nervosa (modifiable for other eating disorders) *(continued)*

Stage 2 *(continued)*

Generating lists of novel places and circumstances in which to eat, especially those that were avoided as a result of the eating disorder:

Start introducing eating experiences in safe places and circumstances to break up the rigid patterns of social eating that may have evolved during the course of the disorder.

Increasing and extending use of alternative activities and tactics for delaying and resisting binge eating and purging.

Cognitive restructuring—reshaping thoughts and attitudes:

The cognitive restructuring includes attention to dysfunctional body shape and weight concerns and depressive, self-defeating cognitions.

Identify specific, detailed problematic thoughts and the context in which they occur in order to objectify, externalize, and scrutinize them

Assist the patient to write detailed thought diaries to collect evidence to verify or help dispute, challenge, and disconfirm the assumptions of the negative, maladaptive thoughts. These strategies include enumerating the pros and cons of maintaining these thoughts and imagining potential "win-win" situations or other changes that would permit the patient to revise or surrender these maladaptive thoughts.

Challenge patient as to whether she judges others by the same criteria that she harshly employs on herself.

Stop negative self-labeling (using the "stop" technique employed in the treatment of obsession thoughts).

Use worry and exposure, conjuring up certain types of feared thoughts and their imagined outcomes, and having the patient stay with them for 5–30 minutes to experience the emotion, in effort to extinguish the fear. This is similar to the methods employed in treatment of anxiety disorders and obsessive-compulsive disorders (Fisher and Wells 2005).

Improving the patient's problem-solving skills by means of the following:

Improve *problem identification* through reflection, journaling, and assigning words and labels to deconstruct unclear, distressing, frustrating, and dysphoric feeling states. Help identify, clarify, elucidate, and objectify negativistic, maladaptive cognitions and associated schemas.

Identify specific *interpersonal problems* that may contribute to the chronic and specific sources of frustration, feelings of loss of control, anger, and frustration that trigger eating disorder–related maladaptive cognitions and behaviors.

Table 11–1.   Prototypical cognitive-behavioral therapy (CBT) program elements for bulimia nervosa (modifiable for other eating disorders) *(continued)*

Stage 2 *(continued)*

Assist *option identification and selection,* helping patient to identify alternative emotional, behavioral, and interpersonal responses to negative and maladaptive cognitive self-statements, and then to analyze the pros and cons of the behavioral and cognitive responses she has identified.

Assist patient in *anticipating and subsequently assessing the outcomes of various courses of action.*

Encourage patient to *record her attempts at problem solving* and to compare anticipated with actual outcomes.

Stage 3 (approximately three to four sessions)

Aims

Preparing patient for termination by helping her to review what she has accomplished; considering the strategies that work best for her; identifying and framing remaining behavioral, cognitive, emotional, and interpersonal issues; and developing a plan for relapse prevention.

Techniques

Focusing on future rather than on the present:

The patient is asked to anticipate and imagine predictable high-risk and high-stakes situations, circumstances, and settings that may provoke her to relapse in the future.

Instructing patient to write out anticipated strategies to deal with these situations, using the techniques she has learned during treatment, including new coping strategies; cognitive immunizations (i.e., the very fact that the patient anticipates and is forewarned and forearmed may diminish the intensity of the emerging threat); well-worn protective thoughts, mantras, and self-statements; and avoidance of certain circumstances during vulnerable periods if necessary.

Instructing patient in the perspective that a "lapse" is not a "relapse." She is asked to write out "maintenance plans," specifying what she would do if a "lapse" were to occur, starting with mindfulness, reinstituting self-monitoring, and reinstituting structured meal plans including snacks.

Instructing patient on how to reconnect with caregivers should the need arise.

Source.   Synthesized from programs described by Agras and Apple 1997; Fairburn et al. 1993; Garner et al. 1997; Wilson et al. 1997, among others.

week initially, and toward the end may be scheduled less frequently. The first stage focuses on education and on self-monitoring. The very act of self-monitoring increases awareness of eating and its associated settings, triggers to maladaptive behaviors, and their emotional and cognitive consequences, and may help patients gain additional self-control. A typical self-monitoring worksheet page for a patient with bulimia nervosa is illustrated in Figure 11–1.

Clinician and patient will both benefit when a specific protocol is followed systematically. Fortunately, a number of these manuals have been published, including several that offer separate versions for patients and the clinicians working with them. Several of the more popular illustrative resources are listed in Table 11–2.

The success of CBT is directly related to the fidelity with which the clinician applies the treatment. For example, if the patient is asked to complete detailed self-monitoring diaries of her pathological eating-related behaviors, harmful thoughts, and the circumstances preceding and succeeding them, during sessions with the patient the clinician must devote sufficient time and interest to going over these records in sufficient detail to reinforce the patient's enthusiasm for continuing to do the considerable work required to produce them. The clinician's enthusiasm and appreciation for the good efforts the patient makes will ordinarily generate continued application. However, if the clinician seems disinterested, the patient will usually follow suit quickly, sabotaging potential gains that might be obtained from this approach.

In a commonly employed session-by-session schedule, the clinician devotes the first 10 minutes to a review of what is transpiring in the patient's day-to-day life and assesses for any overriding issues or concerns; the next 10 minutes to reviewing the self-monitoring diary sheets, picking up important patterns and themes; and the next 20 minutes to setting the agenda and dealing with the cognitive or behavioral issues claiming focus for the day via education, Socratic discussion, and/or strategy formation. Finally, there is a summary of what has been discussed and the assignment of homework for the next appointment. To continue with the clinical story of Heather begun earlier:

> By age 21 Heather had been binge eating and purging several times each week for 4 years. When she started her first-ever serious relationship with a boyfriend, and it appeared that they wanted to live together, she sought treatment

for the first time. She had concealed her bulimic problems from her boyfriend and wanted to be rid of them before she moved in with him. With this motivation Heather diligently applied herself to the tasks set forth by CBT. With her therapist's help and the use of a CBT workbook, she learned about the psychological and physiological aspects of bulimia nervosa and started to record a daily diary of her eating behaviors and associated thoughts and feelings, and other behaviors. Within 2 weeks her eating patterns had improved and her purging episodes decreased correspondingly. Within a month her episodes of binge eating and purging had diminished to about once weekly. After several months they remitted entirely. At 6-month follow-up Heather remained free of binge-eating and purging episodes and reported that she and her boyfriend were getting engaged and doing well. She required no psychotropic medication.

When CBT Is Insufficient or Does Not Work

Despite CBT's demonstrated effectiveness for the treatment of bulimia nervosa, there are clearly many patients who do not take to CBT or for whom a course of CBT is insufficient or ineffective. Several of the clinical circumstances in which these limitations are more likely to occur were described in the preceding sections. For the psychotherapeutic treatment of patients with bulimia nervosa, several additional strategies have been designed and are the subject of current research. As discussed in greater detail in Chapter 16 ("Management of Patients With Chronic, Intractable Eating Disorders"), treatment impasses and so-called treatment resistance always call for a thorough reassessment and rethinking of the clinical situation. Only a few points will be considered here. When the difficulty appears to be with the basic motivational status of the patient toward treatment and recovery, *motivational interviewing* and motivational enhancement techniques are applied (Dunn et al. 2006; Feld et al. 2001; Vitousek et al. 1998). The basic premise of the intervention is to help patients formulate their own detailed lists of pros and cons for staying in their current conditions or attempting change. The clinician maintains an empathic, nonpreachy, Socratic stance.

For patients who concurrently demonstrate significant degrees of behavioral chaos, including self-harming behaviors, several programs are studying the potential utility of *dialectical behavior therapy* (Palmer et al. 2003; Telch et al. 2001).

Table 11–2.   Illustrative cognitive-behavioral therapy (CBT) manuals and related materials for clinicians and patients

CBT manuals for professionals

Fairburn CG, Wilson GT: *Binge Eating: Nature, Assessment, and Treatment.* New York, Guilford, 1993

Cooper Z, Fairburn CG, Hawker DM: *Cognitive-Behavioral Treatment of Obesity: A Clinician's Guide.* New York, Guilford, 2003

CBT manuals and self-help manuals for patients

Cash TF: *The Body Image Workbook.* Oakland, CA, New Harbinger Publications, 1997

Cooper PJ, Fairburn CG: *Bulimia Nervosa and Binge Eating: A Guide to Recovery.* London, Constable & Robinson, 1993

Fairburn CG: *Overcoming Binge Eating.* New York, Guilford, 1995

Freeman C: *Overcoming Anorexia Nervosa: A Self-Help Guide Using Cognitive Behavioural Techniques.* London, Robinson, 2002

McCabe R, McFarlane T, Olmsted M: *Overcoming Bulimia Workbook.* Oakland, CA, New Harbinger Publications, 2004

Heffner M, Eifert GH: *Overcoming Anorexia Workbook.* Oakland, CA, New Harbinger Publications, 2004

Paired manual sets for patients and clinicians

Treasure J, Schmidt U: *Getting Better Bit(e) by Bit(e): A Survival Kit for Sufferers of Bulimia Nervosa and Binge Eating Disorders.* Hove, East Sussex, UK, Psychology Press, 1993

Schmidt U, Treasure J: *Clinician's Guide to Getting Better Bit(e) by Bit(e).* Hove, East Sussex, UK, Psychology Press, 1997

Goodman LG, Villapiano M: *Eating Disorders: The Journey to Recovery Workbook.* New York, Brunner-Routledge, 2001

Villapiano M, Goodman LJ: *Eating Disorders—Time for Change: Plans, Strategies, Worksheets.* New York, Brunner-Routledge, 2001

Apple RF, Agras WS: *Overcoming Eating Disorder (ED): A Cognitive-Behavioral Treatment for Binge-Eating Disorder.* Client Kit. Oxford, UK, Oxford University Press, 1997

Agras WS, Apple RF: *Overcoming Eating Disorder (ED): A Cognitive-Behavioral Treatment for Binge-Eating Disorder.* Therapists' Edition. Oxford, UK, Oxford University Press, 1997

Table 11–2.   Illustrative cognitive-behavioral therapy (CBT) manuals and related materials for clinicians and patients *(continued)*

CD-ROM and Internet-based CBT programs for eating disorders

Commercial: self-help CBT for bulimia nervosa:

Take Control of Bulimia (http://www.myselfhelp.com/Programs/TCB.html)

Overcoming Bulimia by Drs. Chris Williams, Ulrike Schmidt (http://www.calipso.co.uk/mainframe.htm)

Current research using CD-ROM or Internet-based CBT programs:

Dr. Ulrike Schmidt et al., Institute of Psychiatry Eating Disorders Unit at the Maudsley Hospital, King's College, London (http://www.iop.kcl.ac.uk/IoP/Departments/PsychMed/EDU/index.shtml)

Dr. Chris Williams et al., University of Glasgow (http://www.gla.ac.uk/departments/psychologicalmedicine/staff/chriswilliams.html)

Dr. Jennifer Shapiro et al., University of North Carolina–NIMH–funded study of CD-ROM–based CBT for binge-eating disorder and obesity (http://www.unceatingdisorders.org)

Dr. Fernando Fernández Aranda et al., University Hospital of Bellvitge, Barcelona, Internet-based self-help: Guide for Treatment of Bulimia

For patients whose eating disorder–related or other dysfunctional core beliefs appear to be more deeply entrenched, a modified form of CBT called *schema-focused CBT* has been developed but has not yet been tested (Waller and Kennerley 2003). This therapy employs several additional cognitive techniques in an attempt to help patients modify and reframe their cognitive stances. As a way to help reduce "all or none," "black and white" thinking, patients are asked to rate their dysfunctional thoughts via a scaling/continuum technique that basically requires them to assign dimensional ratings to these thoughts, estimating the extent to which they are true. By means of positive data logs, patients are asked to produce objective evidence to support their distorted beliefs. (In the absence of supporting evidence, it is assumed, some patients may be able to revise their thinking.) A historical review—essentially a detailed thought record including ABCs (*a*ntecedents, *B*ehaviors, *C*onsequences)—is used to drill down more specifically on distorted thoughts and dysfunctional beliefs and schemas. Finally, visual restructuring is employed; this approach is essentially a form of guided imagery through which it is posited that nonverbal negative schemes may be assessed and modified.

Time/ Setting	Foods consumed	Eating disorder behavior (Behaviors)	Prior thoughts, feelings, and setting (Antecedents)	Subsequent thoughts, feelings, and setting (Consequences)
8:30 A.M.— home, breakfast	Coffee, bagel, cream cheese, 4 oz OJ	—	—	—
Noon— school, lunch	Turkey sandwich on wheat bread, apple, diet soda	—		
4 P.M.— home, snack	Glass of milk, chocolate chip cookie	—		
7 P.M.— dinner with family	Grilled chicken breast, salad, baked potato, small ice cream			
8 P.M.	Eating binge—bag of chips, pint of ice cream, 10 cookies	Vomit 3 times, plus take 2 laxatives	Mother was screaming at me—I couldn't stop her and couldn't handle it	After I vomited I was able to go back into the room and let her screaming bounce off me

Figure 11–1.   Illustrative self-monitoring diary of a patient in cognitive-behavioral therapy (CBT) for bulimia nervosa.

For eating disorder patients with significant comorbid complex personality disturbance, and particularly those who are prone to all-or-none thinking and splitting, cognitive-analytic therapy, a manual-based relatively brief psychotherapy, combines elements of cognitive therapy and a psychoanalytic therapy based on object relations hypotheses (Dare et al. 2001). In this model, eating disorder patients who experienced early parental traumas became more likely to develop splitting, with all-or-none thinking, revolving around "good/bad" schemes of the world. This model suggests that those who were in abusive/abused relationships with early figures are more likely to experience terror and rage, while those who experienced early parenting as controlling and felt crushed are likely to exhibit rebellious anger. The premise is that dealing with these issues will permit patients to reformulate their experiences, recognize their inner processes, and revise their thinking (Ryle 2004).

As described in Chapter 12 ("Psychodynamic Management of Eating Disorders") and Chapter 16, although they generally lack the research support of CBT, other psychotherapeutic approaches to eating disorders stemming from long-standing clinical traditions may help individual patients. In the final analysis, we require a more extensive and better-tested array of psychotherapies for patients with eating disorders, and we have to learn to use those strategies currently available to us with wisdom and compassion so that each individual patient who entrusts us with her care receives the best that we currently have to offer.

References

Agras WS, Apple RF: Overcoming Eating Disorder (ED): A Cognitive-Behavioral Treatment for Binge-Eating Disorder. Client Kit. Oxford, UK, Oxford University Press, 1997

Dare C, Eisler I, Russell G, et al: Psychological therapies for adults with anorexia nervosa: randomised controlled trial of out-patient treatments. Br J Psychiatry 178:216–221, 2001

Dunn EC, Neighbors C, Larimer ME: Motivational enhancement therapy and self-help treatment for binge eaters. Psychol Addict Behav 20:44–52, 2006

Fairburn CG: Body checking, body avoidance and "feeling fat." Presentation at the Academy for Eating Disorders International Conference on Eating Disorders, Barcelona, Spain, June 1, 2006

Fairburn CG, Marcus MD, Wilson GT:. Cognitive-behavior therapy for binge eating and bulimia nervosa: a comprehensive treatment manual, in Binge Eating: Nature, Assessment, and Treatment. Edited by Fairburn CG, Wilson GT. New York, Guilford, 1993, pp 361–404

Fairburn CG, Cooper Z, Shafran R: Cognitive behaviour therapy for eating disorders: a "transdiagnostic" theory and treatment. Behav Res Ther 41:509–528, 2003

Feld R, Woodside DB, Kaplan AS, et al: Pretreatment motivational enhancement therapy for eating disorders: a pilot study. Int J Eat Disord 29:393–400, 2001

Fisher PL, Wells A: Experimental modification of beliefs in obsessive-compulsive disorder: a test of the metacognitive model. Behav Res Ther 43:821–829, 2005

Garner DM, Vitousek KM, Pike KM: Cognitive-behavioral therapy for anorexia nervosa, in Handbook of Treatment for Eating Disorders, 2nd Edition. Edited by Garner DM, Garfinkel PE. New York, Guilford, 1997, pp 94–144

Halmi KA, Agras WS, Crow S, et al: Predictors of treatment acceptance and completion in anorexia nervosa: implications for future study designs. Arch Gen Psychiatry 62:776–781, 2005

McIntosh VV, Jordan J, Carter FA, et al: Three psychotherapies for anorexia nervosa: a randomized, controlled trial. Am J Psychiatry 162:741–747, 2005

McKenna PJ: Disorders with overvalued ideas. Br J Psychiatry 145:579–585, 1984

Miller WR, Rollnick S: Motivational Interviewing: Preparing People for Change, 2nd Edition. New York, Guilford, 2002

Palmer RL, Birchall H, Damani S, et al: A dialectical behavior therapy program for people with an eating disorder and borderline personality disorder—description and outcome. Int J Eat Disord 33:281–286, 2003

Pike KM, Walsh BT, Vitousek K, et al: Cognitive behavior therapy in the posthospitalization treatment of anorexia nervosa. Am J Psychiatry 160:2046–2049, 2003

Ryle A: The contributions of cognitive analytic therapy to the treatment of borderline personality disorder. J Pers Disord 18:3–35, 2004

Safran JD, Segal ZV: Interpersonal Process in Cognitive Therapy. New York, Basic Books, 1990

Shafran R, Teachman BA, Kerry S, et al: Br J Clin Psychol 38:167–179, 1999

Telch CF, Agras WS, Linehan MM: Dialectical behavior therapy for binge eating disorder. J Consult Clin Psychol 69:1061–1065, 2001

Vitousek K, Watson S, Wilson GT: Enhancing motivation for change in treatment-resistant eating disorders. Clin Psychol Rev 18:391–420, 1998

Waller G, Kennerley H: Cognitive-behavioural treatments, in Handbook of Eating Disorders, 2nd Edition. Edited by Treasure J, Schmidt U, van Furth E. Chichester, West Sussex, UK, Penguin, 2003, pp 233–251

Walsh BT, Kaplan AS, Attia E, et al: Fluoxetine after weight restoration in anorexia nervosa: a randomized controlled trial. JAMA 295:2605–2612, 2006

Wilson GT, Fairburn CG, Agras WS: Cognitive-behavioral therapy for bulimia nervosa, in Handbook of Treatment for Eating Disorders, 2nd Edition. Edited by Garner DM, Garfinkel PE. New York, Guilford, 1997, pp 67–93

12

Psychodynamic Management of Eating Disorders

Kathryn J. Zerbe, M.D.

From the patient's point of view, psychoanalysis does several things you can't get any other way. It provides support during the process of working through conscious and deeply unconscious separations and for bearing the pain that such losses entail. It maintains a sense of being listened to intently by a thoughtful person who will not let you be self-destructive without at least asking a question, but who will also, unblamingly, let you accept the consequences of your mistakes.... This results in something I've labeled "The Chamber of Truth," a condition where thoughts and feelings expressed freely allow reality to emerge.

Lucy Daniels, *With a Woman's Voice:*
A Writer's Struggle for Emotional Freedom

Lucy Daniels is a novelist and clinical psychologist living in North Carolina. When reviewing her list of professional and personal accomplishments, one would never suspect she also struggled for many years with a severe eating disorder. In her autobiography *With a Woman's Voice: A Writer's Struggle for Emotional Freedom* (Daniels 2001), she describes her journey out of the abyss of enormous emotional suffering.

Daniels' tale is remarkable, but clinicians who work in the subspecialty of eating disorders will not be surprised by the history she describes or the toll that a 45-year battle with anorexia nervosa took on her quality of life. She endured not only a 5-year psychiatric hospitalization for her anorexia but also a number of failed or marginally helpful therapeutic procedures, including forced feedings, electroconvulsive therapy and insulin therapy, and low-intensity supportive psychotherapies. Those personal dynamics that she believes played a significant role in her starvation—obsession with body-checking rituals, feelings of demoralization and disgrace, and antipathy toward her female body— are amply, and painfully, described in her memoir.

Daniels was born to a life of privilege. Her parents were wealthy, highly educated, ambitious, and driven. How could they miss the fact that their gifted, preadolescent daughter was severely depressed and emaciated and found it impossible in her misery to communicate with anyone? The reader can turn to almost any page and read a vignette about egregious empathic failures, glaring psychological impingements, and severe maltreatment in her family of origin. Like parents of many of our patients, Daniels' parents also tried to provide good things, and did so in many respects. What is unique about Daniels' tale is not the symptom profile of anorexia or even the family dynamic constellation of the depersonified child. Her odyssey is important for clinicians because it charts how she was able to disengage from her severe eating disorder to cultivate a fuller life and sense of self.

Daniels credits her success to her work in middle age with her psychoanalyst, Dr. Howie, with whom she found the words to describe her remarkable story, then reconstruct her life, and finally put childhood neglect, parental misattunement, and a range of disappointments into perspective in order to move forward. A clinician will quickly read between the lines and assume that even now Daniels has struggles with which to contend. Nonetheless, the memoir is full of hope about how an individual can come to survive, even thrive, even after years of marginal help managing a severe eating disorder. Daniels' autobiography is also a testament to how a psychoanalytically based therapy works, why it is supposed to work, and where it may succeed in ways that are qualitatively different from other important, and useful, treatment modalities described in this volume.

Psychodynamic psychotherapy as practiced in the twenty-first century is derived from psychoanalysis and shares many of the features. Differentiating between the two forms of treatment is beyond the scope of this chapter (see Blatt and Shahar 2005; Wallerstein 1986) and currently a matter of significant debate and ongoing research within the analytic community. For my purposes, the agreed-on commonalities between the therapeutic mechanisms of psychoanalysis and psychodynamic psychotherapy are highlighted as I seek to show how clinicians may pragmatically employ important concepts derived from this body of work in the psychosocial treatment of patients.

Key Aspects of Psychodynamic Therapy

A significant majority of patients with eating disorders do not respond to either medication or less-intensive psychotherapy but may benefit from more intensive, frequent, psychodynamic work (Hamburg et al. 1996; Thompson-Brenner and Westen 2005; Westen 2000; Yager 1988, 1992, Zerbe 1996, 2001a, 2001b, in press). I agree wholeheartedly with Lucy Daniels that psychodynamic treatment does "several things you can't get any other way" (p. 240). Her personal history provides a unique case example for a clinical paper because it is highly detailed; her voice speaks directly in a way that eludes cursory summaries and statistics.

I begin by expanding on five pivotal issues that Daniels found essential in her own treatment, which she comments on in the epigraph to this chapter: 1) providing support during the process of working through separation and loss; 2) listening intently as the patient reveals personal history; 3) confronting self-destructive behavior in order to develop better modes of coping; 4) sticking with the patient for a sufficient period of time, especially during times of perceived failure or weakness; and 5) creating a safe haven that is nonintrusive and helps the patient bear even the most difficult feelings or embarrassing experiences. These core aspects of psychodynamic psychotherapy and psychoanalysis lead, in the best of circumstances, to a patient's feeling a greater sense of "thrilling freedom" (Daniels 2001, p. 319) that paradoxically accompanies "the sensation—even if painful—of definitely being alive" (Daniels 2001, p. 302).

Providing Support During Working Through of Separation and Loss

No human being can traverse the stages of life without sustaining loss. Each real (e.g., abandonment, trauma, death, divorce, unachieved personal goal) and perceived (e.g., sense of failure for not having a perfect body; belief that one can never have a significant relationship; suspicion that one has failed one's parents) loss puts particular strain on the individual already suffering from an emotional or physical illness. Patients with eating disorders are faced with a complicated array of psychological and physical difficulties that underlie their specific problem, yet they must also negotiate normative developmental steps that entail dealing with loss. In particular, to recover from the eating disorder, the patient must eventually let go of (e.g., mourn) the role the eating disorder has played in her life as a pivotal aspect of identity (Boris 1984; Kearney-Cooke 1991; Zerbe 1993a, 2001a, in press). In addition, the patient must come to grips with common but painful losses that affect us all (e.g., empathic failures on the part of significant people in our lives; sense of not always being loved for the person one is or the real talents one brings to the world; moving out of one's home to attend college or get a job; growing up and separating from the family of origin; actual death of a beloved parent, grandparent, primary caretaker, sibling, friend, mentor, or spouse). The acquisition of autonomy and separation is founded on a capacity to mourn. As Daniels (2001) summarizes, asserting one's personhood is "costly," and "[c]laiming my voice has separated me from people with whom I once had a semblance of belonging" (p. 319).

Regardless of the actual cause of a given person's eating disorder, the multifarious tolls it takes on the psyche place the individual in a state of compromise in dealing with these psychological realities. As Daniels alludes to in her statement, the psychodynamic therapist who accompanies the patient on her journey into better health will hear many tales over a prolonged period of time and in a safe place of losses that must be successfully worked through in order to grow and give up the coping mechanism of disordered eating (see Bowlby 1988). This process leads to substantially greater "emotional freedom" but requires significant time and patience. And, as Daniels further describes, growing up and moving away from the eating problem always comes with an added price tag of eventually leaving treatment, because "it has brought a new form of aloneness" that "reminds me sadly that the time is coming when the next step in this freedom march will require me to leave Dr. Howie" (p. 319). Ultimately, therapist and patient are both required to bear the feelings of letting go lest an unproductive sense of dependency or treatment impasse stymie autonomy (Kearney-Cooke 1991; Rinsley 1982; Zerbe, in press).

Each of us knows from personal experience that loss is not worked through quickly, hence one of the reasons that a psychodynamic process takes significant time (usually 2–5 years, and sometimes even longer, as in Daniels' case). Some contemporary therapies—for example, interpersonal psychotherapy (IPT)—also emphasize the importance of working on loss as a pivotal aspect of treatment, and research has documented the benefit that IPT has for a wide array of persons working with an acute loss (Weissman et al. 2000). What is different for the person with an eating problem, and hence the need for a more in-depth process that evolves over time, is that the losses are neither clear nor relatively simple, nor does the patient have the internal emotional ballast to work with them on her own.

The regular, frequent meetings (one to four times per week) form a cocoon around the patient so that the losses can be processed and worked through until the butterfly (e.g., a nascent sense of self that can deal with loss and begin to perceive oneself as functioning without the eating disorder) can emerge. Also implicit in this model is how the patient has the time and space to move through the normative stages of separation and individuation (Mahler et al. 1975), frequently "checking back" with the therapist as the child does during the rapprochement subphase. In so doing, the sense of becoming oneself as an individuated human being emerges over time, along with the "ineluctable urge" (Rinsley 1980, 1982) to eventually separate. The patient practices the range of feelings that inevitably arise during times of separation from the therapist, such as interruptions between sessions, weekend and vacation separations, and even unplanned absences. These normative separations become a speakable and meaningful part of the work, helping to form an emotional ballast as the patient internalizes the therapist.

Part of the "chamber of truth" that our patients have missed is the opportunity to speak truth to power growing up. How often have we heard adults confide that their childhood feelings of anger, resentment, shame, mortification, disappointment, or simple disagreement with parents, siblings, teachers, and other important people in their lives were unwelcome (see Bowlby 1988; Miller 1981; Zerbe 1993a, 1999, 2001a, 2001b)? Revealing their vulnerable feelings led to minimization, devaluation, punishment, and reprimands. They appear to have never experienced being taken seriously or recognized for their unique selves. Consequently, their powerful feelings remained unspoken but subsequently make their appearance in dysregulated affect states, manifesting themselves in eating disorder symptoms or other psychological disorder (e.g., personality disorder) (Thompson-Brenner and Westen 2005). Experiencing and processing these long-suppressed, split-off affects in the therapeutic relationship results in a sense of knowing oneself better, feeling understood, and being permitted, even encouraged, to speak one's own truth, the telltale therapeutic marker that an individuated human being is emerging and able to engage more fully in life (see also Knapp 2003 for another autobiographical account of these principles in the treatment of an eating disorder).

Imparting a Sense of Being Listened to Intently

When Daniels shares the value of being listened to intently, she pinpoints a value and tradition of psychodynamic work: the creation of the individual life narrative (Schafer 1983, 1992; Spence 1982). The treatment frame of a regular time and "safe place" where the patient's individual life story can unfold at its own pace is one of the central tenets of psychodynamic work because it harbors the mechanism for therapeutic change. Self-reflective capacities expand (Fonagy et al. 2000, 2002; Mitrani 1995) as patients "begin to consider issues of self-definition and sense of agency" (Blatt and Shahar 2005, p. 429). Lucy Daniels captures these scientific principles embedded in the dyadic patient–therapist relationship poetically: "Listening...Listening...LISTENING in a way that filled the whole room with me. Making me what mattered, in pain and confused at first and then later clearer and more confident or sometimes even amazed at hearing myself" (p. 270).

As the story is told and retold, the individual becomes more comfortable with her own humanness and with those around her. Even the internal objects paradigms in the patient's world undergo modification. Psychodynamic psychotherapy thus proceeds from surface to depth, with the patient gradually revealing new facets of herself as she engages in the work and overcomes her difficulties (e.g., resistances) to telling more about herself.

In an atmosphere of relative neutrality, the psychodynamic therapist refrains from exhortations or directives regarding the patient's eating disorder, at least as much as possible. Conventional wisdom encourages an atmosphere of neutrality because it provides an ambiance in which the patient can develop her own life story or narrative with as few encumbrances as possible. Maintaining neutrality in the face of a life-threatening eating disorder is always quite difficult, and sometimes impossible, because the clinician is placed in a position where the patient's life must be saved first. Consequently, it is important that the adjective *relative* be used as a modifier before the noun *neutrality*. Nonetheless, as much as possible, a listening stance that seeks to draw out the patient through empathy, reflection, and patience serves the double purpose of helping the patient define who she is and who she is not. In this way, the self of the person with an eating disorder expands in its capacity to weather affect storms and to deal constructively with reality without regressing as frequently in the direction of the eating disorder.

Confronting Self-Destructive Behavior

All eating disorder behaviors, almost by definition, are self-destructive and potentially life-threatening. Each therapeutic modality (e.g., cognitive-behavioral therapy, hospitalization, patient education, medication) addresses this dimension of illness to ensure patient improvement and eventual relinquishment of the eating disorder. Psychodynamic psychotherapy seeks to understand why the patient must attack her body and thereby relentlessly preclude a sense of basic pleasure (i.e., eating, sexuality) in life. Significant developmental deficits (brought about by, e.g., constitutional diathesis, childhood maltreatment, sexual abuse, parental misattunement and narcissism, and compromised boundaries within the family of origin) undergird severe eating disorders and make it unlikely that manifest symptoms will come under control quickly. Research and long-term outcome studies certainly bear this out. Hence, any clinician who works with eating disorder patients must develop his or her own style for confronting and working with the ongoing plethora of self-destructive behaviors that accompany the process of healing.

In psychodynamic psychotherapy, the patient will play out in the transference the needs to undo forward movement by acting out, usually in the direction of a recrudescence of the eating problem or other self-destructive behavior (e.g., not coming to sessions, self-mutilation, refusing to take medications or meet with other team members such as a nutritionist or internist). The psychodynamic therapist takes an active role in seeing these behaviors as ultimately self-defeating and in "asking the question" about the patient's understanding of why this undermining of the self is happening at this time in the treatment.

Herein lies the moment when treatment becomes most alive, and most dicey, for patient and therapist. On a conscious level, the patient says she wants to improve, and she may have already made excellent use of a range of therapeutic tools such as education or cognitive-behavioral therapy, a circumstance that implies that she is making strides. How can her relapse be productively worked with, especially if she has an unconscious need to defeat herself? In some cases, the individual seeks to defy the therapist, because by being helped to overcome the eating problem, the patient has the unconscious notion that the therapist is "taking over my body" and "making me into somebody just like you" (Bromberg 1996, 2001; McDougall 1989; Zerbe 1993b, 1996). This common transference pattern derives from the dynamic wish to both separate from and punish the primary caretaker (usually the mother) and reflects profound conflict in separation–individuation and pathological enmeshment in the family of origin. The patient may also feel guilty about moving forward because it means doing better than others and puts her in a loyalty bind.

Psychodynamic psychotherapy will "reactivate a previously disrupted developmental process" (Blatt and Shichman 1983, p. 249) in order for the patient to achieve a sense of greater self-definition and sense of relatedness. By repeatedly pointing out the undermining tendencies and poor self-care ubiquitous among eating disorder patients, is not the therapist helping to correct a developmental deficit that eventuates in more mature, autonomous functioning? Deficits of this kind are frequently seen in families in which there have been turmoil, abuse, and continual bickering; sometimes the child is placed in the role of the parent's caretaker (the so-called parentified or depersonified child), which necessitates leaving the needful parent behind if one is to lead one's own life. Whatever the particular dynamic at play, the patient must develop new modes of coping given the real and perceived impingements on her life or she will likely backslide into her old coping strategies of self-destructive behavior. Repeatedly raising questions about the meaning of the patient's progress and relapses helps set the stage for mastery, ultimately leading to enhanced sense of autonomy and mature dependency.

Once again, an example from Daniels' memoir documents this process. Although the patient did not mention that she was developing a severe writing block while other forward leaps were being made with respect to her anorexia, her analyst questioned her about the absence of comments about her work and what a slowdown in her creative process might be pointing toward in her emotional life. Daniels valued the confrontation, explaining a range of reactions to the query about her block: "Sometimes I would remain silent. Sometimes I'd make excuses or express doubt. But over time I came to welcome those questions and to feel grateful for Dr. Howie's 'challenge'" (p. 273).

Sticking With the Patient During Times of Perceived Weakness

All human beings on the trajectory of growth must inevitably weather disappointment, experience backslides, confront weaknesses, and become more aware of aspects of themselves of which they are not proud. Paradoxically, achievement of any kind is often met with a sense of loss of what or whom one is leaving behind in order to move to a new plateau; anxiety about taking on and mastering the new role or identity propels a backslide. In psychodynamic parlance, this disquieting pattern is termed a "success neurosis" and is familiar to some degree in anyone who closely observes himself or herself. This propensity to "grab defeat from the jaws of victory" can range from being downright embarrassing to being seriously self-defeating. Take, for example, the proverbial student who never finishes the thesis and so never graduates, or the pining romantic who says she desperately wants to marry but always manages to choose the "wrong type" of partner and never makes it to the altar. In both examples, the person consciously wants so much to have something better in life but on another level stays entrenched in self-defeating patterns.

During long-term psychodynamic psychotherapy, the clinician inevitably witnesses surges of progress that are often followed by expectable but temporary regressions because development is never a linear process. Patients with eating disorders frequently relapse even as they move forward and are likely to feel a sense of shame, worthlessness, and defeat; these relapses frequently herald a partial return of the original eating disorder symptoms (e.g., purging, dieting, overuse of exercise) or may take on a more global form of emotional illness (e.g., becoming seriously depressed or anxious, having significant interpersonal conflicts). At these pivotal moments patients need the therapist more than ever to provide a sense of stability, hopefulness, and perspective lest they become inundated with a sense of defeat and paralyzed by shame or guilt.

In the history a range of dynamics may be found to play a role in the patient's perception of failure or weakness. The therapist may find high family expectations or absent caretakers who were not available to shepherd the patient through normative life transitions. By sticking with a person at times of defeat or disappointment, the therapist helps the patient achieve a new level of mastery in at least two ways. The patient has the "corrective emotional experience" (Alexander and French 1946; Friedman 1978) of learning that support is available and constructive, even when one is feeling flawed or deficient. The patient also has the essential opportunity to grasp that reversals of fortune and feelings of inadequacy happen to each of us and are more likely to be conquered when they can be met head on. The emotions encountered are thereby consciously processed as opposed to being split off, leading to further integration of a sense of self as someone who has both strengths and weaknesses (Bromberg 1996, 2001; A. Goldberg 1999; Zerbe 1993b, 2001b).

Lucy Daniels (2001) explains that her writing block was overcome quite gradually because it derived from conflicting feelings of attraction and repulsion she harbored toward her psychologically abusive father. Her analyst's patience ("continual listening" [p. 273], "saying useful things along the way" [p. 302]) permitted her the emotional space to eventually cleave creative inhibitions and romantic yearnings, all worked through in a series of dream images she analyzed that revealed her feelings of shame and inadequacy as a woman. Psychodynamic psychotherapy seeks to make all of the inevitable ups and downs of life something that can be spoken about so that they will not have to be enacted by more unconsciously based, self-destructive symptoms. Little wonder it takes longer than other modes of treatment. In psychodynamic psychotherapy, regressions and "perceived failure" are actually welcomed as an essential part of the work of becoming a real person who can more honestly and directly deal with crisis, frustration, failure, setbacks, and normative transitions over the life cycle and emerge the stronger person for having done so.

Creating a Safe Haven Where the "Private Self" Can Grow

In families in which there has been discord, impingement, anxiety, or trauma, the child often emerges with difficulties in self-soothing and failures in object constancy. Infant research demonstrates how babies regulate periods of engagement and disengagement from their caretakers and so develop the sense of "being fueled from within" (Edelman 1992; Schore 2001, 2003, 2005). That is, in order for normative development to continue, the child must achieve the capacity to hold the caretaker in mind during times of distress. One important outcome of this process is the attainment of a sense of emotional equilibrium in times of angst and eventual mastery over uncomfortable, potentially painful situations.

Each school of psychotherapy implicitly recognizes that a failure to regulate affect and soothe the self in times of distress is a major difficulty encountered in the treatment of eating disorders. Various techniques are suggested (e.g., challenging core beliefs; using affirmations, meditation, yoga, or relaxation exercises; writing in a journal) to rectify the problem. The cultivation of a "private self" that has the capacity to find comfort in solitude and to process experience and find meaning in it is an essential feature of psychodynamic psychotherapy (Modell 1993; Winnicott 1960/1965). These are particularly important qualities for the patient with an eating disorder to cultivate because she must learn to withstand being alone and coping without turning to her manifest symptom. Indeed, when questioned about the prelude to a binge or a relapse into excessive exercise, restriction, or purging, the patient will often tell the clinician, "I just cannot stand to be alone."

To live successfully, all persons must develop the capacity to be alone (Winnicott 1960/1965), and the "companionable solitude" of psychodynamic psychotherapy provides the "private space and private time" where the individual can practice doing just that. As psychoanalyst Arnold Modell (1993) further explains, this capacity is "the mirror image of relatedness" that "affords the individual a certain degree of freedom from the domination of the past" (p. 185). The capacity to be alone inevitably signals greater opportunity for the patient to be able to make successful interpersonal separations from her family of origin that will eventuate in termination of treatment. Lucy Daniels believes that her psychoanalysis "brought a new form of aloneness" and "solitary freedom" (p. 319) that could be borne because she internalized Dr. Howie.

Additional Psychodynamic Considerations

In the sections that follow, I use clinical examples from practice and supervisory sessions to illustrate some other principles of psychodynamic theory that help effect change in the therapy of patients with severe eating disorders. The selected issues appear with relative frequency in longer-term therapy with patients. I have found that thinking about each of these areas helps to conceptualize treatment, particularly if an impasse in the treatment seems to have been reached. Working within each domain also appears to have a relatively high yield in moving therapy forward and enabling therapist and patient to gain greater understanding of the individual's psychic reality, with beneficial results.

Understanding the Ubiquitous Role of Conflict

Understanding and teasing apart overt or subtle intrapsychic conflict has always played a pivotal role in psychodynamic psychotherapy. Initially, even anorexia was formulated as a woman's conflict between her wish to become pregnant and her defense against it (Freud 1892–1899/1962; see also Battegay 1991; Farrell 2000). While this formulation may be relevant in a minority of cases, clinical experience demonstrates that the array of conflicts patients struggle with is much greater than inhibitions in expressing their libidinal impulses alone. In the late twentieth century, eating disorders were understood, by Hilde Bruch, also as resulting from developmental deficits and family enmeshment (Bruch 1973, 1978). In essence, Bruch emphasized the patient's conflict about staying in the role of a child or growing up and leaving the family of origin.

This emphasis on failure to achieve a sense of separateness led to other kinds of psychological conflict being minimized in therapy. Because the important formulation of "enmeshment" did not address all core concerns of patients, working with intrapsychic conflicts is finding new application in a large list of psychiatric conditions, including eating disorders (Abend 2005; Brenner 1982, 1994; Smith 2005; Zerbe 2001b, in press). When unacknowledged longings are uncovered, inhibitions in expressing anger or showing appropriate aggression are made expressible, and the self-destructive forces propelling the individual toward death are interpreted, demonstrable shifts in the patient's functioning are sometimes observed. Thus, the clinician must consider how aspects of anorexia, bulimia, and binge-eating disorder might be disguises of overt or subtle conflict, as the following examples attest.

Clinical Examples

Lindsay, now age 21, entered puberty early. Peers would make fun of her, and she would naturally feel overtly embarrassed but unconsciously angry. She also struggled with her maturation, remembering that as she developed breasts and achieved menarche, her father spent less time with her. Sometimes he would also tease, which led her to feel she "needed to hide." Lindsay retreated from competitive swimming and debate, and gained 50 pounds between ages 12 and 16. In psychodynamic psychotherapy, she talked about development of her eating disorder but made no connection between the changes in her body image and other people's negative reactions.

Lindsay denied any history of sexual or physical abuse. When it was pointed out that she tended to hesitate when talking about her father's pulling away from her, she became curious about the pattern. Over time she was able to link periods of turning toward food as a way of managing her feelings about her father's negative attention. Interpretations centered on the conflict Lindsay felt between her love for her father and anger at him for what she experienced as making fun of her. Teasing apart elements of her conflict between love and hate led to a notable shift in her affect regulation and her eating disorder management by facilitating individuation and self-assertion (Blum 2003).

Lindsay began to talk straightforwardly about her experiences and turn to food less often. In her case, food was much less a modality of self-soothing than it is for others. Her weight gain signified an inner battle about growing up and her relationship to her father and peers. Lindsay's binge eating and adolescent weight ensured that she did not act out sexually, thereby maintaining a close, albeit unconscious, tie to her father. As this conflict about separation from her father was worked with in the psychotherapy process, she came to recognize that her fears about sex and expressing frustration and irritation were linked to her unconscious anxieties about alienating, and potentially losing, her father.

Devon was an 18-year-old compulsive exerciser with anorexia nervosa. He was determined to become a professional soccer player and practiced relentlessly despite family interventions and multimodal outpatient care (e.g., psychotropic medication, nutritional counseling, individual psychotherapy, professional physical training to help regulate the amount of exercise). After a successful inpatient hospitalization in which Devon gained enough weight and control over his symptoms to return to college, his individual psychotherapy process deepened.

While genetic and biological factors were clearly implicated in Devon's case (his younger sister suffered from facial tics and obsessive-compulsive disorder), he confided that he worried about the state of his parents' marriage and was preoccupied by his sister's psychiatric disorder. According to Devon, everyone in the nuclear family was always "mad about something but never able to talk about it." When encouraged to speak openly about why he felt so burdened, Devon remarked that he was angry because he never seemed to be able to please his father. Interestingly, this was also Devon's mother's complaint about her husband.

The intrapsychic conflicts that this young man struggled with played a significant role in the development of his anorexia, as evidenced by the fact that his need to exercise all of the time diminished when his annoyance and disappointment regarding his father brought to the fore. In essence, Devon's major conflict centered on unexpressed anger and worry about his father's role and lack of responsibility in the family; Devon "ran off" his rage on the soccer field. But Devon also had loving feelings, as evidenced by his pursuit of a goal (e.g., career in sports) from which he felt he would win his father's coveted affection. In his illness lay the embedded wish to both acquire approval and show his aggression and disappointment to the object of his affection, his father.

Devon's illness also hinged on an unresolved conflict in growing up in a household where he felt responsible for his mother's and sister's well-being. His commitment to sports represented a libidinal investment in moving forward in life, doing something he wanted that was productive for himself. On the other hand, his illness ensured the attention of his parents and kept him in the role of a youngster who needed support and help. Needless to say, family therapy was also an essential component in addressing the interpersonal conflicts that paralyzed Devon. In individual therapy, additional conflicts he felt between his loyalty and love for his family and the immobilizing nature of his anger were repeatedly pointed out, leading to a diminishment over time of his exercise addiction. He became more able to put into words the intense feeling states heretofore embedded in his food restriction and overexercise, leading to increased emotional freedom and sense of self.

Decreasing the Need for Self-Punishment

Another characteristic of a psychodynamic psychotherapy process is explicit work with the patient's sense of guilt and self-recrimination. Self-starvation, various means of purging, excessive exercise, and the like all paradoxically serve as ways the person organizes and punishes the self. As ego organization consolidates over time, healthier coping mechanisms must come into play wherein the person displays better self-care. A marker for the therapist is not only improved control of eating symptoms but also the patient's concomitant enhanced capacity to feel that she has a right to live her own life with less guilt and need to punish herself for having good things.

At the conclusion of a successful psychodynamic psychotherapy, the patient should have an increased capacity for realistic gratification outside of the eating disorder. Most clinicians are struck by how individuals equate their eating disorder with their identity and cling to it. As treatment proceeds the patient has the in vivo experience of not being punished for living her own life. The patient is encouraged to have areas of interests and movement into new realms where realistic gratification is possible. As Weiss and Sampson (Weiss et al. 1986) have pointed out, patients often engage in a series of tests of the therapist when they are attempting to move forward. They expect the therapist to have a negative reaction to their resolve to think their own thoughts and live autonomously. The therapist's neutrality, and sometimes even encouragement, will be important technical devices in helping a patient to work through an unconscious sense of guilt, especially guilt for living one's own life.

Clinical Example

Bette was the second child and only daughter of an alcoholic businessman and his anxiety-ridden, agoraphobic spouse. Bette grew up sacrificing many of her own desires in order to take care of her mother, who was inhibited from leaving the family home. Bette was able to attend a small community college and finished her degree as a dental assistant by managing her own anxiety by stuffing herself with baked goods from local coffee shops and delicatessens. By the time she sought treatment, Bette was clinically depressed, anxiety ridden, and dangerously out of control with her eating.

In one notable segment of a treatment that took 3 years, Bette explained that she was able to put more limits on herself when taking care of her mother (and, by inference, in the transference, the therapist). She became silent after talking about her goals and seemed to be worried about what was going to happen next. Her thoughts proceeded in a stop-start fashion as if she were trying to hold back her sense of accomplishment lest she be punished for moving ahead. Her therapist was aware that Bette was experiencing more realistic gratification in her life but that she was likely terrified by the guilt she felt in moving away from her caretaking functions. Repeated interpretations of Bette's fear of being left alone and/or punished for doing better became a cornerstone of the work.

Demonstrating How and Why History Repeats Itself

Repetition of themes is also central to the work of psychodynamic psychotherapy. Over time, the patient comes to gain perspective by witnessing "the repetition and reenactment of wish, intent, and sentiment" (Galatzer-Levy and Cohler 1993) play themselves out over and over again. The sense of self grows when, with each retelling, the focus shifts and deepens, leading to greater mastery of maturity, integrity, and self-coherence. With each retelling the role of therapist is central, because the very act of being listened to intently helps one hear additional details of one's own story with new meaning, perspective, and compassion.

Clinical Example

Lauren was a 39-year-old woman who entered treatment for bulimia. Soon other problems also became apparent. "It's the same story all over again," Lauren said well into the sixth year of an expressive process. She was beginning to see how her difficulties in the workplace were caused by problems with affective regulation, the very same type of affect problem that had led her to seek treatment for her eating disorder in the first place.

Instead of speaking directly to her angry feelings, she would binge eat and then overexercise. Lauren did not believe that others would hear her complaints and be able to come to some kind of accommodation or compromise. Consequently, she withdrew into a solitary life, convinced that no job or person could ever be fulfilling.

Determined that no one would see into her loneliness, she stayed quiet and aloof from others, being a better caretaker than a care receiver. Beneath the facade of a hard-working, concerned wife and daughter stood an emotionally emaciated individual who was bitter and angry about the nurturance she felt she should have gotten but was denied. Her cycles of angry withdrawal followed by obsequious importuning put everyone on notice that her emotional reactions could not be trusted.

What convinced the patient of her need to change was seeing the repetition play itself out time and time again under different circumstances in the creation of her personal life narrative. The surface story was her eating disorder, but only hearing the backstory led to a more in-depth appraisal of her internal object world and eventual control of bulimia. Through it all, central themes repeated themselves time and time again, but with new additions and more mastery every time she discussed her life.

Working With Negative Transference and the Ability to Be the "Bad Object"

The capacity to hate as well as love is a developmental achievement (Blum 1997; Winnicott 1960/1965). For those individuals who have not had the experience in childhood of trusting their caretakers to be with them during outbursts of anger or angry withdrawal, for fear of punishment or abandonment, being able to feel hatred or become enraged with the therapist is a sign of significant progress. Allowing the patient to integrate both positive and negative transference is one of the most time-consuming and personally demanding aspects of psychodynamic therapy because the process requires reworking of the patient's entire internal object world.

None of us went into this field to be disliked by our patients, so containing and working with their hatred is demanding. It feels assaultive (Zerbe 1993a, 2001a, in press). Yet progress is frequently observed in what transpires outside of the therapy hours, as when a patient has improved capacity to handle strains at work or in relationships without turning to the eating disorder. By making negative transference feelings discussable or by taking on the role of the "bad object" (Fairbairn 1943) without becoming defensive, the therapist enables the patient to move into a new developmental position where love and hate can be more freely experienced and integrated.

Clinical Example

When Lissa entered treatment for bulimia nervosa, everything in her life seemed to have a negative valence. She collected injustices. She came to every session on time and seemed to work hard, only to do an about-face after the hour and let the therapist know in no uncertain terms that nothing that was said or done was helping very much. For 4 years she railed against every intervention the therapist made. What the therapist said or did not say, her office location, the décor of the office, the therapist's physique, and even the therapist's pets (she had once seen the therapist walking her dogs in a neighborhood park and gleefully taunted her by saying how "ugly" they were) were fodder for her projections of how poorly she felt about herself.

The therapist sought consultation and decided to take on the role of the "bad object," allowing the patient to project these hated aspects of herself out onto "the other" for a reasonable period of time. Theoretically, the patient would take back these noxious aspects of herself over time and integrate them into herself as a whole person, a self that views others ambivalently and is more fully human. When one's own strengths and weaknesses can be taken into account, one has less psychological need to make someone else the bad object and thereby rid oneself of imperfections and flaws.

As the therapy unfolded, the patient came to appreciate that others, especially her parents, had done the best they could with what they were given. No wonder the patient struggled so mightily with an eating disorder—it was clearly a multigenerational issue. The patient learned in discussions with her mother that her grandmother had regaled the mother during adolescence and adulthood with stories of her own body image problems and had made the patient's mother feel guilty and depleted for her own desires to live away from the family of origin.

The therapist's capacity to withstand Lissa's onslaught over time resulted in a "reworking" of the patient's internal object world. She no longer spoiled relationships by making others into the enemy. Moreover, she had less need to perceive her body as her enemy, the ultimate "bad object." She was able to take in the good that the therapist, and others, had to offer her, becoming more of a "true self" (Winnicott 1960/1965, 1988) who no longer required perfection of herself or others.

Integrating Sensory Data

Clinicians who work with eating disorder patients know how sensitive these patients can be to disturbances in the external environment, even an apparently small change such as in the arrangement of furniture in the therapist's office. These sensitivities are difficult to understand at first and to appropriately respond to clinically. The late Francis Tustin was a British analyst who described preoccupation with raw sensory experience as an autistic phenomenon that begins in infancy as a way of organizing sensory data, particularly on the skin surface (Hunter 1994; Tustin 1986, 1990). Shifts in the physical environment cause perturbation on the body surface that lead eating disorder patients to "compulsively repair leaks in their sensory self" (Schneider 1995, p. 181) by turning to eating symptoms.

All human beings have reactions to changes in their environment that reflect sensitivity to their surrounds, but the developmental arrest of anorexic and bulimic patients impairs their sense of feeling physically contained in their own bodies. They do not adjust to changes readily and seek physical, as opposed to emotional, grounding. Hence, they will turn to the "compulsive and rhythmic" nature of their symptoms on a quest for maternal soothing and calming. Their sensitivity to objects in the therapist's office or remarks about the feel or touch of food in their mouths denote a primitive way these patients find a sense of safety. Theoretically, as one proceeds up the developmental ladder, words are used to describe experiences, and higher-level defenses come into play to help one deal with one's "bad feelings" (Schafer 2003).

Individuals with eating disorders attempt to "repair" themselves through their eating disorder symptoms. Their bingeing or restriction is "the 'glue' to hold these persons together" (Schneider 1995, p. 181) and speaks to a developmental arrest at the autistic-contiguous position (Ogden 1989). In effect, experiences like gorging, evacuations, and relentless exercising that accompany some eating disorders can form a kind of protection that helps hold unintegrated parts of the person together. As the patient develops words to describe experiences and comes to trust the regularity of the therapeutic environment and master separations, new developmental levels are reached.

Early in treatment the therapist must listen carefully for the sensory data revealed in the patient's communication about food or the environment and attempt to help the patient integrate these experiences into life. The therapist must also consider how the patient may be using food as a transitional experience to separate from or to be close to those in her object world.

Clinical Example

Marie was a 17-year-old college freshman with subclinical anorexia and severe depression. In the second month of treatment this gaunt, brilliant woman asked her therapist if it was "bad or good" that she ate a gallon of ice cream every day, since she was starting to feel less depressed. While pleased that the therapy and medication seemed to be working, the therapist knew that more was going on that Marie wanted—but needed—to put into words. Sensing it was important to get in touch with the sensory experience of the patient, he wondered if the patient ate the ice cream "for taste or flavor." The patient replied that it was not the taste itself but rather the experience of cold in the mouth, "like an ice cube."

The therapist went on to help the patient describe exactly how the "smooth, creamy, soft, and cold" sensations felt in the patient's mouth and as they traveled down her esophagus. In a family therapy session, the patient's mother spoke about how she was exasperated with the patient and "would have never left the carton on the cabinet" if she had known that the patient would eat all of the ice cream. In this situation the patient was using the ice cream as a primitive form of separation from mother. She was starting to eat what she wanted instead of following her mother's advice. By wondering if the ice cream is "bad or good," she actually conveyed in a sensory mode a new capacity for new self-definition. Contained in her act of eating and feeling the ice cream was a primitive boundary she was establishing between her and her mother.

Evolving Psychodynamic Research: Implications for Therapeutic Change

Studies of the efficacy of psychodynamic psychotherapy in the treatment of patients with eating disorders are growing but still limited. Most of the studies to date are of small samples or individual case reports (Dare et al. 2001). As Dare and Crowther (1995) opined, from their years of experience doing psychodynamic psychotherapy at the Maudsley Hospital in London, psychoanalytic psychotherapy has clear benefit for a select number of patients, but trials are challenging to execute and to fund.

In Dare and Crowther's (1995) study of a time-limited approach (i.e., 1 year), the authors confirmed their hypothesis that the patient–therapist alliance and a formulation of a "focal hypothesis" about the patient's difficulties are essential to good outcomes. Specifically, the therapists in their study attempted to help the patient understand the role the symptoms held in life. They found that the eating disorder served multiple functions, including helping the patient suppress affect, retain a sense of powerlessness in interpersonal relationships, and sabotage forward movement in life. Even though the therapists were all novices to the psychodynamic approach and the cohort of very ill patients presented formidable resistances to engaging in treatment, notable gains were observed over the course of the year.

Dare and Crowther concluded that while more research with longer follow-up is essential to ascertain the circumstances in which a psychodynamic approach will be most useful and cost-effective, for a sizable number of patients this approach has substantial benefit for symptom control. Interestingly, the factors they found most important to outcome were also ones embedded in Lucy Daniels' memoir and quotations I selected for this chapter. Dare and Crowther (1995) summarized their findings thus: "Psychotherapy can open the door on a particular way of thinking, can provide a new view of oneself in the world, and as an understanding of relationships can be a resource that the patient carries away into the future" (p. 307).

Dare and Crowther's research also confirmed some other long-held clinical wisdom about applying psychodynamic psychotherapy to eating disorders:
the therapist needs to deviate from the traditional shibboleth of absolute ano-
nymity, be prepared to be a real person and show feeling, and not fear employing
interpretation. Other key constituents found in the research were the role of
the therapist–patient relationship (i.e., transference and countertransference
paradigms), demonstrating the influential role of the past on the present,
making use of the insights derived from contemporary self psychology and object relations therapy, and facilitating expression of and understanding of the
patient's core conflicts and family history. In order to *gradually* expand awareness, Dare and Crowther contend, the therapist acts as a good container of the
patient's terrifying inner world. This silent tolerance of powerful feelings on
the part of the therapist promotes the development of autonomy in the patient. Later on, more direct confrontation of resistances and defenses, particularly
related to guilt and shame, can go on to ensure expansion of the patient's healthy
ego.

Contemporary psychodynamic psychotherapy is also a "life stage" theory,
one that grounds itself in early infancy and the life of the child but does not
stop there. Attachment patterns (see Fonagy et al. 2000, 2002; S. Goldberg et
al. 1995) and Margaret Mahler's (Mahler et al. 1975) stages of separation/in-
dividuation are being applied to patients with eating disorders on the basis of
infant research findings. For example, in some centers eating disorders have
been linked to disorganized, dismissing, and insecure attachment patterns
(Candelori and Ciocca 1998; Fonagy et al. 2002; S. Goldberg et al. 1995).
The European Collaborative Longitudinal Study on Eating Disorders (i.e.,
European Union Research COST Programme) is drawing on contemporary
attachment research designs to test the effectiveness and efficacy of a broad array of psychotherapy treatment programs. This Europe-wide research will likely
yield data to help clinicians stage-match patients with interventions for eating
disorders depending on a range of specific factors. Those patients who need
only a low-intensity treatment will be supplied a manual-based treatment and
differentiated from those whose interpersonal difficulties and underlying attachment problems are likely to require a longer-term, and significantly greater-
intensity, treatment (Treasure 1998; Treasure and Schmidt-1997, 1999).
These treatments are bound to have a significant focus on interpersonal fac-

tors and development of self, thereby making use of some of the implicitly long-held psychodynamic psychotherapy principles described in this chapter.

Finally, a series of articles have been published in the past few years based on intricate analysis of the observations of experienced clinicians. These clinician-reported data are being studied in aggregate form, and inferences made from them will inform the treatment of eating disorders (Betan et al. 2005; Thompson-Brenner and Westen 2005; Westen 2000; Westen and Harnden-Fischer 2001; Westen et al. 2004). These studies are not only demonstrating the different personality subtypes of eating disorders that can predict treatment length and outcome but also suggesting the range of interventions that can be commonly applied "to help regulate emotions, contain impulsivity, and resolve crises with more dysregulated patients" (Thompson-Brenner and Westen 2005, p. 522).

Like all research studies, this practice network approach of clinician reported data has strengths and limitations. However, one yield is documenting what practitioners actually do and how clinicians adjust their strategies for the so-called difficult-to-treat patient. According to these reports, psychodynamic therapists make greater use of cognitive-behavioral therapy interventions, and cognitive-behavioral therapists employ more psychodynamic interventions, for patients with the "difficult," dysregulated, more treatment-refractory subtypes. These reports bear ongoing scrutiny because they will help practitioners determine more of the specific constituents of a truly integrated treatment plan (Westen 2005). The data will also likely add evidence to the assumption that most clinicians make use of dynamic principles, even when they may not realize it consciously, and augur for greater emphasis in the teaching of dynamic therapy in graduate and residency programs.

Conclusion

Psychodynamic psychotherapy as practiced in the twenty-first century is optimistic about the individual's capacity to grow and develop over the life cycle and to move beyond seemingly intractable, potentially fatal symptoms as found in a severe eating disorder. Beginning with comments taken from the autobiography of Dr. Lucy Daniels, a survivor of a 45-year battle with anorexia who undertook a psychodynamic process, I elaborated on certain characteristics of dynamic therapy that can be employed in daily clinical work. This noninclusive list includes 1) providing support during the process of working through separation and loss; 2) imparting a sense of being listened to intently; 3) confronting self-destructive behavior; 4) sticking with the patient during times of perceived weakness; and 5) creating a safe haven where the patient can come to know herself more fully. Other important considerations in psychodynamic psychotherapy of eating disorders are 6) understanding the role of conflict; 7) decreasing the need for self-punishment; 8) repetition of themes; 9) working through negative transference; and 10) integrating sensory data. Contemporary research based on attachment theory, observation of clinicians immersed in the field, and follow-up data of patient samples is beginning to demonstrate the conditions under which a psychodynamic approach is particularly useful and is providing insight into when these types of interventions are so important.

Psychological pain, interpersonal deficits, impaired ability to regulate emotions, and a diminished or absent sense of self are the subjects of the psychodynamic treatment of eating disorders. As in other psychiatric illnesses, a person with an eating disorder expresses somatically what cannot yet be expressed in words. Psychodynamic psychotherapy offers to help the individual with his or her problems by putting conflicts and interpersonal struggles that are manifested in the body into words; a mutative force in this treatment is helping the patient make sense of his or her personal history, the life narrative. For most patients, a psychodynamic approach should be integrated with nutritional, educational, cognitive-behavioral, and pharmacological approaches. However, the humanistic and existential underpinnings of psychodynamic psychotherapy are particularly useful in helping the person with anorexia nervosa, bulimia nervosa, or binge-eating disorder consolidate a sense of agency and identity in order to traverse the normative transitions of life with greater fulfillment and meaning. As Daniels further explains, progress in laying claim to one's unique life in this manner is not without ongoing struggle or the problems and disappointments that confront all human beings. As she faces down the message of demise embedded in the eating disorder, the patient must come to terms with "change, to almost expect it and to know that it can only be weathered, not stopped" (Daniels 2001, p. 258) if she is to embrace what it means to be fully alive.

References

Abend S: Analyzing intrapsychic conflict: compromise formation as an organizing principle. Psychoanal Q 74:5–26, 2005

Alexander F, French TM: Psychoanalytic Therapy: Principles and Application. New York, WW Norton, 1946

Battegay R: The Hunger Diseases. Lewiston, NY, Hogrefe & Huber, 1991

Betan E, Kegley-Heim A, Conklin C, et al: Countertransference phenomena and personality. Am J Psychiatry 162:890–898, 2005

Blatt SJ, Shahar G: Psychoanalysis with whom, for what, and how? Comparisons with psychotherapy. J Am Psychoanal Assoc 52:393–447, 2005

Blatt SJ, Shichman S: Two primary configurations of psychopathology. Psychoanalysis and Contemporary Thought 6:187–254, 1983

Blum HP: Clinical and developmental dimensions of hate. J Am Psychoanal Assoc 45:358–375, 1997

Blum HP: Psychic trauma and traumatic object loss. J Am Psychoanal Assoc 51:415–431, 2003

Boris HN: On the treatment of anorexia nervosa. Int J Psychoanal 65:435–442, 1984

Bowlby J: A Secure Base: Clinical Applications of Attachment Theory. London, Routledge, 1988

Brenner C: The Mind in Conflict. Madison, CT, International Universities Press, 1982

Brenner C: The mind as conflict and compromise formation. Journal of Clinical Psychoanalysis 3:473–488, 1994

Bromberg P: Standing in the Spaces: Essays on Clinical Process, Trauma, and Dissociation. Hillsdale, NJ, Analytic Press, 1996

Bromberg P: Out of body, out of mind, out of danger: some reflections on shame, dissociation, and eating disorders, in Hungers and Compulsion: The Psychodynamic Treatment of Eating Disorders and Addictions. Edited by Petrucelli J, Stuart C. Northvale, NJ, Jason Aronson, 2001, pp 65–80

Bruch H: Eating Disorders: Obesity, Anorexia Nervosa, and the Person Within. New York, Basic Books, 1973

Bruch H: The Golden Cage: The Enigma of Anorexia Nervosa. Cambridge, MA, Harvard University Press, 1978

Candelori C, Ciocca A: Attachment and eating disorders, in Psychotherapeutic Issues on Eating Disorders: Models, Methods, and Results. Edited by Bria P, Ciocca A, De Risio S. Rome, Società Editrice Universo, 1998, pp 139–154

Daniels L: With a Woman's Voice: A Writer's Struggle for Emotional Freedom. Lanham, MD, Madison Books, 2001

Dare C, Crowther C: Living dangerously: psychoanalytic psychotherapy of anorexia nervosa, in Handbook of Eating Disorders: Theory, Treatment, and Research. Edited by Szmukler G, Dare C, Treasure T. New York, Wiley, 1995, pp 293–308

Dare C, Eisler I, Russell G, et al: Psychological therapies for adults with anorexia nervosa: randomised controlled trial of out-patient treatments. Br J Psychiatry 178: 216–221, 2001

Edelman G: Bright Air, Brilliant Fire. New York, Basic Books, 1992

Fairbairn WRD: The repression and return of bad objects (with special reference to the war neuroses), in Psychoanalytic Studies of the Personality. London, Routledge & Kegan Paul, 1943, pp 59–81

Farrell EM: Lost for Words: The Psychoanalysis of Anorexia and Bulimia. New York, Other Press, 2000

Fonagy P: Attachment Theory and Psychoanalysis. New York, Other Press, 1999

Fonagy P, Target M, Gergely G: Attachment and borderline personality disorder: a theory and some evidence. Psychiatr Clin North Am 23:103–122, 2000

Fonagy P, Gergely G, Jurist M, et al: Affect Regulation, Mentalization, and the Development of the Self. New York, Other Press, 2002

Freud S: Extracts from the Fliess papers (1892–1899), in The Standard Edition of the Complete Psychological Works of Sigmund Freud, Vol 1. Translated and edited by Strachey J. London, Hogarth Press, 1962, pp 175–280

Friedman L: Trends in psychoanalytic theory of treatment. Psychoanal Q 47:524–567, 1978

Galatzer-Levy RM, Cohler BJ: The Essential Other: A Developmental Psychology of the Self. New York, Basic Books, 1993

Goldberg A: Being of Two Minds: The Vertical Split in Psychoanalysis and Psychotherapy. Hillsdale, NJ, Analytic Press, 1999

Goldberg S, Muir R, Kerr J: Attachment Theory: Social, Developmental, and Clinical Perspectives. Hillsdale, NJ, Analytic Press, 1995

Hamburg P, Herzog D, Brotman A: Treatment resistance in eating disorders: psychodynamic and pharmacologic perspectives, in Challenges in Clinical Practice: Pharmacologic and Psychosocial Strategies. Edited by Pollack M, Otto M, Rosenbaum J. New York, Guilford, 1996, pp 263–275

Hunter V: Psychoanalysts Talk. New York, Guilford, 1994

Kearney-Cooke A: The role of the therapist in the treatment of eating disorders: a feminist psychodynamic approach, in Psychodynamic Treatment of Anorexia Nervosa and Bulimia. Edited by Johnson CL. New York, Guilford, 1991, pp 295–319

Knapp C: Appetites: Why Women Want. New York, Counterpoint, 2003

Mahler M, Pine F, Bergman A: The Psychological Birth of the Human Infant. New York, Basic Books, 1975

McDougall J: Theaters of the Body: A Psychoanalytic Approach to Psychosomatic Illness. New York, WW Norton, 1989

Miller A: Prisoners of Childhood: The Drama of the Gifted Child and the Search for the True Self. New York, Basic Books, 1981

Mitrani JL: Toward an understanding of unmentalized experience. Psychoanal Q 64:68–111, 1995

Modell AH: The Private Self. Cambridge, MA, Harvard University Press, 1993

Ogden TH: The Primitive Edge of Experience. Northvale, NJ, Jason Aronson, 1989

Rinsley DB: Treatment of the Severely Disturbed Adolescent. New York, Jason Aronson, 1980

Rinsley DB: Borderline and Other Self Disorders: A Developmental and Object Relations Perspective. New York, Jason Aronson, 1982

Schafer R: The Analytic Attitude. New York, Basic Books, 1983

Schafer R: Retelling a Life: Narration and Dialogue in Psychoanalysis. New York, Basic Books, 1992

Schafer R: Bad Feelings. New York, Other Press, 2003

Schneider JA: Eating disorders, addictions, and unconscious fantasy. Bull Menninger Clin 59:177–190, 1995

Schore AN: The effects of a secure attachment relationship on right brain development, affect regulation, and infant mental health. Infant Ment Health J 22:7–66, 2001

Schore AN: Affect Dysregulation and Disorders of the Self. New York, WW Norton, 2003

Schore AN: Attachment, affect regulation, and the developing right brain: linking developmental neuroscience to pediatrics. Pediatr Rev 26(8):204–216 2005

Smith H: Dialogue in conflict: toward an integration of methods. Psychoanal Q 74: 327–363, 2005

Spence D: Narrative Truth and Historical Truth: Meaning and Interpretation in Psychoanalysis. New York, WW Norton, 1982

Thompson-Brenner H, Westen D: Personality subtypes in eating disorders: validation of a classification in a naturalistic sample. Br J Psychiatry 186:516–524, 2005

Treasure J: Staged matched interventions for eating disorders, in Psychotherapeutic Issues on Eating Disorders: Models, Methods, and Results. Edited by Bria P, Ciocca A, De Risio S. Rome, Società Editrice Universo, 1998, pp 59–66

Treasure J, Schmidt U: Clinician's Guide to Getting Better Bit(e) by Bit(e): A Survival Kit for Sufferers of Bulimia Nervosa and Binge Eating. Hove, East Sussex, UK, Psychology Press, 1997

Treasure J, Schmidt U: Beyond effectiveness and efficiency lies quality in services for eating disorders. European Eating Disorders Review 7:162–178, 1999

Tustin F: Autistic Barriers in Neurotic Patients. New Haven, CT, Yale University Press, 1986

Tustin F: The Protective Shell in Children and Adults. London, Karnac, 1990

Wallerstein RS: Forty-Two Lives in Treatment: A Study of Psychoanalysis and Psychotherapy. New York, Guilford, 1986

Weiss J, Sampson H, and Mount Zion Psychotherapy Research Group: The Psychoanalytic Process: Theory, Clinical Observations, and Empirical Research. New York, Guilford, 1986

Weissman MM, Markowitz JC, Klerman GL: Comprehensive Guide to Interpersonal Psychotherapy. New York, Basic Books, 2000

Westen D: Integrative psychotherapy: integrating psychodynamic and cognitive-behavioral therapy and technique, in Handbook of Psychological Change: Psychotherapy Processes and Practices for the 21st Century. Edited by Snyder CR, Ingram R. New York, Wiley, 2000, pp 217–242

Westen D, Harnden-Fischer J: Personality profiles in eating disorders: rethinking the distinction between Axis I and Axis II. Am J Psychiatry 158:247–255, 2001

Westen D, Novotny CM, Thompson-Brenner H: The empirical status of empirically supported psychotherapies: assumptions, findings, and reporting in controlled clinical trials. Psychol Bull 130:631–663, 2004

Winnicott DW: Ego distortion in terms of true and false self (1960), in The Maturational Processes and the Facilitating Environment: Studies in the Theory of Emotional Development. New York, International Universities Press, 1965, pp 140–152

Winnicott DW: Human Nature. London, Free Association Books, 1988

Yager J: The treatment of eating disorders. J Clin Psychiatry 49 (suppl 9):18–25, 1988

Yager J: Psychotherapeutic strategies for bulimia nervosa. J Psychother Pract Res 1:91–102, 1992

Zerbe K: The Body Betrayed: Women, Eating Disorders, and Treatment. Washington, DC, American Psychiatric Press, 1993a

Zerbe K: Whose body is it anyway? Understanding and treating psychosomatic aspects of eating disorders. Bull Menninger Clin 57:161–177, 1993b

Zerbe K: Feminist psychodynamic psychotherapy of eating disorders: theoretic integration informing clinical practice. Psychiatr Clin North Am 19(4):811–827, 1996

Zerbe KJ: The crucial role of psychodynamic understanding in the treatment of eating disorders. Psychiatr Clin North Am 24:305–313, 2001a

Zerbe K: When the self starves: alliance and outcome in the treatment of eating disorders, in Hungers and Compulsions: The Psychodynamic Treatment of Eating Disorders and Addictions. Edited by Petrucelli J, Stuart C. New York, Jason Aronson, 2001b, pp 183–208

Zerbe K: Women's Mental Health in Primary Care. Philadelphia, PA, WB Saunders, 1999

Zerbe KJ: Integrated Treatment of Eating Disorders: Beyond the Body Betrayed. New York, WW Norton (in press)

13

Eating Disorders in Special Populations

Medical Comorbidities and Complicating or Unusual Conditions

Stephanie L. Berg, M.D.

Arnold E. Andersen, M.D.

In this chapter, we describe typical eating disorders, occurring in a variety of populations, that may not ordinarily be considered because eating disorders are usually and stereotypically associated with teenage girls. Clinicians will not diagnose eating disorders if they do not think of them; when the usual epidemiological cues are absent, considerations of eating disorders may be far from clinicians' awareness. While eating disorders are most common in young Western females (Hsu 1996), it is important to appreciate that other populations are also at risk. We focus here on eating disorders in persons with diabetes mellitus, pregnant women, older-age women, and males. Additionally, we consider the value of potentially broadening current diagnostic concepts of anorexia nervosa so that certain types of conditions that clearly fall within the general category of this disorder are not excluded or misidentified as atypical.

Diabetes Mellitus

> Ms. D., a 40-year-old woman with history of a cycle of bingeing/purging alternating with restriction of food since age 14, has had type 1 (insulin-dependent) diabetes for the past 10 years. She was first seen by a psychiatrist after being admitted to a general medicine unit for diabetic ketoacidosis related to dehydration four times in the course of 2 years. During her last admission for ketoacidosis, a psychiatric evaluation requested by her internist revealed that she had been bingeing, vomiting, and restricting her food intake in order to keep her weight low. The psychiatrist was so concerned with her lack of insight that he felt it appropriate to file for commitment and have her transferred to the eating disorders unit at the state university hospital. There she was determined to be at 86% of ideal body weight, her blood sugars were brittle, and she required almost daily adjustment of her insulin regimen. Throughout her hospitalization she complained that her stomach felt full. When her blood sugar levels were high, she often felt depressed and irritable. Her weight was restored to 100% of ideal, and her blood glucose level was stabilized such that she was transferred to the eating disorder program's partial hospitalization program, while she lived at the local residential care facility.

With diabetes mellitus affecting 7% of the U.S. population (Engelgau et al. 2004), a substantial subpopulation will inevitably have both an eating disorder and either type 1 (insulin-dependent) or type 2 (non-insulin-dependent) diabetes mellitus.

While overall the literature is inconclusive, some recent research suggests an increased likelihood of an eating disorder in patients with diabetes mellitus. A study of 3,000 individuals identified from primary care found an increased likelihood (odds ratio = 2.4) of eating disorder in patients with diabetes mellitus (Goodwin et al. 2003). Diagnosis of frank eating disorders is more difficult than usual in these patients because overvaluation of body weight and shape often overlaps with the adaptive close monitoring of diet and exercise necessarily practiced by patients with diabetes to control their blood glucose levels.

Theories associating eating disorder with type 1 diabetes include the emphases given by medical professionals to healthy eating and exercise. Patients with perfectionistic or obsessional overemphasis on these concerns, compounded by the usual overvaluation of shape and weight among adolescents and their peers, may be more prone to disordered eating behaviors. Additionally, state-of-the-art treatment for glucose regulation, such as an insulin pump, involves minute-to-minute evaluation of blood glucose and promotes a mindful, conscious, and continuous effort to regulate the body's metabolism (Rubin and Peyrot 2001). The additional psychological stress imposed by this sort of hypervigilance, compounded by dread of potential sequelae of diabetes mellitus, may render otherwise typically anxious individuals even more prone to psychiatric illnesses, including anorexia nervosa (Rubin and Peyrot 2001).

Although the prevalence of eating disorders in type 1 and type 2 diabetes mellitus does not appear to differ, each type may be associated with a specific eating disorder psychopathology (Herpertz et al. 2001). Patients with type 2 diabetes have been demonstrated to have more depression and are more likely to be overweight and to have difficulty losing weight. Distress may stem both from medically related pressures and from eating disorder–related cognitions to lose weight, thereby exacerbating symptoms (Figure 13–1). Additionally, patients who omit insulin as a form of purging seem to have more pronounced difficulties with retinopathy (Rydall et al. 1997), neuropathy, and other complications of hyperglycemia. These findings suggest that detecting and intervening with this population is of the utmost importance.

Detection may be particularly difficult in patients with diabetes mellitus. Possible clues to underlying eating disorders in these patients are unexplained episodes of ketoacidosis or hypoglycemia, persistently elevated hemoglobin A1c (HgbA1c) levels (which may indicate omission of insulin to promote weight loss), and easy control in inpatient settings of blood glucose levels that were previously difficult to manage in outpatient settings.

Rates of medical complications in patients with comorbid eating disorders and diabetes mellitus are significantly higher than those in patients without these comorbidities. Patients who regulate their bodies' insulin levels exogenously have many opportunities for abuse: they can allow glucose levels to remain high and thereby lose weight through glycosuria, inadvertently provoke hypoglycemia by failing to adjust insulin while restricting intake, or gain weight by increasing their insulin doses during binge episodes (Garner and Garfinkel 1997).

Treatment issues include proper management of insulin regimens, often requiring inpatient hospitalizations for initial stabilization. Dehydration and

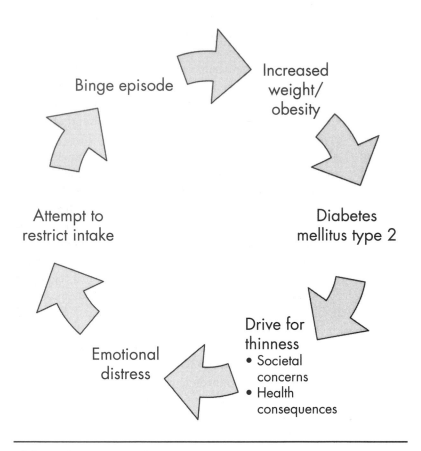

Figure 13–1.   Cycle of disorder in bulimia nervosa/anorexia nervosa, binge-purge subtype and diabetes mellitus.

hypokalemia are particular risks. Basic tenets of nutrition for diabetes mellitus are applicable in prescribing diets for patients with eating disorders—namely, using complex rather than simple carbohydrates, avoiding saturated fats, and coordinating meals with onset of insulin action (Gearhart and Forbes 1995). A thorough physical examination on admission should focus particularly on sequelae of long-term hyperglycemia (Table 13–1).

Selective serotonin reuptake inhibitor antidepressants have been demonstrated to be safe and effective in patients with both diabetes mellitus and de-

Table 13–1. Complications of diabetes mellitus

Microvascular

Retinopathy

Nephropathy

Neuropathy

    Distal sensory polyneuropathy

    Mononeuropathy

    Autonomic neuropathy

        Orthostatic hypotension

        Gastroparesis

        Silent myocardial infarction

        Erectile dysfunction

Macrovascular

Coronary artery disease

Cerebrovascular disease

Peripheral vascular disease

pression (Lustman and Clouse 2002) and beneficial in the maintenance treatment of patients with eating disorders (Mayer and Walsh 1998). Because the depression seen in large numbers of individuals with eating disorders may further hamper glycemic control, it is prudent to treat depression vigorously. Issues to be addressed in psychotherapy include body dissatisfaction (with regard to both shape and impaired function), frustrations related to diabetes management, and issues generated by having a chronic, life-threatening medical condition requiring significant lifestyle management that inevitably sets these patients at least to some extent apart from their peers (Rubin and Peyrot 2001).

Nonadherence to medication regimens, dietary management, and other aspects of self-care is common among diabetic patients with eating disorders. The nonadherence is often related to impaired insight and fostered by unpleasantness of many aspects of diabetes treatment, including invasive procedures (e.g., fingersticks for use of blood glucose meter, insulin injections) and various unpleasant adverse medication effects (e.g., possible gastrointestinal upset resulting from medications such as metformin). Therefore, adherence and self-control are key and critical issues in the psychological management of diabetic patients with eating disorders.

Pregnancy

> Ms. B., a 28-year-old woman with a 6-month-old daughter, had difficulty in be-coming pregnant due to anovulation. In an effort to keep her weight at 110 pounds (at a height of 5 feet, 7 inches), she had eaten very restrictively and had exercised for 2 hours daily for many years. Because she was unable to get preg-nant, she was seen in a reproductive endocrinology clinic, where she was not identified as having an eating disorder and was given clomiphene citrate to stimulate ovulation. She then conceived and suffered severe vomiting during the first 17 weeks of the pregnancy, which led to one hospitalization for de-hydration. During the pregnancy, she gained only 14 pounds as she continued to restrict her food intake relative to her requirements. Although she ate an in-creased amount—for her—she also continued to eat only foods she consid-ered "safe." Her daughter was born at 37 weeks, small for gestational age. Ms. B. had difficulty breast-feeding and started to bottle-feed her daughter exclu-sively when she was 4 days old. She also experienced significant depression starting 2 weeks after the birth of her child, which she attributed to then weigh-ing 124 pounds and to the changes in her body shape. She then started exer-cising for 3 hours daily, to the marked detriment of her relationship with her hus-band and daughters. Ms. B. came to treatment when her daughter was 5 months old, recognizing that the intrusive thoughts she was having about her daugh-ter being "too fat" were problematic.

Eating disorders most commonly affect women of childbearing age. There-fore, clinicians should fully appreciate how eating disorders can impact pregnancy, since eating disorders can cause long-term adverse effects for both the mother and the child. Many women who have never had an eating disorder may develop concerns regarding changes in body shape and eating-related physical symptoms during pregnancy, so some experiences along these lines may be normative— a finding that can occasionally complicate diagnosing patients with frank pregnancy-associated eating disorders.

Approximately 5% of pregnant women have significant levels of eating disorder symptoms. Factors such as lower education, younger age, a history of previous eating disorder symptoms, and depression increase the risk of having eating disorder symptoms (Conti et al. 1998; Turton et al. 1999). Eating disorders are extremely common in infertility clinics; in one study 17% of women treated for infertility were found to have eating disorder difficulties (Stewart et al. 1991). In counseling women with eating disorders who desire to have children, the best recommendation is that the eating disorder be treated prior to attempts to conceive, because poor response to treatment predicts greater difficulties in being able to conceive and higher risks of complications during pregnancy and in the perinatal period.

In pregnancy the impact of anorexia nervosa differs from that of bulimia nervosa in several ways. In anorexia nervosa it is thought that fertility may be impaired because of anovulation associated with hypogonadism induced by malnutrition, but this conjecture remains controversial (Bulik et al. 1999). Women with anorexia nervosa may have fertility rates approximately one-third of expected (Brinch et al. 1988). Bulimia nervosa is less often associated with altered menstrual cycles and decreased fertility (Crow et al. 2002). In fact, pregnancy rates in bulimia nervosa may theoretically be increased because of risk-taking behaviors such as sexual promiscuity and the mistaken belief that amenorrhea or menstrual irregularity confer infertility (Morgan et al. 1999). However, similarities regarding complications, treatments, and outcomes of anorexia nervosa and bulimia nervosa in pregnancy are considerably greater than differences.

Studies examining outcome of eating disorder symptoms in pregnancy have yielded varied results (Figure 13–2). Some studies have found that symptoms improve during pregnancy (Brinch et al. 1988; Crow et al. 2004; Turton et al. 1999), with either sustained improvement in the postpartum or, alternatively, a return to symptoms (Morgan et al. 1999). Other studies have found increased symptoms in pregnancy, thought to occur in reaction to altered body shape and increased weight (Abraham 1998; Kouba et al. 2005), whereas still others have found no change in symptoms (Carter et al. 2003). Some individuals have new-onset eating disorders during pregnancy (Turton et al. 1999) or in the postpartum period (Mazzeo et al. 2006).

Potential medical complications in pregnant women with eating disorders vary and are dependent on the degree of malnutrition and specific symptoms of the eating disorder itself (Table 13–2). Complications in pregnancy include higher rates of miscarriages, cesarean deliveries (approximately 25%), hypertension, preeclampsia, vaginal bleeding, increased or decreased weight gain, anemia, and postepisiotomy suture tearing (Bulik et al. 1999; Franko and Spurrell 2000; Franko et al. 2001; Kouba et al. 2005). While the baseline rate in the general population for hyperemesis gravidarum is low (approximately 1%), this syndrome is seen in up to 67% of women with eating disorders (Kouba et al. 2005).

One of the most striking and consistent findings in women with eating disorders is an increased incidence of postpartum depression, occurring in ap-

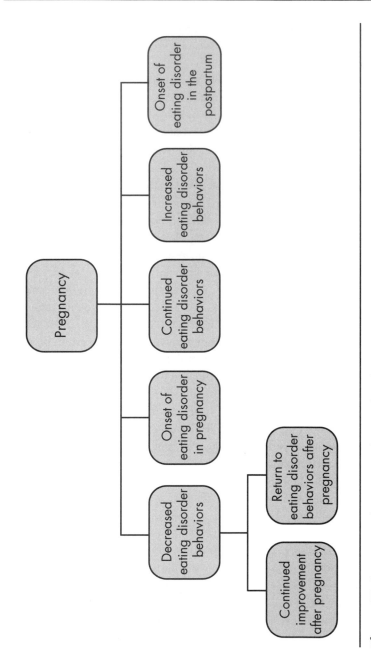

Figure 13–2.   Potential outcomes of eating disorders in pregnancy.

Table 13–2.   Complications of eating disorders in pregnancy

Hypotension (anorexia nervosa and bulimia nervosa)/hypertension (bulimia nervosa)

Lower- or higher-than-expected weight gain

Anemia (anorexia nervosa)

Increased risks of

- Postpartum depression
- Cesarean section
- Hyperemesis gravidarum
- Pregnancy termination (either therapeutic or spontaneous)
- Stillbirth
- Breech pregnancy
- Preeclampsia
- Postepisiotomy suture tearing
- Vaginal bleeding

proximately 33% (Franko et al. 2001; Morgan et al. 1999), a prevalence far in excess of the general population's estimated prevalence of 13% (O'Hara and Swain 1996). The increased risk may result both from concerns about weight after delivery and from much greater predispositions to mood disorders (Abraham et al. 2001). In turn, postpartum depression may then contribute to relapse of eating disorder symptoms, particularly in patients with bulimia nervosa (Morgan et al. 1999). Babies born to mothers with eating disorder are at higher risk for lower birth weight, prematurity, lower Apgar scores, microcephaly, and increased malformations, including cleft lip and palate (Conti et al. 1998; Kouba et al. 2005; Lacey and Smith 1987; Park et al. 2003) (Table 13–3).

Furthermore, children born to mothers with eating disorders have higher rates of psychiatric illness, including depression and alcoholism. Feeding behaviors in children of parents with eating disorders tend to be abnormal and include increased fussiness, body dissatisfaction, and imitative eating disorder behavior (Park et al. 2003). Seventeen percent of children born to mothers with eating disorders have failure to thrive in the first year of life (Brinch et al. 1988). Relationships between mother and child may be disturbed in several ways—for example, the relationship may be overly distant or enmeshed, or there may be a reversal in the caretaker relationship. Disturbed parenting in mothers with eating disorders and later development of abnormal behaviors

Table 13–3.   Potential risks to children of mothers with eating disorders

Premature birth
Perinatal mortality (sixfold increase)
Cleft palate
Epilepsy
Developmental delays
Abnormal growth
Food fussiness
Low birth weight
Microcephaly
Low Apgar scores

in children may result from genetic factors, modeling of eating disorders in parents, disrupted parenting due to eating disorder behaviors, imitative behavior, and/or abnormal family relationships (Park et al. 2003).

Medically, cardiovascular status must be closely monitored in pregnant women with active eating disorders. Impairments resulting from ipecac cardiomyopathy, bradycardia, or hypokalemia can decrease cardiac output and compromise fetal circulation. Pregnant women with eating disorders also risk hypocalcemia and lower body fat that can impair milk production and ability to breast-feed (James 2001). Other commonly occurring medical issues, such as renal disease, hyperamylasemia, hypo- or hypernatremia, and skin fragility, should be treated carefully. Table 13–4 lists laboratory values to be monitored closely in pregnant women with eating disorders. Treating pregnant patients with eating disorders requires a team approach, including coordinated care by obstetricians, dietitians, psychiatrists, and therapists. Early detection is vital for proper treatment.

Table 13–5 suggests points of evaluation that will help screen all women seen for prenatal and antenatal care and identify at-risk individuals. Psychotherapy of the pregnant patient should focus on encouraging the health of the fetus and the mother. The treatment team must agree on weight restoration and expected healthy targets for weight. While close outpatient monitoring may suffice, inpatient treatment—preferably voluntarily but in severe cases involuntarily—may be safest for mother and fetus,. Red flags include 1) insufficient weight gain in the second trimester during two consecutive weeks and 2) hyperemesis gravidarum (Franko and Spurrell 2000).

Table 13–4.   Abnormal laboratory values found in pregnant women with eating disorders

Hypokalemia

Hypophosphatemia

Hyponatremia

Hypochloremia

Elevated bicarbonate level

Hypomagnesemia

Increased urine specific gravity

Alkaline urine (due to laxative abuse, diuretic abuse, or vomiting)

Ketonuria

Leukopenia

Thrombocytopenia

Normochromic, normocytic anemia

Hypercarotenemia

Increased liver function tests

Increased salivary amylase

Hyperaldosteronemia

Decreased T_4 levels, normal TSH level

Hypercortisolemia

Decreased erythrocyte sedimentation rate

Note. T_4 = thyroxine; TSH = thyroid-stimulating hormone.
Source.   Adapted from James 2001.

Table 13–5.   Screening evaluation for early detection of eating disorders in women receiving prenatal and antenatal care

1.   Current food intake

2.   Dietary regimen or food rituals

3.   Presence of binge eating episodes

4.   Body weight history (e.g., significant fluctuations)

5.   Current concern about body weight/fear of weight gain in pregnancy

6.   Frequency of weighing self

7.   Purging and compensatory behaviors

8.   Exercise and fasting behaviors

9.   History of current presence of menstrual cycle abnormalities

Source.   Adapted from Wolfe 2005.

Nontraditional-Age Population

> Ms. S., a 60-year-old woman, was admitted to the inpatient eating disorder service at only 70% of ideal body weight. Her first eating disorder–related difficulties occurred when she became pregnant at the age of 18 years and began restricting food intake in order to hide her pregnancy. Her baby was born without complications, but shortly after delivery, Ms. S. started bingeing and purging because she was concerned that she was not losing her pregnancy weight quickly enough. She then started using laxatives multiple times daily, a routine that continued for decades until this admission. In her 40s, she had the first of a series of recurrent depressive episodes, which were treated intermittently with antidepressant medications by her primary care physician. Her husband died 7 years ago, and since that time the frequency of her bingeing and purging had increased to twice a day. On admission she had a complete medical workup to evaluate her weight loss and was found to have diffuse brain atrophy and significant osteoporosis. She required transfer to a medical unit for a short time for treatment of bowel obstruction due to severe constipation.

While eating disorders occur most commonly in young females ages 13 through 18 years (Halmi et al. 1979), approximately 5% of patients with eating disorders are between the ages of 30 and 40 years, and even older patients with eating disorders are being seen in increasing numbers. In 1979 Carrier introduced the term "anorexia tardive" to describe the condition of older individuals with anorexia nervosa. The anorexia nervosa in these older patients either may have had an earlier onset (e.g., during adolescence) or may have initially developed at an older age (Nicholson and Ballance 1998). Dally (1984) described a frequently observed interpersonal relationship pattern in women with "anorexia tardive" in which the patient's eating disorder behaviors foster dependence on her husband, which he then enables and perpetuates. Additionally, as in many individuals with eating disorders, these women show continued development conflicts. The limited literature suggests vulnerability to illness throughout the life span during significant life transitions, such as childbirth, widowhood, or menopause (Fornari et al. 1994). Figure 13–3 describes the cycle of perpetuation in the older population, similar to that in others with eating disorders but with additional emphasis on reactions to later life-transitions, including grieving after the loss of a partner.

At any age the presence of unexplained weight loss requires a full medical evaluation, but such evaluation is especially important in the older population,

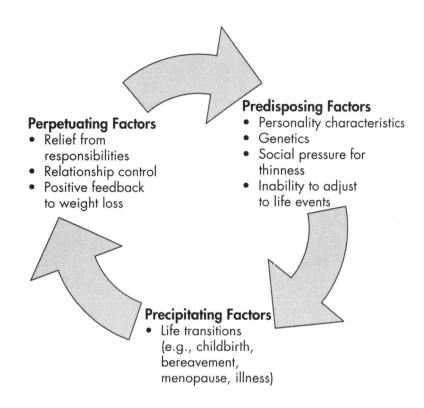

Perpetuating Factors
- Relief from responsibilities
- Relationship control
- Positive feedback to weight loss

Predisposing Factors
- Personality characteristics
- Genetics
- Social pressure for thinness
- Inability to adjust to life events

Precipitating Factors
- Life transitions (e.g., childbirth, bereavement, menopause, illness)

Figure 13–3.   Cycle of symptoms of eating disorders in the older compared with the traditional-age population.
Source.   Adapted from Nicholson and Ballance 1998.

in whom physical causes of weight loss are more likely (Kasper et al. 2004). Concerns regarding weight loss in older populations drawn from several sources are presented in Table 13–6.

Medical complications of eating disorders in older patients are similar to those occurring in patients at younger ages, but it is thought that older patients are more vulnerable to medical complications. Table 13–7 lists possible medical complications in this population. In particular, cerebral atrophy has been associated with decreased attention, decreased concentration, impaired judgment, and

Table 13–6.   Differential diagnosis of weight loss in the older population

Weight loss due to increased energy consumption

Cardiovascular (e.g., increased protein turnover in some patients with chronic heart failure)

Diabetes mellitus

Hyperthyroidism

Infection

Malabsorption

Medications (e.g., L-dopa, stimulants)

Nicotine

Neoplasm

Parkinson's disease

Pheochromocytoma

Weight loss due to decreased nutritional intake[a]

Benign gastrointestinal disorders* (e.g., hepatic disease due to cirrhosis or hepatitis, with associated nausea and bloating)

Depression* (especially in nursing home residents)

Neoplasm* (e.g., lung, gastric, colon, esophageal)

Adrenal insufficiency

Anemia

Cardiovascular disorders (e.g., congestive heart failure)

Chronic obstructive pulmonary disease (e.g., emphysema)

Dementia (e.g., Alzheimer's disease)

Hypercalcemia

Infection (e.g., HIV, urinary tract infection, endocarditis)

Medication-induced nausea, dysgeusia, dysphagia

Neurological disorders inducing dysphagias

Poor access to food due to limited finances, limited mobility, and poor social supports

Uremia

---

[a]Asterisk indicates most common causes.

Source.   Compiled from Gazewood and Mehr 1998; Huffman 2002; Kasper et al. 2004; Lorefalt et al. 2004, among other sources.

inability to think abstractly (Nicholson and Ballance 1998). Basic laboratory evaluations, guided by physical examinations, should be performed, and special attention should be paid to ruling out other causes of weight loss in older individuals (Table 13–8). Depression often occurs comorbidly in patients with eating disorders (Herzog 1984). In the elderly, a distinguishing feature between the eating disorder per se and depression may be loss of appetite in individuals with depression but preservation of appetite in individuals with eating disorders (Nicholson and Ballance 1998). Other psychiatric conditions that must be ruled out include obsessive-compulsive disorder, psychosis, and dementia.

While not systematically studied or reported, the general approaches to treating eating disorders in the elderly are similar to those in younger patients and include structured psychotherapy and prescribed refeeding, if necessary, with proper treatment of medical concerns (e.g., osteoporosis, electrolyte imbalance, B_{12} or folate deficiency) and family involvement when possible and indicated.

Males With Eating Disorders

> Mr. G., an 18-year-old male, was admitted to the inpatient eating disorder service because he had been having difficulty with involuntary purging of all food that he had eaten over the 3 months before admission. A year previous to admission, he had gained 10 pounds from his baseline weight of 175 pounds (Mr. G. was 5 feet, 11 inches). He had been a star wrestler with his high school team but, because of his weight gain, was told by his wrestling coach to take "whatever measures necessary" to return to his previous weight class. He then started vomiting after every meal in the week before wrestling tournaments, running outside for five miles in insulated track suits, and spitting into cans on the days of tournaments. He was able to lose the 10 pounds. Even after wrestling season ended, Mr. G. was unable to stop these behaviors, transitioning to binge eating followed by self-induced vomiting. He presented to the Eating and Weight Disorders Evaluation Clinic, where he was diagnosed with bulimia nervosa. He responded well to 10 sessions of CBT and nutritional prescription.

Appreciation of the fact that males also present with eating disorders has increased in recent decades. "Gender-specific medicine" has highlighted males with eating disorders. Eating disorders occur more commonly in males than previously appreciated and exhibit some diagnostic features, social contextual

Table 13–7.   Medical complications of eating disorders in the older population

Vitamin deficiencies (e.g., B_{12}, folate)

Low albumin or prealbumin

Electrolyte disturbances (e.g., hypokalemia)

Anemia

Leukopenia

Osteoporosis, pathological fractures, kyphosis

Electrocardiographic changes

Mitral or triscupid valve insufficiency

Decreased gastrointestinal motility

aspects, and subtypes relatively exclusive to males. Although the phenomenology of the disorders in males remains secure as the basis for confident identification, social stereotypes, valid clinical disagreements about diagnostic criteria, and wide variations in prevalence data all remain open for lively discussion (Andersen 1990).

Despite the fact that the two cases commonly accepted as the first accurate clinical accounts of anorexia nervosa in 1689 included one male and one female, males were subsequently neglected for a number of reasons. During the heyday of the initial recognition of endocrine disorders in the late nineteenth century, anorexia nervosa was thought to result from postpartum pituitary necrosis, a presumed etiology that obviously excluded males. Males were also excluded during the reign of early psychoanalytic theories because they did not meet the core dynamic thematic criterion of "fear of oral impregnation." Since the current diagnostic criteria for anorexia nervosa in DSM-IV-TR (American Psychiatric Association 2000) include amenorrhea as a criterion, males are again excluded or, at best, seem to be somewhat grudgingly recognized. ICD-10 (World Health Organization 1992), more gender neutral, cites "abnormality of gonadotropin functioning." Bulimia nervosa, recognized as a diagnostic entity for only the past 25 years, is more behaviorally based and neutral toward gender. The core diagnostic features of anorexia nervosa for *both* males and females are 1) abnormal eating behavior—self-starvation driven by the internalization and overvaluation of the socioculturally touted benefits of slimness or shape change; 2) abnormal core psychopathology—a morbid fear of fatness

Table 13–8. Suggested routine laboratory assessments for older patients with weight loss

Electrolytes
Complete blood cell count
B_{12}
Folate
Thyroid function tests
Liver function tests
Urinalysis and culture
Electrocardiogram
Chest radiograph
Pelvic examination in females
Stool guaiac

(emphasized by the British psychopathologists) and/or the relentless pursuit of thinness (emphasized historically in the United States by Hilde Bruch), both included in the underrecognized psychopathological category of "overvalued beliefs"; and 3) medical signs and symptoms of starvation enduring more than 3 months (to avoid overdiagnoses that might result if short-term intensive diets were to slip under the diagnostic screen).

The most detailed study estimating the prevalence of eating disorders in males in the general population suggested that the community male-female ratio is between 1:2 and 1:3, which is far higher than ratios based on clinic admissions (usually reported as 1:10 to 1:20) (Woodside et al. 2001). Several reasons may account for the far lower prevalence figures derived from clinic-based estimates for males:

1. Low clinician awareness of eating disorders in males may result in low detection rates.
2. Anorexia nervosa and bulimia nervosa are both highly ego-dystonic and more shameful for males, whereas although shame is still significant, females may more readily accept that they have an eating disorder.
3. Certain nonessential clinical features of eating disorders in males may reduce the likelihood of their being diagnosed with an eating disorder: males focus more on their upper rather than lower bodies and are con-

cerned almost as much about shape change (toward extreme lean muscularity) as weight loss, so they may have less regard for common benchmark goals of weight, such as the less than 100 pounds sought in many women. Among males, in the absence of a good personal reason, dieting is atypical, whereas *not* dieting is atypical among females in Westernized societies.

4. Certain forms of male-dominated eating disorders, such as the poorly phrased "reverse anorexia nervosa," overlapping with muscle dysmorphia, are associated with the distorted perception that one can never be big or muscular enough. As is common with anorexia nervosa, this syndrome is characterized by perverse distortion of the entire body image and by overvalued beliefs.

5. Commonly used assessments and clinical severity measures, such as the Eating Attitudes Test and the Eating Disorder Inventory, were normed on females. Studies have shown that because of the female skew of the questions incorporated into these instruments, males with clinical eating disorders score lower than females with comparable levels of clinical impairment.

6. Current DSM criteria (i.e., DSM-IV-TR criteria)—particularly those for anorexia nervosa—are outmoded because of built-in gender bias.

Once an eating disorder has been recognized in a male, treatment can proceed on the basis current treatment guidelines, with a few modifications based on gender-specific needs: Males appear to do better if they are admitted to specialized hospital programs where available that both accept males and develop special male-oriented tracks. (Many eating disorder programs exclude males, a practice that seems unacceptable for patients with other psychiatric diagnoses.) Having a cluster of males for a male-only group decreases a sense of isolation. Males report that strength training, beginning very modestly with emphasis on good form and low weights, serves as an important morale booster during weight restoration, emphasizing the desirability of increased lean muscle mass.

Although systematic evidence-based studies are lacking to date, we have sometimes treated males older than 18 years, who signed informed consents, with exogenous testosterone to achieve normal testosterone levels and hence, presumably, a more normal hormonal environment until their own gonadotropin production returned, during the phase of weight restoration. Such restoration may also promote building more lean muscle mass and mood improvement, and patients have commented positively on the subjective effects of such treatment combined with a physical activity program. In these regimens, limited to males at or close to complete axial growth, exogenous testosterone is discontinued once the patients have attained a fully normal body weight.

The psychotherapeutic needs of males often include discussions of sexuality in general and questions that patients may have about their own sexual orientation, but gay males still constitute a minority of males with eating disorders, and clinicians should make no assumptions about sexual orientation. Asexuality is actually the most common sexual state of teenage males with anorexia nervosa.

Overall, the recognition and treatment of males with eating disorders are improving, but both still lag behind the status of increasingly well-recognized, -diagnosed, and -treated eating disorders in females.

Beyond the Narrow Diagnostic Boundaries in Anorexia Nervosa

Despite improvements in the diagnostic schemes for eating disorders over the past several decades through several iterations of DSM, DSM criteria for eating disorders are still too rigid and narrow, or are interpreted in too narrow a fashion, leading to mislabeling of very typical cases of anorexia nervosa as atypical cases or eating disorder not otherwise specified (EDNOS). For example, the criterion in DSM-IV-TR that weight be below 85% for a diagnosis of anorexia nervosa is given as exempli gratia, for example, not as commandment. In practice, this weight criterion is often taken as a requirement. The results of mislabeling patients as having an "atypical" eating disorder or an EDNOS are sometimes quite serious: some insurance companies deny benefits for diagnostic assessment and treatment for "atypical" cases, considering them less serious, although several studies have disproven this misapprehension. Clinicians may feel less confident about treating patients with eating disorders considered "atypical." If clinicians stick with the core diagnostic features for anorexia nervosa described earlier, true cases will be recognized without the danger of excluding, for example, males due to requiring gender-biased amenorrhea, or "less than 85%" of expected weight, when in fact *sustained features of medical starvation persisting from self-starvation driven by overvalued beliefs* are all that is required (Watson and Andersen 2003).

References

Abraham S: Sexuality and reproduction in bulimia nervosa patients over 10 years. J Psychosom Res 44:491–502, 1998

Abraham S, Taylor A, Conti J: Postnatal depression, eating, exercise, and vomiting before and during pregnancy. Int J Eat Disord 29:482–487, 2001

American Psychiatric Association: Diagnostic and Statistical Manual of Mental Disorders, 4th Edition, Text Revision. Washington, DC, American Psychiatric Association, 2000

Andersen AE: Males With Eating Disorders. Philadelphia, PA, Brunner/Mazel, 1990

Brinch M, Isager T, Tolstrup K: Anorexia nervosa and motherhood: reproduction pattern and mother behavior of 50 women. Acta Psychiatr Scand 77:98–104, 1988

Bulik CM, Sullivan PF, Fear JL, et al: Fertility and reproduction in women with anorexia nervosa: a controlled study. J Clin Psychiatry 60:130–135, 1999

Carrier J: L'anorexie mentale. Paris, Librairie E Le François, 1979

Carter FA, McIntosh VVW, Joyce PR, et al: Bulimia nervosa, childbirth, and psychopathology. J Psychosom Res 55:357–361, 2003

Conti J, Abraham S, Taylor A: Eating behavior and pregnancy outcome. J Psychosom Res 44:465–477, 1998

Crow SJ, Thuras P, Keel PK, et al: Long-term menstrual and reproductive function in patients with bulimia nervosa. Am J Psychiatry 159:1048–1050, 2002

Crow SJ, Keel PK, Thuras P, et al: Bulimia symptoms and other risk behaviors during pregnancy in women with bulimia nervosa. Int J Eat Disord 36:220–223, 2004

Dally P: Anorexia tardive—late onset marital anorexia nervosa. J Psychosom Res 28:423–428, 1984

Engelgau MM, Geiss LS, Saaddine JB, et al: The evolving diabetes burden in the United States. Ann Intern Med 140:945–950, 2004

Fornari V, Kent J, Kabo L, et al: Anorexia nervosa: "thirty something." J Subst Abuse Treat 11:45–54, 1994

Franko DL, Spurrell EB: Detection and management of eating disorders during pregnancy. Obstet Gynecol 95:942–946, 2000

Franko DL, Blais MA, Becker AE, et al: Pregnancy complications and neonatal outcomes in women with eating disorders. Am J Psychiatry 158:1461–1466, 2001

Garner DM, Garfinkel PE (eds): Handbook of Treatment for Eating Disorders, 2nd Edition. New York, Guilford, 1997

Gazewood JD, Mehr DR: Diagnosis and management of weight loss in the elderly. J Fam Pract 47:19–25, 1998

Gearhart JG, Forbes RC: Initial management of the patient with newly diagnosed diabetes. Am Fam Physician 51:1953–1968, 1995

Goodwin RD, Hoven CW, Spitzer RL: Diabetes and eating disorders in primary care. Int J Eat Disord 33:85–91, 2003

Halmi KA, Casper RC, Eckert ED, et al: Unique features associated with age of onset of anorexia nervosa. Psychiatry Res 1:209–215, 1979

Herpertz S, Albus C, Kielmann R, et al: Comorbidity of diabetes and eating disorders: a follow-up study. J Psychosom Res 51:673–678, 2001

Herzog DB: Are anorexic and bulimic patients depressed? Am J Psychiatry 141:1594–1597, 1984

Hsu LK: Epidemiology of the eating disorders. Psychiatr Clin North Am 19:681–700, 1996

Huffman GB: Evaluating and treating unintentional weight loss in the elderly. Am Fam Physician 65:640–650, 2002

James DC: Eating disorders, fertility, and pregnancy: relationships and complications. J Perinat Neonatal Nurs 15(2):36–48, 2001

Kasper DL, Braunwald E, Fauci A, et al (eds): Harrison's Principles of Internal Medicine, 16th Edition. New York, McGraw-Hill Professional, 2004

Kouba S, Hallstrom T, Lindholm C, et al: Pregnancy and neonatal outcomes in women with eating disorders. Obstet Gynecol 105:255–260, 2005

Lacey JH, Smith G: Bulimia nervosa: the impact of pregnancy on mother and baby. Br J Psychiatry 150:777–781, 1987

Lorefalt B, Ganowiak W, Palhagen S, et al: Factors of importance for weight loss in elderly patients with Parkinson's disease. Acta Neurol Scand 110:180–187, 2004

Lustman PJ, Clouse RE: Treatment of depression in diabetes: impact on mood and medical outcome. J Psychosom Res 53:917–924, 2002

Mayer LE, Walsh BT: The use of selective serotonin reuptake inhibitors in eating disorders. J Clin Psychiatry 59 (suppl 15):28–34, 1998

Mazzeo SE, Slof-Op't Landt MCT, Jones I, et al: Associations among postpartum depression, eating disorders, and perfectionism in a population-based sample of adult women. Int J Eat Disord 39:202–211, 2006

Morgan JF, Lacey JH, Sedgwick PM: Impact of pregnancy on bulimia nervosa. Br J Psychiatry 174:135–140, 1999

Nicholson SD, Ballance E: Anorexia nervosa in later life: an overview. Hosp Med 59:268–272, 1998

O'Hara MW, Swain AM: Rates and risk of postpartum depression: a meta-analysis. Int Rev Psychiatry 8:37–54, 1996

Park RJ, Senior R, Stein A: The offspring of mothers with eating disorders. Eur Child Adolesc Psychiatry 12 (suppl 1):110–119, 2003

Rubin RR, Peyrot M: Psychological issues and treatments for people with diabetes. J Clin Psychol 57:457–478, 2001

Rydall AC, Rodin GM, Olmsted MP, et al: Disordered eating behavior and microvascular complications in young women with insulin-dependent diabetes mellitus. N Engl J Med 336:1905–1906, 1997

Stewart DE, Robinson E. Goldbloom DS, et al: Infertility and eating disorders. Am J Obstet Gynecol 165:1576–1577, 1991

Turton P, Hughes P, Bolton H, et al: Incidence and demographic correlates of eating disorder symptoms in a pregnant population. Int J Eat Disord 26:448–452, 1999

Watson TL, Andersen AE: A critical examination of the amenorrhea and weight criteria for diagnosing anorexia nervosa. Acta Psychiatr Scand 108:175–182, 2003

Wolfe BE: Reproductive health in women with eating disorders. J Obstet Gynecol Neonatal Nurs 34:255–263, 2005

Woodside DB, Garfinkel PE, Lin E, et al: Comparisons of men with full or partial eating disorders, men without eating disorders, and women with eating disorders in the community. Am J Psychiatry 158:570–574, 2001

World Health Organization: International Classification of Diseases, 10th Revision. Geneva, World Health Organization, 1992

14

Athletes and Eating Disorders

Pauline S. Powers, M.D.
Ron A. Thompson, Ph.D.

Considerable evidence suggests that competitive athletes in certain sports are at greater risk for disordered eating and eating disorders than the general population. Multiple factors appear to increase the risk. In the last few years the sport world has recognized that eating disorders are serious illnesses and has taken steps to decrease identifiable risks. In this chapter, we examine the relationship between athletes and eating disorders and review the risks that are unique to the athletic environment. We highlight difficulties in identifying the athlete with an eating disorder; discuss controversial questions regarding whether or not the athlete can continue in his or her sport during treatment; review key elements of treatment, particularly as they differ for the athlete; describe the meager evidence available on prevention of eating disorders among athletes; and, finally, offer commonsense guidelines for athletes, families, and sport and health care teams.

Role of the Athletic Environment in Predisposing Athletes to Eating Disorders

For many individuals, sports and sport participation can provide a very healthy and enjoyable experience that helps build self-esteem and self-efficacy and, at the same time, can provide a buffer against eating disorders (Fulkerson et al. 1999). This is not to say, however, that at least some sport environments are without their special, if not unique, risks to the athlete regarding such disorders (Thompson and Sherman 1999a, 1999b). A meta-analysis of 34 studies involving the relationship between sport participation and eating problems suggested that sport participation might serve as a protective factor for some athletes, whereas it might constitute a risk factor for others (Smolak et al. 2000). These findings imply that it is not sport participation per se that creates the risk for the athlete but rather certain aspects of at least some sports and/or sport environments. Because athletes are exposed to the same risk factors as their nonathlete counterparts in addition to those specific to the athletic environment, athletes are assumed to be at greater risk than nonathletes. Several specific aspects of sport environments and of specific sports pose these additional risks for the athlete.

Emphasis on Leanness and Thinness

Because of pressures to lose weight or body fat, athletes who participate in sports that emphasize a thin shape, small size, or low weight appear to be most at risk for eating disturbances (Brownell and Rodin 1992) and related problems such as the female athlete triad (Torstveit and Sundgot-Borgen 2005a, 2005b) (i.e., disordered eating, amenorrhea, and osteoporosis). These pressures are in large part related to a prevailing notion in the sport environment that thinness or leanness can enhance athletic performance (Wilmore 1992). This notion is embraced by coaches and athletes, despite the fact that the research in this area is, at best, equivocal. Its endorsement leads many athletes to engage in dietary restriction and/or excessive training in efforts to be leaner for the purpose of enhancing performance. However, high-risk sports appear to include not only those that emphasize thinness as it relates to enhanced performance, but almost any sport with a potentially unhealthy body emphasis or focus.

Revealing Uniforms and Sport Attire

An unhealthy body focus can result from revealing uniforms (National Collegiate Athletic Association 2005). If an athlete, especially a female athlete, is dissatisfied or uncomfortable with her body, she may feel too exposed in her uniform. As a consequence, she may be more apt to resort to weight loss as a means of coping, thereby increasing her risk for an eating disorder. However, the risk is not only related to her appearance or size. Such conditions can also play a role in competitive thinness.

Competitive Thinness

Some athletes engage in competitive thinness. They notice others who look thinner and feel a competitive need to lose weight for the same reasons as their nonathlete counterparts. But they also tend to be more competitive than others, both with respect to body comparisons related to thinness and appearance and in sport competition (Thompson and Sherman 1999b). We previously discussed the belief in the sport world that the leaner/thinner athlete performs better. If an athlete perceives that a better-performing competitor is also thinner, this perception may provide another rationale for losing weight (International Olympic Committee Medical Commission 2005; National Collegiate Athletic Association 2005). Revealing uniforms further increase the likelihood of competitive thinness by facilitating unhealthy body comparisons.

Unhealthy Subcultural Aspects

Some sports contain unhealthy beliefs, attitudes, and behaviors that appear to be embedded in that particular sport's subculture. To illustrate, the sport of horse racing not only accepts but facilitates unhealthy, pathogenic weight-loss methods used by jockeys to "make weight" (King and Mezey 1987). These include risky weight-loss procedures involving saunas (sweatboxes) and special oversized toilets at racetracks to foster dehydration and self-induced vomiting by jockeys who try to lose weight rapidly in order to make their weight limits. The Kentucky Derby Museum features a large display of photographs of jockeys with eating disorders (and a detailed description of how jockeys maintain a very low weight) without any suggestion that these behaviors are pathological or that attempts should be made to modify the risky environment for these men.

Perhaps the most obvious and well-known example of a subculture related to eating disturbances involves the sport of wrestling and the issue of "weight cutting." Wrestlers often will "wrestle down" one or two weight classes below their usual body weight. The guiding belief in the sport is that wrestlers who can lose enough weight (mostly through dehydration) to wrestle down to a lower weight class but maintain strength will have a decided advantage over their opponents. (Of course, this "rationale" fails to take into account that the wrestler's opponent is following the exact same set of beliefs and behaviors.) In the past, such prematch weight loss had been accomplished by "cutting weight" until the weigh-in prior to a match, usually by means of dietary restriction and excessive exercise in addition to a variety of behaviors and techniques that were essentially dehydration techniques, a battery of techniques well known to wrestlers and their coaches. Usually, immediately after the weigh-in and prior to the match, the wrestler would rehydrate and eat (often overeat or binge eat) in order to restore his strength (and weight). These beliefs and behaviors regarding weight cutting seemed to be an accepted part of the sport, at least until 1998, when three collegiate wrestlers died in a 33-day period as a result of complications related to weight cutting (Thompson 1998). As a consequence, at least at the collegiate level, more safeguards were put in place to protect athletes. Given the strength of the weight-cutting subculture, however, it would be naive to assume that such procedures are no longer used.

Role of the Coach

We began this section by discussing the fact that sport participation can positively affect athletes or be a risk factor. The same undoubtedly holds true for coaches. Since coaches have considerable power and influence with their athletes (e.g., LeUnes and Nation 1989; Sherman and Thompson 2001; Zimmerman 1999), depending on how that power and influence are used, a coach's effect on the athlete's eating attitudes and behaviors can be positive or negative. Certainly, accounts in the popular press (e.g., Ryan 2000), as well as in the professional literature (e.g., Rosen and Hough 1988; Thompson 1998), suggest that coaches can precipitate disordered eating or exacerbate an existing eating disorder in athletes. In their role as powerful authority figures, some coaches transmit messages to athletes that may actually foster or favor certain eating disorder behaviors, another risk factor. On the other hand, a recent survey of collegiate coaches indicated that most coaches have had some education or training regarding eating disorders, that they do not want their athletes undereating, and that they are aware of the seriousness of eating disorder behaviors/symptoms for both the athlete's health and performance (Trattner Sherman et al. 2005). These coaches can play a positive role in facilitating the identification, management, treatment, and prevention of eating disorders (National Collegiate Athletic Association 2005).

Risk and Type of Sport

Although eating disorders probably occur in all sports, at least among female athletes (Trattner Sherman et al. 2005), not all athletes are at the same risk. Substantial evidence suggests that athletes in sports that focus on leanness or low weight are at greater risk for eating disorders and disordered eating than those in "nonlean" sports (Beals and Manore 2002; Sundgot-Borgen 1993; Sundgot-Borgen and Larsen 1993; Sundgot-Borgen and Torstveit 2004; Torstveit and Sundgot-Borgen 2005a, 2005b). Included in the category of "lean" sports are those characterized as "aesthetic," "endurance," and "weight-class" sports (Torstveit and Sundgot-Borgen 2005a, 2005b). Some evidence also suggests that athletes in judged sports are at greater risk than athletes in refereed sports (Zucker et al. 1999). Thus, athletes who appear to be most at risk participate in sports that emphasize leanness/thinness (e.g., distance running, ski jumping), as well as aesthetic sports in which athletes are judged (e.g., diving, figure skating, gymnastics) or that have an appearance component (e.g., ballet, cheerleading), sports employing weight classes (e.g., lightweight rowing, wrestling), and sports that use revealing sport attire (e.g., swimming, volleyball).

Identification and Assessment of Eating Disorders in Athletes

Significant difficulties hamper easy identification of the athlete with an eating disorder. To start, although disordered eating is very common among athletes, many fewer of these athletes actually meet formal DSM-IV-TR criteria (American Psychiatric Association 2000) for an eating disorder (Johnson et al. 1999). However, this concern may not actually be too critical, because disordered eating sometimes can be as dangerous as full-syndromal anorexia nervosa or bulimia nervosa. Therefore, it may be more important to identify the entire gamut of disordered eating in athletes than to determine whether or not they meet formal diagnostic criteria. In this section, we describe methods available to detect disordered eating and eating disorders in athletes.

Difficulties in Recognition: Role of Potentially Misguided Health-Athletic Performance Beliefs

One important problem facing athletes is the unsubstantiated belief that weight loss will invariably improve athletic performance. More accurately, weight loss in *some* athletes will *sometimes* improve performance, but weight loss in other athletes will *sometimes hinder* performance. Factors that appear to be more important than weight loss in determining athletic performance are genetic inheritance (Wolfarth et al. 2005), muscle mass (Arslan 2005), and motivation (Orlick 2000). Evidence suggests that some very talented athletes are genetically endowed with certain types of muscle fibers that enhance certain types of athletic performances (e.g., Roger Bannister, who was the first person to run a mile in under 4 minutes) (Kyrolainen et al. 2003). Nonetheless, the belief that weight loss invariably improves performance is widely accepted in the sport world.

Another challenge in identifying eating disorders in athletes is the ease of misperceiving eating disorder symptoms such as amenorrhea and excessive exercise as being "normal" or even desirable (Trattner Sherman et al. 2005). Clearly, excessive exercise, sometimes difficult to identify for nonathletes, can be even harder to recognize in athletes. Thus, key eating disorder symptoms such as excessive dieting, weight loss, amenorrhea, and excessive exercise may be overlooked or even be considered positive developments.

Another important factor is the presumption that anyone who can perform well must be healthy. However, athletes with eating disorders are often able to perform well even if they are binge eating, purging, or restricting their food intake. Good performance may make it difficult for sport personnel, family, or friends to recognize the eating disorder. Unfortunately, many of the most serious physiological complications emerge silently or without warning, and sometimes the most dangerous signs and symptoms are not seen during the person's athletic career. One clearly undesirable physical complication that can develop without warning is sudden cardiac death associated with a prolonged QT interval (Roden 2006). Athletes who are genetically prone to a prolonged QT interval and who exercise excessively, eat restrictively, and/or purge habitually may suffer potentially lethal cardiac arrhythmias such as torsades de pointes associated with prolonged QT intervals (see Figure 14–1). Certain medications can also induce torsades de pointes in the context of the long QT syndrome (Abriel et al. 2004). A physiological complication that may become apparent later in life is osteoporosis. Although long-term studies have not been done among former athletes, many recovered eating disorder patients still have osteoporosis years later (Lucas et al. 1999).

Risk Factors

Many studies have attempted to find risk factors to identify athletes who might be particularly prone to develop disordered eating or a frank eating disorder. Among factors that may especially predispose women athletes, Sundgot-Borgen (1994) and Williamson and colleagues (1995) identified involvement in a sport that emphasizes body appearance; pressure from influential people (coaches or parents) to lose weight to improve performance; overinvolvement in sports, with few other social or recreational activities; training even when sick or injured; training outside of scheduled practice times or more than other athletes in the same sport or team; a traumatic event; injury; poor performance; or change in coaching personnel. Some researchers studying coaching styles have concluded that critical coaches or trainers may contribute to the development of disordered eating (Ryan 2000).

Thompson and Sherman (1999b) have proposed that "overcommitment" and "overcompliance" may represent additional risk factors. They noted many similarities between what are considered "good athlete" traits and personality characteristics seen in patients with anorexia nervosa (Table 14–1). A good athlete is usually considered to have a commitment to training, which in the individual with anorexia nervosa may be viewed as excessive exercise. A good athlete is described as coachable, whereas this same characteristic in anorexia nervosa is often called "over-compliance." These similarities may both predispose the athlete to an eating disorder and make it more difficult to identify the athlete who is developing an eating disorder.

Related to these risk factors are obsessive-compulsive traits, particularly those related to perfectionism. Several studies suggest that these traits may

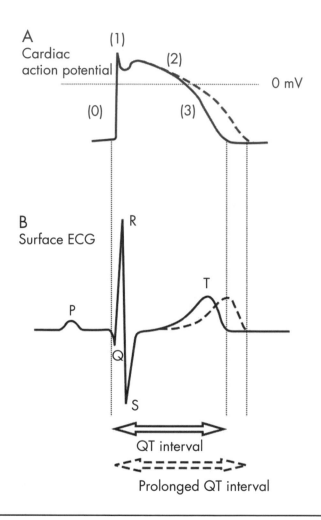

Figure 14–1.   Illustration of prolonged QT interval that can predispose to torsades de pointes arrhythmia.

Note.   ECG = electrocardiogram.

Source.   Reprinted from Abriel H, Schlapfer J, Keller DI, et al.: "Molecular and Clinical Determinants of Drug-Induced Long QT Syndrome: An Iatrogenic Channelopathy." *Swiss Medicine Weekly* 123:685–694, 2004. Used with permission.

Table 14–1. Similarities between "good athlete" traits and anorexia characteristics

Good athlete	Anorexic individual
Mental toughness	Asceticism
Commitment to training	Excessive exercise
Pursuit of excellence	Perfectionism
Coachability	Overcompliance
Unselfishness	Selflessness
Performance despite pain	Denial of discomfort

Source. Reprinted from Thompson RA, Sherman RT: "'Good' Athlete Traits and Characteristics of Anorexia Nervosa: Are They Similar? *Eating Disorders* 7:181–190, 1999b. Used with permission.

predispose to anorexia nervosa (and perhaps to bulimia nervosa) (Anderluth et al. 2003). Among patients with a formal diagnosis of anorexia nervosa, at least one-fourth meet the criteria for obsessive-compulsive disorder or obsessive-compulsive personality disorder (Kaye et al. 2004). With respect to athletics, having both a competitive nature and perfectionistic tendencies may predispose to the development of an eating disorder in an athlete and may contribute to why a person enters athletics in the first place.

Detection of an Eating Disorder in Athletes

Although the risk factors noted in the previous subsection may be associated with disordered eating even in the absence of a formal eating disorder, certain additional signs and symptoms may indicate that the athlete is developing a more severe disorder. These include fatigue, depressed mood, inability to concentrate, social withdrawal, cold intolerance, abdominal pain and bloating, constipation, light-headedness, irritability, insomnia, and withdrawal from social activities.

Screening tools devised to detect eating disorders include the Eating Disorder Inventory (both versions 2 and 3) (Garner 1994, 2003) and the Bulimia Test—Revised (Brelsford et al. 1992). However, these tests are not specific to athletes with eating disorders and are not adequately sensitive for athletes, perhaps because these instruments are obviously probing for eating disorder symptoms—and the athlete may not be willing or able to acknowledge the eating disorder. The Eating Disorder Examination (Fairburn and Cooper 1993) is considered to be the gold standard for detecting eating disorders, but administration requires lengthy training and the test requires about an hour to administer by trained personnel. The Athletic Milieu Direct Questionnaire (Nagel et al. 2000) is a newer test specifically designed to detect eating disorders in athletes, but, as with the other instruments thus far described, respondents immediately know what the test is looking for and may opt not to answer truthfully.

Black and colleagues (2003) have described the Physiologic Screening Test for Eating Disorders/Disordered Eating Among Female Collegiate Athletes. This test has the advantage of including physiological symptoms and signs, some of which can be directly measured or which are not obviously related to eating disorders. The 18 items include 4 physiological measurements (percent body fat, waist-hip ratio, standing systolic blood pressure, parotid gland enlargement), 6 interviewer questions (e.g., dizziness and abdominal bloating), and 8 self-report items (e.g., hours exercised outside of practice, menstrual irregularity). The authors report this test to be highly sensitive (87%) and highly specific (78%) for detecting athletes who have either disordered eating or eating disorders, and to not falsely detect those without disordered eating or eating disorders. Although this test does not solve the problem of identifying athletes who meet formal diagnostic criteria for eating disorders, it may offer a sensible first screening step. After athletes with eating disorder issues are identified through screening, a more complete evaluation by an eating disorder specialist or assessment with the Eating Disorder Examination can establish a formal diagnosis of anorexia nervosa or bulimia nervosa.

Sport Participation for Symptomatic Patients: Evaluation Criteria

When an athlete is identified as having an eating disorder, the question of whether an athlete can continue participating in a sport is inevitably raised by the athlete, coach, athletic trainer, team physician, and/or parent. How this question is considered and dealt with by the treatment and sport teams can play an important role in the athlete's overall health and academic and athletic management.

Reasons to Consider Sport Participation

From a health care perspective, clinicians might reasonably ask why one should even consider sport participation (training and/or competition) for a symptomatic athlete. The most conservative or "safest" response might argue that the athlete cannot train or compete as long as eating disorder signs or symptoms are present. However, there are actually several reasons to consider permitting athletes with eating disorders to continue participating, but only if many health maintenance criteria are first put in place to protect the athlete.

Identity and Self-Esteem

The importance of sport in the life of some athletes should not be underestimated. Being an athlete may constitute the individual's primary or sole role identity and may provide the person's primary source of self-esteem. As one athlete said, "I'm an anorexic basketball player; without basketball, I'm just an anorexic." Without sport, the athlete may become (more) depressed and suffer further exacerbation of eating disorder symptoms.

Attachment and Support

Allowing athletes to train and compete affords them the opportunity to remain attached to teammates, team, and sport. This sense of attachment and the possibilities for support from coaches and teammates—the athlete's "sport family"—can be beneficial to the athlete's recovery.

Monitoring and Safety

If sport participation is withheld, the ability to monitor the athlete's condition may be significantly decreased. Beumont and colleagues (1994) suggested that it is difficult, if not impossible, to keep eating disorder patients from exercising. Athletes with eating disorders may, in fact, be more apt than their teammates to exercise, citing their need to maintain conditioning as an excuse and rationale for their extra exercise. When the athlete is allowed to train and compete as part of a team, the athlete's symptoms and condition can more easily be monitored by appropriate sport (i.e., coaches) and sport medicine (e.g., athletic trainer, team physician) personnel and perhaps better controlled.

Facilitation of Eating

Exercise (sport participation in this case) can facilitate the eating and weight changes that may be necessary in treatment (Beumont et al. 1994).

Motivation

Sport participation can be used to motivate the athlete in treatment. If the athlete-patient is not progressing in treatment or, worse yet, refuses treatment, the threat of withholding training and competition may be raised, and, ultimately, these privileges can be withheld. Many athletes, at least those who truly want to participate, will work harder in treatment in order to maintain or regain sport participation. In the event that training and competition are withheld, the athlete should remain a part of the team and attend all team/sport activities as is feasible and safe (e.g., competitions, practices, team meetings). This arrangement allows for a continuing sense of attachment and opportunities to at least observe and monitor the athlete's medical and psychological condition.

Sport Participation Decisions

Several issues should be considered when determining the sport participation status for an athlete with an eating disorder.

Diagnosis

As long as the athlete meets formal diagnostic criteria for anorexia nervosa, sport participation (training, practice, and competition) should be withheld (International Olympic Committee Medical Commission 2005; Sherman and Thompson 2001). The athlete with frank anorexia nervosa is simply too ill to be training or competing. Withholding sport participation in such a situation communicates to the athlete that health will not be subordinated to athletics. Athletes with eating disorder diagnoses other than anorexia nervosa may be considered for sport participation if they meet several criteria. They must first be "cleared" by the treatment team. That is, responsible clinicians must determine that sport participation would not place the athlete at additional risk medically or psychologically. Also, the treatment team needs to be specific regarding the activities for which the athlete is cleared to perform.

Relationship Between Eating Disorders and Sport Participation

In determining how and whether an athlete should continue to train and compete, the nature of the relationship of the eating disorder to the sport must be carefully examined (Sherman and Thompson 2001). This relationship can be a direct one, in which pressures associated with the sport are exerted on the athlete to lose weight, engage in pathogenic weight-loss methods, or exercise excessively. In the sport of wrestling, this type of pressure has been referred to as "sports-induced disturbances in eating" (Enns et al. 1987). Similarly, consider the situation of a distance runner who uses her sport to create an energy deficit and weight loss, because she, her coach, and her sport subscribe to the belief that a thinner, leaner body will perform better. In most of these environments, training and competing while symptomatic is probably contraindicated, at least until the athlete can make progress in treatment and can protect herself from the potentially unhealthy aspects of participating in her sport.

In other situations, the relationship between the athlete's eating disorder and sport participation may be indirect or the disorder may be unrelated to sport. In these situations the sport does not involve losing weight, decreasing body fat, or exercising excessively in order to perform better. In such cases the athlete might engage in eating disorder symptoms to alleviate pressure or anxiety associated with sport performance or to alleviate uncomfortable emotions associated with poor performance. Some athletes in this group would most likely have had an eating disorder even without having been an athlete. Athletes in this group can be considered for sport participation when symptomatic as long as they meet certain health maintenance criteria.

The Athlete's Desire to Participate in Sport

Individuals with eating disorders are often motivated to please (or at least not displease) significant others. As a consequence, they often make their decisions on the basis what they think others would want. Athletes are no different than their nonathlete counterparts in this regard. In fact, they want to please not only family and friends but also their coaches, teammates, and fans. Providing athletes with the opportunity to make their own decisions in this regard can be a first step in helping them establish internal standards by which to make decisions, and in providing what may feel like a more acceptable way to discontinue their sport. Some athletes with eating disorders who actually do not want to continue in sport may not be psychologically strong enough to actively make that choice known to their coaches, teammates or parents, fearing that they would be letting them down by quitting. In this regard, the treatment team can offer to take that pressure off the athlete by taking responsibility for the decision, and by informing those who have a need to know that continued sport participation is contraindicated.

Treatment Progress

Once the treatment team has determined that participation in sport will not increase the medical or psychological risks and that the eating disorder is not directly related to sport participation, and once the athlete chooses to participate in sport and has been cleared medically, the next criterion is that the athlete must be in treatment. After a reasonable period of time the treatment team must know not only that the athlete is in treatment but that he or she is improving. If the athlete is not improving, the athlete should be informed that sport participation will be withdrawn unless acceptable levels of improvement occur. Then, if progress is not made, sport participation should be withdrawn (International Olympic Committee Medical Commission 2005; Sherman and Thompson 2006). In this event, the athlete should be informed that this change is meant for his or her protection and is not intended as a punishment. The athlete should be explicitly informed of the specific changes that must be made in order to regain sport participation.

Health Maintenance Criteria

In addition to meeting the aforementioned criteria, athletes are expected to meet other health maintenance criteria designed to protect the individual. Some are general in nature and should be applied to all athlete-patients, such as maintenance of a body mass index (BMI) of at least 19, ingestion of sufficient calories to meet nutritional goals regarding weight gain or maintenance, and compliance with all treatment appointments and recommendations. Other criteria can be tailored to meet the unique needs of a particular individual (e.g., following a prescribed exercise/activity regimen).

The following case example illustrates some of the issues that may arise during the evaluation of athletes with eating disorders.

> Amy, a 20-year-old distance runner, was referred for an eating disorder evaluation by the team physician of her collegiate cross-country team. At the evaluation, she told the eating disorder specialist that she did not want to be weighed, but that if she had to be weighed she did not want to know her weight. Her weight was 111 pounds at 5 feet, 4 inches tall (BMI = 19.1), which according to the team physician represented a decrease of 8 pounds during the last year. Amy's training as prescribed by her coach involved workouts 6 days per week, which included running 45–50 miles per week. She admitted that she occa-

sionally ran more on her own. Amy indicated that she thought she was "fat," especially for a distance runner, and needed to lose weight. She denied the current use of any pathogenic weight-loss methods, although she admitted that she had occasionally vomited while in high school. She reported her daily caloric intake to be 1,500–1,600 calories. When asked about her menstrual cycle, she indicated that her periods had been irregular for the past 4–5 months. Amy was given a diagnosis of eating disorder not otherwise specified and was told that she would need to return for outpatient treatment. Amy asked if she would be allowed to continue in her sport during treatment. She was told sport participation would be considered if it was determined by her healthcare team that sport participation would not increase her physical or psychological risk, if she was progressing in treatment, if she maintained a BMI of at least 19, and if she complied fully with all treatment recommendations. Amy was informed that a decision to permit sport participation could be withdrawn at any time by the health care team if any of these healthcare maintenance conditions were not met.

A Final Thought on Sport Participation for Symptomatic Athletes

Deciding to allow an athlete with an eating disorder to continue training and competing while symptomatic has everything to do with guarding and enhancing the psychological health and treatment of the athlete; it has nothing to do with sport performance. Even though sport personnel should be consulted when appropriate, decisions regarding training and competition must be the responsibility of the clinical treatment team. If doubt exists at any time regarding the appropriateness of sport participation, the athlete should be withheld from sport. This explicitly stated value provides a clear message to athletes that although their treatment providers understand and appreciate the importance of sport in their lives, their health is paramount to sport.

Treatment for Athletes With Eating Disorders

The general principles of treatment for athletes with eating disorders are similar to those for patients who are not athletes, but some special considerations demand attention. For athletes with eating disorders, there are also often specific concerns regarding confidentiality and communication between the sport and health care teams.

Anorexia Nervosa and the Female Athlete Triad

Anorexia nervosa and the *female athlete triad*—disordered eating, amenorrhea, and osteoporosis—have important similarities. The term was chosen, in part, to emphasize to the sport team the importance of eating disorders (particularly anorexia nervosa). But the term can be confusing. For example, male athletes often develop eating disorders and may develop analogous symptoms; instead of low estrogen levels and amenorrhea they may suffer decreases in testosterone and estrogen that may also predispose to osteoporosis. Also, some people who have the female athlete triad may not develop all the symptoms that are required in DSM-IV-TR for anorexia nervosa or bulimia nervosa, and their condition may fall into the category termed *eating disorder not otherwise specified*. Often, the underweight athlete with the triad may not be 15% or more below ideal body weight. Many athletes with the triad have a subsyndromal form of anorexia nervosa. These patients usually need a weight restoration program coupled with nutritional counseling and psychotherapy as described elsewhere in this volume (see, particularly, Chapter 2, "Assessment and Determination of Initial Treatment Approaches for Patients With Eating Disorders"; Chapter 4, "Management of Anorexia Nervosa in Inpatient and Partial Hospitalization Settings"; and Chapter 5, "Management of Anorexia Nervosa in an Ambulatory Setting").

Weight Restoration

During this stage of treatment, the initial activity level should be very limited until a full assessment of the athlete's physical condition has been completed. In addition to a complete physical examination and laboratory assessment, the clinician should obtain an electrocardiogram to assess for the presence of arrhythmias and prolonged QT intervals, which are particularly dangerous in this population. Similarly, the clinician should order a dual-energy X-ray absorptiometry (DEXA) to detect abnormalities in bone density, since this group of eating disorder patients is at particular risk for osteopenia or osteoporosis (Waldrop 2005).

Activity Levels

Shifting levels of activity may be permitted as the patient with the triad or anorexia nervosa begins to progress in treatment and gain weight. In the initial stage of treatment, the athlete's prescribed level of activity would not necessarily be different from that of a nonathlete patient. Decisions regarding activity for the athlete depend on her physical and psychological health status and her progress in treatment.

If the athlete with the triad or anorexia nervosa is to be permitted to increase her activity to levels approaching her habitual activity prior to diagnosis and prior to attaining at least 90% of her expected healthy body weight (based on height, weight history, age, and genetics), she should probably be in inpatient or residential treatment. Although allowing such activity for these patients is still controversial, controlled exercise or increased physical activity in a controlled therapeutic environment has become an accepted and effective part of some treatment programs (e.g., Calogero and Pedrotty 2004). However, in these programs the decision to permit the patient to participate in such activity has little or nothing to do with the patient's being an athlete. Rather, the decision is based on what her treatment team regards as being safe and therapeutic given her current condition.

In the event that the athlete with anorexia nervosa is being treated on an outpatient basis, we recommend that she meet the criteria outlined earlier in the subsection "Sport Participation Decisions" regarding decisions concerning permission to train or compete. Even if the athlete's condition and progress in treatment will not permit engagement in full training and competition, treatment staff might want to consider a return to modified training—for example, sport-related skills training that does not require activities that might increase the athlete's risk for physical complications. For example, a basketball player might be allowed to practice shooting, or if free-form shooting seems too vigorous, the player might be restricted to shooting free throws. Volleyball or tennis players might be allowed to practice serving. For other sports or for decisions about higher levels of acceptable activity, the treatment staff might want to consult with the athlete's sports medicine staff (i.e., athletic trainer, team physician, sport psychologist, exercise physiologist). Again, the primary concern of sports medicine professionals involved in such a consultation must be the athlete's mental and physical health rather than her performance (Sherman and Thompson 2006).

The rationale for allowing the patient to participate in some degree of activity has little to do with sport participation per se. Participation in activities should be permitted primarily because this may facilitate the necessary eating and weight changes. And, as mentioned earlier (see "Identity and Self-Esteem"), the athlete who is allowed to participate in modified or partial sport skills training may retain more self-esteem through her valued sense of identity as an athlete and be able to sustain a sense of attachment to and support from her team. Granting or withholding of such training activities can serve to motivate the athlete in treatment.

Nutritional Counseling

Numerous myths abound regarding appropriate nutritional intake for athletes in various sports. At the start of treatment, the initial focus should be on consumption of adequate calories, and as improvement in intake and weight occurs, focus may turn to the appropriate balance of protein, carbohydrates, and fats. There is little evidence that athletes require a significantly different nutritional composition than nonathletes. In fact, well-documented nutritional guidelines for athletes usually recommend the use of the food guide pyramid, along with the general concepts of moderation and variety (e.g., Clark 2003; Girard Eberle 2000). Nonetheless, the registered dietitian must be aware of the nutritional misconceptions commonly held by athletes and be prepared to provide corrective information.

Psychotherapy

The type and focus of psychotherapy depend in part on the athlete's age and developmental stage. Adolescents and younger children usually require significant family therapy, and among athletes the discussion may revolve around the patient's sport. Some athletes may need help to balance their lives with interests and activities in addition to sport. Others may want to stop participating in their sport and need help doing so. Still others may be unsuited to the sport they have initially chosen and may need to recognize that they face inevitable and continued disappointment if they continue to focus exclusively on this sport. Consider, for example, an athlete who has been an outstanding gymnast but who becomes quite tall as she develops and will therefore be unable to perform the maneuvers in which she previously excelled.

Adult athletes are likely to need individual psychotherapy and may need assistance in emancipating from their parents. This goal can be complicated if family members are excessively invested in the athlete's performance or success. Athletes who have habitually used excessive exercise to cope with emotions may need to learn alternative ways to cope with stress.

Bulimia Nervosa

Bulimia nervosa may be particularly difficult to recognize because the person may be at a normal weight and may have few physical symptoms or signs. The term *exercise bulimia* has been employed to describe people who overexercise to compensate for normal eating or binge eating, but this is not a DSM-IV-TR diagnosis. Patients who use exercise to compensate for binge eating are more correctly classified as having bulimia nervosa, nonpurging type, using the current DSM criteria (American Psychiatric Association 2000).

Often the coach or fellow teammates initially recognize bulimia nervosa, and they may be the ones who confront the athlete and ask him or her to seek evaluation and treatment. The basic elements of treatment are similar to those required for nonathlete patients. The most effective treatment is cognitive-behavioral therapy (CBT). Since many athletes with bulimia nervosa may compulsively exercise rather than vomit as a way to compensate for overeating, the focus of CBT may differ from that for nonathletes—that is, the focus may be on binge-eating episodes and overexercise. The athlete will need to identify triggers to both the binge eating and the overexercise. Unlike patients who purge by vomiting, for whom response preventions techniques immediately following binge eating may be effective, the athlete who purges by overexercising can overexercise at any time, not just during the hour or so after a binge. Interrupting excessive exercise can be very challenging.

Although the U.S. Food and Drug Administration has approved the use of fluoxetine for the treatment of bulimia nervosa based on a large multicenter trial ("Fluoxetine in the Treatment of Bulimia Nervosa" 1992), there may be special considerations concerning use of this medication among athletes, especially those who use exercise as a purge method. For athletes who demonstrate obsessive-compulsive characteristics, fluoxetine may be a good choice. However, since some patients develop sedation and a few gain weight while taking this medication, these potential adverse effects should be discussed with the patient before fluoxetine is prescribed. But the main problem, especially for athletes who demonstrate "exercise bulimia," is that the potential effect of fluoxetine on reducing episodes of overexercise is unknown.

Binge-Eating Disorder

Although the precise prevalence of binge-eating disorder among athletes is unknown, it may be quite common.. High caloric requirements are notable for certain sports that involve sustained muscular effort, such as soccer or football, and some sports may overvalue larger-than-normal body sizes. In one large National Collegiate Athletic Association study (Johnson et al. 1999), football players were more likely to describe frequent overeating episodes than athletes in other sports. Overeating among athletes is likely to promote weight gain and may lead to full syndromal binge eating disorder if the athlete begins to feel guilty and out of control of his or her eating.

Prevention of Eating Disorders in Athletes

Because eating disorders occur at different ages and stages of development and among groups with very different skills and stresses, it is likely that differing strategies for prevention will be needed for various groups of athletes. Thus far, although most interest has focused on collegiate and elite athletes, since eating disorders often begin in early to midadolescence, prevention strategies in this younger age group are urgently needed.

Emerging evidence suggests that a curriculum taught to middle school students in the context of team practices can be helpful. For example, in a research study involving the ATHENA (Athletes Targeting Healthy Exercise and Nutrition Alternatives) program, 928 young female high school athletes in 40 sport teams at 18 schools participated in 8 weekly 45-minute sessions incorporated into the team's usual practice activities. Athletes involved in the program reported less ongoing and new use of diet pills and less new use of athletic-enhancing substances, positive changes in strength-training self-efficacy, and healthy eating behaviors (Elliot et al. 2004).

Coaches

Although prevention requires appropriate education of athletes regarding eating disorders, educating coaches may be as, or even more, important. Coaches have such power and influence with their athletes that prevention programs for athletes are unlikely to work without the support of coaches (National Collegiate Athletic Association 2005; Trattner Sherman et al. 2005). Thus, prevention programming for coaches should be a priority.

First, coaches must become better informed about eating, nutrition, weight, the risks of dieting, the female athlete triad, and how these affect the athlete's health and performance. Unfortunately, coaches not only harbor many of the same misconceptions regarding weight and eating as the lay public, but also often embrace myths about weight and eating associated with their particular sports.

Second, coaches must recognize the power and influence they have with their athletes, and that this power and influence can be helpful or harmful. Many coaches appear to serve as surrogate parents (Zimmerman 1999) for the athlete's "sport family."

Third, since coaches understandably tend to focus on athletic performance, they need to recognize and remember that performance is multidimensional and determined by multiple factors, not simply weight or leanness. Certainly, coaches all know heavier athletes who perform well and leaner athletes who do not. Coaches need to emphasize health and good nutrition rather than weight. They can do so by reminding their athletes that good health is most likely the primary contributor to good performance and that good nutrition is likely to be a primary contributor to good health. To better understand and work with these issues, coaches should be using well-documented sources of evidence-based information and strongly recommend that their athletes and sports medicine staff rely on such information. Coaches should also become more familiar with the many successful non-weight-focused strategies for enhancing performance, many of which involve psychological approaches or mental training to improve motivation, concentration, and confidence (Orlick 2000).

Fourth, coaches need to encourage and support appropriate, effective, and early identification and treatment. Coaches' support, encouragement, and participation in an eating disorder patient's treatment may be facilitative and as important as family involvement.

Fifth, some coaches need to focus on establishing better interpersonal relationships with their athletes. Some athletes complain that coaches treat them as "athletes" or "bodies" rather than "people." Better relationships are apt to improve communication regarding important issues such as healthy eating and training, as well as facilitate early identification. Some athletes suggest that improved relationships may also enhance performance, an added bonus.

Families

Although recommendations that families be involved in the prevention of eating disorders among student athletes are common, little research describes effective strategies that a family might take. Suggestions for families that may help prevent or detect eating disorders among their adolescents and young adult children (Powers 2000) are presented in the appendix to this chapter. Although predisposing risk factors for eating disorders among athletes and nonathletes are likely to begin long before middle school, these suggestions may permit the family to detect developing eating disorders in their student athletes.

Conclusion

Athletes in sports that emphasize leanness or appearance or sports that have certain weight classes are more likely to develop eating disorders, but identifying athletes with eating disorders in these groups can be challenging. Once an eating disorder is identified, the health care team needs to consider whether or not the symptomatic athlete can continue in his or her sport. The athlete's mental and physical health are more important than athletic performance and should be the guiding concern in deciding the extent to which athletic performance can be permitted. Exercise should be incorporated into treatment in a way that is mindful of the meaning of sport and exercise to the patient. Although few proven prevention strategies have been developed for athletes, some promising approaches exist, and the role of the coach and the athletic environment in prevention efforts offers some very promising avenues for further research.

References

Abriel H, Schlapfer J, Keller DI, et al: Molecular and clinical determinants of drug-induced long QT syndrome: an iatrogenic channelopathy. Swiss Med Wkly 123:685–694, 2004

American Psychiatric Association: Diagnostic and Statistical Manual of Mental Disorders, 4th Edition, Text Revision. Washington, DC, American Psychiatric Association, 2000

American Psychiatric Association: Practice Guideline for the Treatment of Patients With Eating Disorders, 3rd Edition. Arlington, VA, American Psychiatric Association, 2006. Available at: http://www.psych.org/psych_pract/treatg/pg/Eating Disorders3ePG_04-28-06.pdf. Accessed January 10, 2007.

Anderluth MB, Tchanturia K, Rabe-Heskethd S, et al: Childhood obsessive-compulsive personality traits in adult women with eating disorders: defining a broader eating disorder phenotype. Am J Psychiatry 160:242–247, 2003

Arslan C: Relationship between the 30-second Wingate test and characteristics of isometric and explosive leg strength in young subjects. J Strength Cond Res 19:658–666, 2005

Beals KA, Manore MM: Disorders of the female athlete triad among collegiate athletes. Int J Sport Nutr Exerc Metab 12:281–293, 2002

Beumont PJV, Arthur B, Russell JD, et al: Excessive physical activity in dieting disorder patients: proposals for a supervised exercise program. Int J Eat Disord 15:21–36, 1994

Black DR, Larkin LJS, Coster DC, et al: Physiologic Screening Test for Eating Disorders/Disordered Eating Among Female Collegiate Athletes. J Athl Train 38:286–297, 2003

Brelsford TN, Hummel RM, Barios BA: The Bulimia Test—Revised: a psychometric investigation. Psychol Assess 4:399–401, 1992

Brownell KD, Rodin J: Prevalence of eating disorders in athletes, in Eating, Body Weight, and Performance in Athletes: Disorders of Modern Society. Edited by Brownell KD, Rodin J, Wilmore JH. Philadelphia, PA, Lea & Febiger, 1992, pp 128–145

Calogero RM, Pedrotty KN: The practice and process of healthy exercise: an investigation of the treatment of exercise abuse in women with eating disorders. Eat Disord 12:273–291, 2004

Clark N: Nancy Clark's Sports Nutrition Guidebook, 3rd Edition. Champaign, IL, Human Kinetics, 2003

Elliot DL, Goldberg L, Moe EL, et al: Preventing substance abuse and disordered eating: initial outcomes of the ATHENA (Athletes Targeting Healthy Exercise and Nutrition Alternatives) program. Arch Pediatr Adolesc Med 158:1043–1049, 2004

Enns MP, Drewnowski A, Grinker JA: Body composition, body size estimation, and attitudes toward eating in male college athletes. Psychosom Med 49:56–64, 1987

Fairburn CG, Cooper Z: The Eating Disorder Examination, 12.0D, in Binge Eating: Nature, Assessment, and Treatment. Edited by Fairburn CG, Wilson GT. New York, Guilford, 1993, pp 317–260

Fluoxetine in the treatment of bulimia nervosa: a multicenter, placebo-controlled, double-blind trial. Fluoxetine Bulimia Nervosa Collaborative Study Group. Arch Gen Psychiatry 49:139–147, 1992

Fulkerson JA, Keel PK, Leon GR, et al: Eating-disordered behaviors and personality characteristics of high school athletes and nonathletes. Int J Eat Disord 26:73–79, 1999

Garner DM: Eating Disorder Inventory–2. Odessa, FL, Psychological Assessment Resources, 1994

Garner DM: Eating Disorder Inventory–3. Odessa, FL, Psychological Assessment Resources, 2003

Girard Eberle S: Endurance Sports Nutrition. Champaign, IL, Human Kinetics, 2000

International Olympic Committee Medical Commission, Working Group Women in Sport: Position stand on the female athlete triad, 2005. Available at: http://multimedia.olympic.org/pdf/en_report_917.pdf. Accessed January 10, 2007.

Johnson C, Powers PS, Dick R: The National Collegiate Athletic Association study. Int J Eat Disord 26:209–220, 1999

Kaye WH, Bulik CM, Thornton L, et al: Comorbidity of anxiety disorders with anorexia and bulimia nervosa. Am J Psychiatry 161:2215–2221, 2004

King MB, Mezey G: Eating behaviour of male racing jockeys. Psychol Med 17:249–253, 1987

Kyrolainen H, Kivela R, Koskinen S, et al: Interrelationships between muscle structure, muscle strength, and running economy. Med Sci Sports Exerc 35:45–49, 2003

LeUnes AD, Nation JR: Sport Psychology: An Introduction. Chicago, IL, Nelson Hall, 1989

Lucas AR, Melton LJ 3rd, Crowson CS, et al: Long-term fracture risk among women with anorexia nervosa: a population-based cohort study. Mayo Clin Proc 74:972–977, 1999

Nagel DL, Black DR, Leverenz LJ, et al: Evaluation of a screening test for female college athletes with eating disorders and disordered eating. J Athl Train 35:431–440, 2000

National Collegiate Athletic Association: NCAA Coaches Handbook: Managing the Female Athlete Triad. Indianapolis, IN, National Collegiate Athletic Association, 2005

Orlick T: In Pursuit of Excellence: How to Win in Sports and Life Through Mental Training. Champaign, IL, Human Kinetics, 2000

Powers PS: Athletes and eating disorders: protective and risk factors. Healthy Weight Journal July/August 2000, pp 59–61

Roden DM: Long QT syndrome: reduced repolarization reserves and the genetic link. J Intern Med 259:59–69, 2006

Rosen L, Hough DO: Pathogenic weight control behaviors of female college gymnasts. Phys Sportsmed 16:141–144, 1988

Ryan J: Little Girls in Pretty Boxes: The Making and Breaking of Elite Gymnasts and Figure Skaters. New York, Warner Books, 2000

Sherman RT, Thompson RA: Athletes with disordered eating: four major issues for the professional psychologist. Prof Psychol 32:27–33, 2001

Sherman RT, DeHass D, Thompson RT, et al: NCAA coaches survey: the role of the coach in identifying and managing athletes with disordered eating. Eat Disord 13:447–466, 2005

Smolak L, Murnen SK, Ruble AE: Female athletes and eating problems: a meta-analysis. Int J Eat Disord 27:371–380, 2000

Sundgot-Borgen J: Prevalence of eating disorders in elite female athletes. Int J Sport Nutr 3:29–40, 1993

Sundgot-Borgen J: Risk and trigger factors for the development of eating disorders in female elite athletes. Med Sci Sports Exerc 26:414–419, 1994

Sundgot-Borgen J, Larsen S: Pathogenic weight-control methods and self-reported eating disorders in female elite athletes and controls. Scand J Med Sci Sports 3:150–155, 1993

Sundgot-Borgen J, Torstveit M: Prevalence of eating disorders in elite athletes is higher than in the general population. Clin J Sport Med 14:25–32, 2004

Thompson RA: The last word: wrestling with death. Eat Disord 6:207–210, 1998

Thompson RA, Sherman RT: Athletes, athletic performance, and eating disorders: healthier alternatives. J Soc Issues 55:317–337, 1999a

Thompson RA, Sherman RT: "Good" athlete traits and characteristics of anorexia nervosa: are they similar? Eat Disord 7:181–190, 1999b

Torstveit MK, Sundgot-Borgen J: The female athlete triad: are elite athletes at increased risk? Med Sci Sports Exerc 37:184–193, 2005a

Torstveit MK, Sundgot-Borgen J: The female athlete triad exists in both elite athletes and controls. Med Sci Sports Exerc 37:1449–1459, 2005b

Trattner Sherman R, Thompson RA: Practical use of the International Olympic Committee Medical Commission Position Stand on the Female Athlete Triad: a case example. Int J Eat Disord 39:193–201, 2006

Waldrop J: Early identification and interventions for female athlete triad. J Pediatr Health Care 19:213–220, 2005

Williamson DA, Netemeyer RG, Jackman LP, et al: Structural equation modeling of risk factors for the development of eating disorder symptoms in female athletes. Int J Eat Disord 17:387–393, 1995

Wilmore JH: Body weight standards and athletic performance, in Eating, Body Weight, and Performance in Athletes: Disorders of Modern Society. Edited by Brownell KD, Rodin J, Wilmore JH. Philadelphia, PA, Lea & Febiger, 1992, pp 315–329

Wolfarth B, Bray MS, Hagberg JM, et al: The human genome for performance and health-related fitness phenotypes: the 2004 update. Med Sci Sports Exerc 37:881–903, 2005

Zimmerman TS: Using family systems theory to counsel the injured athlete, in Counseling in Sports Medicine. Edited by Ray R, Wiese-Bjornstal DM. Champaign, IL, Human Kinetics, 1999, pp 111–126

Zucker NL, Womble LG, Williamson DA, et al: Protective factors for eating disorders in female college athletes. Eat Disord 7:207–218, 1999

Appendix: Student Athletes and Eating Disorders: A Parents' Guide[1]

1. *Weight loss.* Many teens beginning a sport lose some weight. However, if the amount seems to be large, it is helpful to see if the athlete is still on his or her growth curve. During development, there are individual differences in growth. Your youngster's pediatrician keeps track of this development and usually has plotted an individual growth curve. Thus, the pediatrician can determine if the athlete has fallen below his or her usual growth curve.

2. *Resetting of weight goals.* Since the majority of adolescent girls (and perhaps boys) diet at some point, it can be difficult to determine if a small weight loss is an early sign of an emerging eating disorder. In addition, many teenagers lose weight when they first begin an active sport and become part of a team. If your teenager decides to lose a modest amount of weight and he or she does lose this weight and is satisfied, probably there is no problem. On the other hand, if the initial weight goal is achieved and your teenager resets his or her goal to a lower weight, it may indicate a problem.

3. *Amenorrhea.* If your daughter loses her menstrual periods, take it seriously. Although the stress of physical exercise can cause amenorrhea, loss of menses can also be an early sign of an eating disorder. Irrespective of the cause, amenorrhea during adolescence is dangerous since it is associated with the early development of osteoporosis (thinning of the bones and bone fractures).

4. *Excessive exercise.* Although it can be difficult to judge whether exercise is excessive, if your teenager exercises more than is expected by his or her particular sport or particular level in that sport, discussion with your teenager or with the coach may be warranted. For example, if the athlete is part of a basketball team and the coach expects the participants to run a mile on 2 days of the week and your teenager runs 2 miles every day, this could be a problem. On the other hand, an elite athlete in training for a marathon may be exercising many hours per day.

---

[1]Adapted from Powers PS: "Athletes and Eating Disorders: Protective and Risk Factors." *Healthy Weight Journal* July/August 2000, pp. 59–61. Used with permission.

5. *Inappropriate dieting behavior.* If your teenager is in a group of athletes who are following extreme or unusual dieting practices, this requires your attention. If more than one athlete in his or her group has an eating disorder, there may be undue emphasis on dieting by the coach or by the group in general. Use of fat-burning aids, laxatives, or diuretics is also hazardous.

6. *Negative comments by coach or trainer.* If you learn that the coach has made negative comments about the weight, shape, or performance of any of the athletes in the sport, it is wise to schedule a meeting with the coach and ask him or her to refrain from such comments. Also, many coaches of elite athletes have received training about eating disorders. For example, USA Gymnastics sponsors educational programs for coaches to teach them about eating disorders and how to prevent them in their athletes. The National Collegiate Athletic Association (NCAA) has recently published a handbook for coaches regarding the female athlete triad (i.e., disordered eating, amenorrhea, and osteoporosis). It is helpful to determine if the coach has participated in these educational endeavors. If you suspect that the coach is making comments to the athletes that are derogatory, it can be helpful to attend a few practices or competitions to assess the attitudes of the coaches.

7. *Use of exercise to purge.* If your teenager exercises regularly after consuming food, he or she may be using exercise to "burn up" calories, and this may be a form of purge behavior.

8. *Intense use of exercise or pursuit of a sport after a significant disappointment.* For example, if your teenager was usually quite sociable, but then her boyfriend broke up with her, and she no longer sees her friends but devotes many hours daily to exercise, this may be a problem.

9. *Avoidance of tasks of adolescence.* If the athlete becomes preoccupied with exercise such that he or she is no longer socializing, achieving in school, or engaged in the process of emancipation from parents, then exercise may have become an inappropriate solution to a problem in one of these areas.

10. *Athletic performance and weight loss.* The belief that weight loss alone will improve athletic performance is incorrect. Genetic endowment, muscle mass, and motivation are the three factors that most influence performance. If the athlete or coach believes that ever-increasing weight loss

will continue to improve performance, this may place the adolescent at risk for an eating disorder.

11. *Participation in high-risk sports.* Certain sports, such as gymnastics or body building, are judged on both athletic performance and appearance and may place the adolescent athlete at particular risk. Prior to participation in these sports, it is wise to know the attitude of the coach and the training that he or she has in prevention of eating disorders.

12. *Unrealistic sport achievement expectations.* Although it is helpful to encourage an athlete who has the potential to become an elite athlete, it is counterproductive, and perhaps dangerous, to encourage an athlete who is not able to become an elite athlete to try to do so. A realistic appraisal of the athlete's potential by the parent, coach, and athlete will decrease the likelihood of a severe later disappointment.

15

Cultural Considerations in Eating Disorders

Tracy M. Anthony, M.D.

Joel Yager, M.D.

Historically, eating disorders have been viewed as endemic to Western culture and even as culture-bound syndromes (Keel and Klump 2003). For decades, the prototypical eating disorder patient has been, and continues to be, a Caucasian woman of higher socioeconomic status. However, the face of the eating disorder patient is changing. Eating disorders have been increasingly described in both typical and atypical forms in non-Caucasian populations in developed Western countries and in non-Western, developing countries.

Accounts of anorexia nervosa–like syndromes, "holy anorexia," described several hundred years ago, were explained in cultural terms as women who "starved themselves as a route to God" (Pearce 2004). In a review of the history of anorexia, Bemporad (1996) described girls and women who by rigidly adhering to self-denial and mortification of the flesh "secured a sense of superi-

387

ority in their sanctity and beliefs of belonging to God's elect" (p. 223). Today's predominant cultural account focuses on overvaluation of thinness as the physical embodiment of beauty and, correspondingly, success. Such cultural values and pressures in turn lead to dieting behaviors in the service of improved self-image, acceptance, and status. These cultural values have increasingly pervaded all strata and subcultures of society, thanks to the ubiquitous influences of mass media. Media influences have resulted in changing eating, exercise, and fashion practices among the children of recent immigrants, in the United States and Western Europe, contributing to shifts in weight and in the prevalence of eating disorders and obesity. Anyone receiving television is exposed to these messages, so virtually no subculture in the contemporary world, regardless of ethnicity, family influence, peer group, or generational cohort, is untouched. But each of the major subcultures and their corresponding myriad microcultures contend differently with the multiple eating-, weight-, and shape-related messages they receive from the media and from all other points of contact with the dominant Western culture. All of these influences potentially affect how subcultures and the individuals within them appraise, experience, and manifest disordered patterns of eating. These are clearly worldwide phenomena (Becker et al. 2004; Pike and Borovoy 2004; Pike and Walsh 1996).

As a result of globalization, diet and exercise patterns appear to have followed such cultural shifts. Rates of obesity have been increasing worldwide in developing as well as in developed countries as a result of what has been called "nutrition transition" (Popkin 2001; Popkin and Gordon-Larsen 2004). This transition has involved large changes in diet and exercise, particularly the increased consumption of a more Western diet that includes an intake high in saturated fats, sugar, and refined foods, and less physical activity. Popkin (2001) notes that these patterns have been observed throughout America's dominant cultures and subcultures, as well as throughout Asia, Latin America, the Middle East, and parts of Africa. One mechanism by which this transition has occurred is via the aggressive promotion of brand-name fast foods. Correspondingly, rising levels of obesity have been accompanied by the desire for thinness and the propensity toward disordered patterns of eating. As a result, this trend has led to the worldwide recognition of the existence of pathological eating behaviors.

A prime example is described by Becker (2004), who, working with girls in Fiji, found that thinness and body modification were not factors in Fijian culture prior to the introduction of television and that Fijians, historically, "strongly support more robust appetites and body shapes." Furthermore, Fijians had not been traditionally engaged in body reshaping. However, in a series of interviews with Fijian girls conducted 3 years after television was introduced, Becker found that Fijian girls began developing weight and body shape preoccupation. They also began to show disordered eating and dieting behaviors and the desire to modify their bodies.

Focusing primarily on the United States, we explore in this chapter pathological eating behaviors and eating disorders in non-Caucasian populations, discuss culturally sensitive assessments of eating disorders in ethnically minority individuals, and highlight treatment considerations of special note in these populations. We also provide case vignettes that illustrate some of the variety of patients we have encountered.

Epidemiology of Eating Disorders in Non-Caucasian Populations

As described in Chapter 1 ("Diagnosis, Epidemiology, and Clinical Course of Eating Disorders") in this volume, epidemiological data regarding incidence and prevalence rates for eating disorders are limited. Data on rates of eating disorders in non-Caucasian populations are even more limited and do not allow for reliable estimates of the rates in non-Caucasian and ethnic groups. Few systematic data are available to provide good comparisons of rates of disorders among minority individuals compared with Caucasian individuals. Anecdotal impressions from several treatment centers suggest that compared with Caucasians, minority individuals may have an equal risk of binge-eating disorder (BED) and lower risks of bulimia nervosa and anorexia nervosa. However, many studies reveal that consistent with traditional views, disordered eating behaviors and maladaptive body concerns are less frequent in minority than in Caucasian populations.

Body Image and Eating and Dieting Behaviors in Non-Caucasian Women

Western values, which promote autonomy and the success of the individual, suggest that physical beauty provides women with advantages in attaining these goals. For many women, thinness is a primary marker of physical beauty. Women who identify with such mainstream ideas may be particularly vulnerable to developing disordered eating behaviors.

Given these seemingly ubiquitous cultural values and associated pressures, why have minority individuals exposed to Western culture not developed eating disorders at the same rate as Caucasians? Possibly, some minority cultures contain certain protective factors that reduce the risk for development of certain eating disorders. Correspondingly, individuals who maintain strong cultural affiliations and identifications with their cultures of origin may be less vulnerable to eating disorder–promoting influences of the dominant culture.

Two aspects of cultural affiliation, ethnic identity and acculturation, have received attention in the eating disorder literature. Broadly, *ethnic identity* refers to "the psychological relationship of ethnic and racial minority group members to their own group" (Phinney 1990). The *minority identity development model* (Atkinson 2004) defines varying degrees of ethnic identity, with progressively greater identification with one's culture of origin, together with an integration of those roots with experiences of the dominant culture, as one moves toward higher stages. In stage 1, individuals experience *conformity,* preferring the dominant group and rejecting the values of their group of origin. In stage 2, *dissonance,* individuals experience conflicts between values held by the dominant group and those of their group of origin. In stage 3, individuals experience *resistance and immersion,* during which they completely endorse the beliefs and practices of their culture of origin but reject the values of the dominant culture. In stage 4, *introspection,* individuals "experience feelings of discontent and discomfort with group views rigidly held in the resistance and immersion stage." Individuals in this stage begin to seek more individual autonomy. In stage 5, *synergism,* individuals have resolved and integrated the practices and beliefs of their culture of origin with those of the dominant culture.

Each stage of this model carries its own risks for vulnerability to eating disorders. For example, during the first stage, disordered eating may result from strong attempts to become more identified with the practices, values, and beliefs of the dominant group. Such identifications may occur to greater or lesser extent in any of the stages during which individuals feel pulled to assimilate with the dominant group. Furthermore, intragroup racism, self-hate, and attempts to flee from feelings of oppression may lead to further rejection of one's group of origin and a desire to appear more similar to the dominant group.

Acculturation occurs as individuals and their group as a whole accept and buy into the mainstream culture's values and beliefs. The exposure to eating disorder–promoting influences is evident.

African Americans

> Cherise, a 17-year-old African American high school senior, grew up in a predominantly middle-class African American community in a large urban area. Her parents both worked for the federal government. She was determined to do well in her local public high school and go to college, and she socialized with peers who shared her values and perspectives. Cherise and several of her friends were built "on the stocky side," and as a group they determined to lose weight prior to graduating from high school so that they would "look hot" in college the following year. They reinforced one another in "extreme dieting." Cherise found herself unable to eat normally, commenced frequent episodes of binge eating and purging, developed moderate depressive symptoms, and sought help. Her parents were supportive and involved in her care. Through a combination of cognitive-behavioral psychotherapy, fluoxetine 60 mg/day, and dietary counseling, her eating symptoms and mood improved considerably. Cherise was able to graduate from high school with honors and continued into a local college, where her academic and social development continued successfully.

Body Image

Multiple studies show that African American women have greater rates of overweight and obesity than Caucasian women. However, when body mass index (BMI) is controlled for, African American women generally report greater levels of body satisfaction and an overall greater level of positive body image than Caucasian women (Wilfley et al. 1996). In a study using the Eating Disorders Examination Questionnaire, Pernick et al. (2006) found that Caucasian and Latina girls scored higher on a weight concern subscale than African American girls. In Project EAT, a study of weight-related concerns and behaviors among adolescents, African American girls were less likely to perceive themselves as being overweight, to desire to weigh less, and to be dissatisfied with their bodies (Neumark-Sztainer et al. 2002). In a study of eating disturbances and body image in a sample of African American and Caucasian women, D.E Wilfley et al. (unpublished data) found that Caucasian women were significantly more likely to perceive that they were heavier than their best friend and that Caucasian women were more likely to endorse negative attitudes about their weight than African American women. A fuller physique seems to be more acceptable among African American women than among Caucasian women. This suggests that ethnic identity may also be protective for African American women, although studies have been mixed. Further studies should assess the relationship between an African American woman's ethnic identity and her level of body satisfaction.

Eating and Dieting Behaviors

Generally, studies have revealed lower rates of eating disorders in African American than Caucasian women (Pike et al. 2001). In a study comparing 1,061 African American women with 985 Caucasian women, Striegel-Moore et al. (2003) found that no African American women, compared with 15 Caucasian women, met criteria for anorexia nervosa. Similarly, more Caucasian women than African American women met the criteria for bulimia nervosa and BED. However, other studies have been mixed with regard to rates of BED, and some suggest that African American women show rates of binge eating and of BED equivalent to or greater than those of Caucasian women (Regan and Cachelin 2006; Regan and Hersch 2005; Shisslak et al. 2006). These findings are consistent with the higher levels of obesity and a greater acceptance of overweight among African American women.

Latin Americans

> Belinda, a 16-year-old Hispanic American who had dropped out of school, was admitted to a pediatric unit for malnutrition with a BMI of 14 that occurred in the context of self-starvation, binge eating, and purging. She came from an impoverished, abusive home background and had run away to the streets at age 13. She was befriended by a 19-year-old gang member who dealt illicit drugs, and she embarked on a life in which she abused cocaine and methamphetamines and was often physically and sexually abused. She developed symptoms of anorexia nervosa, binge/purge type, at age 14. Belinda intermittently returned to her mother for help when she was feeling particularly down and out, and it was during one of these periods that her mother dragged her to the medical center because of her emaciated condition. During her hospitalization on a pediatric inpatient unit, Belinda was uncooperative and claimed that she really did not want to lose weight. After a semifutile attempt on the part of her pediatricians and consulting mental health workers to institute a structured treatment pro-

gram that ultimately included overnight gastric gavage, and an unsuccessful few weeks on an adolescent mental health unit, Belinda was discharged at a BMI of 17. She halfheartedly participated in follow-up appointments with her mental health system and devoted pediatrician. In her early 20s she entered drug rehabilitation, got a GED, and tried to live a more structured and normalized life, remaining "clean and sober" thereafter. She also sought treatment. However, her eating disorder symptoms persisted throughout, and Belinda ultimately succumbed to malnutrition in her mid-40s.

"Latin American" describes a large and diverse group, also variously labeled as "Hispanic," "Latino," or "Latina." Latin American individuals may originate from any of the countries of South and Central America, the Caribbean, or Europe. Each group has its own unique customs and practices. However, most eating disorder studies have lumped all Latin American individuals together regardless of place of origin.

Body Image

In a thoughtful article on the culturally sensitive assessment and treatment of eating disorders, Kempa and Thomas (2000) suggest that since Latin American culture itself can theoretically put Latin American women at risk for eating disorders, separate from the effects of acculturation, Latin American women may have a double burden of vulnerability for eating disorders. In Kempa and Thomas's view, traditional characteristics that may contribute to such vulnerability include the overriding importance of male domination, self-sacrificing and submissive roles for women, adherence to family customs, maintenance of personal respect, and certain religious practices. In a world of machismo, suppressed female resentment or efforts to assert control by women may further place women at risk for the development of eating disorders. While the more traditional female role and more submissive gender roles generally attributed to Latin American women might be associated with greater body disturbances and greater levels of body dissatisfaction (Kempa and Thomas 2000), greater acculturation into a dominant Western lifestyle may also negatively impact body image among these women.

Given the complexity of these potential influences, it is not surprising that empirical body image studies of Latin American women have yielded mixed findings. In contrast with what Kempa and Thomas (2000) might have predicted, Warren et al. (2005) found that Spanish women and Mexican American women had lower levels of body dissatisfaction than Caucasian women. White and Grilo (2005) also found Latin American women and African American women to have lower levels of body image dissatisfaction than Caucasian women. However, Project EAT found that Latin American girls were most likely to perceive themselves as being overweight and express low levels of body satisfaction (Neumark-Sztainer et al. 2002). These discrepancies may reflect the fact that the Latin American adolescents studied in Project EAT may have been striving harder than Latinas in other studies to assimilate into the dominant culture.

Eating and Dieting Behaviors

Although data are sparse, Latin American women have shown equivalent or greater pathological dieting behaviors than Caucasian women, including excessive dieting and purging (Neumark-Sztainer et al. 2002). Project EAT found that Latin American girls showed the highest rates of current weight-loss attempts, binge eating, and chronic dieting among the different ethnic groups examined. Excessive dieting has been found to be an early marker of eating disorders. In a multiethnic study using the Eating Attitudes Test, Bisaga et al. (2005) found that non-Hispanic whites and Hispanics scored highest for disturbed eating disorder attitudes and behaviors.

Asian Americans

> Tina, a 20-year-old second-generation Japanese-American student at a prominent university, was a second child in a success-oriented professional family. She had developed anorexia nervosa, restricting type, in high school. She was academically driven, a star athlete, and a competitive musician, having internalized the drive to succeed in all areas that characterized her parents and older brother. Her perfectionism was unrelenting, and she became extremely self-derogating whenever she failed to meet her high standards of performance. Hospitalized at the point of exhaustion and decreasing quality of school performance at a BMI of 15, she responded well to treatment in a structured residential program. She expressed gratitude for having the opportunity to rethink her values, goals, and behaviors at that point and resolved to continue treatment.

Body Image

Studies of Asian Americans encounter the same difficulty noted with studies of Latin Americans—namely, the term *Asian American* implies homogeneity, whereas the group is extremely heterogeneous. Therefore, the many studies that lump all Asian Americans under one category are undoubtedly too simplistic. However, as is also true for the Latin American culture, certain shared values and beliefs may permit certain common cultural patterns to be identified regardless of country of origin.

Traditional cultural values, notably an emphasis on community and family that tends to de-emphasize the individual, are important in understanding how Asian American women perceive themselves. Hall (1995) has suggested that maintaining certain standards of physical appearance takes on even greater significance under collective pressure. Acculturation is also a factor for Asian American women. For some, as for Caucasians in the dominant culture, personal success and power may be perceived as linked to a drive for perfection in the expression of thinness as an idealized Western image of beauty. Even though studies show lower rates of overweight and higher rates of underweight in Asian American populations (Neumark-Sztainer et al. 2002), the few studies that exist suggest that body image satisfaction among Asian American women is low. Project EAT found levels of body dissatisfaction among Asian American adolescents to be similar to or greater than those of Caucasians (Neumark-Sztainer et al. 2002). This dissatisfaction was hypothesized to relate to the tendency of Asian Americans to conform to a social norm that emphasizes thinness. In a study by Davis and Katzman (1999) focusing on the effect of acculturation on factors such as self-esteem, depression, and characteristics associated with eating disorders, highly acculturated Chinese American females showed higher rates of body dissatisfaction and "drive for thinness" compared with Caucasians.

Eating and Dieting Behaviors

Davis and Katzman (1999) found that highly acculturated Chinese females scored higher on the Eating Disorder Inventory and on a separate measure of bulimic behaviors than less acculturated Chinese females on the Eating Disorder Inventory that included a measure of bulimia. One report from Project EAT found Asian American girls more likely than Caucasian girls to report chronic dieting, unhealthy weight-control behaviors, and having been told that they have an eating disorder by a health care provider (Neumark-Sztainer et al. 2002). However, using data from that same study, Croll et al. (2002) found that along with African American females, Asian American females reported the lowest rates of disordered eating behaviors.

Native Americans

> Trisha, a 30-year-old Native American, grew up in a rural area of the Southwest, intermittently living on her tribal lands with her family and in nearby towns and villages with a large extended family. As a child she had been emotionally abused in her family and also sexually abused by neighbors and cousins on several occasions. Her father had been in the U.S. military, and her mother had been educated in federal government boarding schools. An older brother had had significant problems with alcohol dependence and had drifted away from the family, to her parents' deep disappointment. She started to gain weight at age 15, became preoccupied with not wanting to become obese, started to severely restrict her intake, but quickly developed a pattern of daily binge eating and purging. She was not able to complete high school. Her area lacked mental health providers, and she was not able to access appropriate care. Throughout her 20s, Trisha remained hampered by anorexia nervosa and lived with various family members, finding marginal employment from time to time.

Body Image

Once again, Native American populations comprise an extremely diverse group of cultures, ethnicities, and degrees of assimilation. That said, few data exist on body image perceptions of Native Americans. The few studies that have looked at body image suggest that Native American females have high levels of body dissatisfaction. Smith and Krejci (1991), using the Eating Disorder Inventory, found that Native American females were significantly less likely than Caucasians or Latin Americans to agree with the statement "I feel satisfied with the shape of my body."

Eating and Dieting Behaviors

Native American girls may engage in greater rates of disordered eating behaviors than do Caucasians. Smith and Krejci (1991) found that Native American adolescent girls scored highest on measures of disturbed eating behaviors and attitudes on the Eating Disorder Inventory and a bulimia measure when compared with Latin American and Caucasian girls. Croll et al. (2002) reported that disordered eating was most prevalent among Native American and Latin American girls. This study also found that Native American females were more likely to engage in behaviors such as skipping meals, smoking cigarettes, taking diet pills, and vomiting to control their weight.

Eating Disorders in Non-Caucasian Men

As in Caucasian populations, eating disorders are seen far less frequently among non-Caucasian males than among non-Caucasian females. Although there are far fewer data and the results have been inconsistent, available data for males have also revealed ethnic differences. Croll et al. (2002) found that Native American males were more likely to show disordered eating behavior compared with Caucasian, African American, and Latin American males. For a more detailed discussion of eating disorders in men, see Chapter 13 ("Eating Disorders in Special Populations: Medical Comorbidities and Complicating or Unusual Conditions") in this volume.

International Trends in Eating and Dieting Behavior

An expanding body of literature is exploring international populations that have experienced varying degrees of Westernization (Gordon et al. 2001; Lee et al. 1996). Most reports have revealed an increase in patterns of disordered eating and clinical eating disorders in the various countries investigated. Sing Lee's work with eating disorder patients in Hong Kong and China has challenged the established criteria used to diagnose eating disorders (Lee et al. 1996). Specifically, according to Lee, the American Psychiatric Association's DSM criteria for anorexia nervosa appear inadequate for a subtype of patients he has identified who show pathologically restrictive eating behaviors and severe weight loss but who do not appear to have the fear of becoming fat ("fat phobia") usually deemed central to the usual construct of anorexia nervosa. Rather, Lee's patients often attribute their disturbed and restrictive eating to a lack of hunger or somatic discomforts associated with food consumption but specifically deny that they fear becoming fat. By DSM criteria for anorexia nervosa, Lee's patients have an atypical presentation of eating disorder. Lee suggests that clinicians should strive to discern each anorexia nervosa patient's own idiosyncratic meanings regarding food consumption and disturbed eating-related behaviors, and how they may be grounded in the complex beliefs and practices of that individual's culture (Lee et al. 1996).

Culturally Sensitive Assessment of Eating Disorders

As should ordinarily be one's practice with patients from dominant Western cultural groups, a clinician assessing members of minority groups for an eating disorder must take into account cultural beliefs, acculturation, and ethnic identity in the context of the individual's personal identity development. Factors indicating the extent to which the individual has become assimilated into the mainstream are important. For immigrants and for first- and second-generation minorities, clinicians should assess, where appropriate, age at time of immigration or generation of immigration, English fluency, and major ethnic and dominant-culture family, extended family, and peer group influences. All these issues should be addressed within the usual eating disorder assessment protocols described in Chapter 2 ("Assessment and Determination of Initial Treatment Approaches for Patients With Eating Disorders") in this volume. However, cultural sensitivity also requires that the clinician understand how an individual's ethnic community and culture conceptualize food, eating, weight, and body image, and, in particular, how the family understands and reacts to eating disorder attitudes and behaviors. Since assessing the family is a key element in the assessment of any child or adolescent, and important in understanding eating disorder issues in all patients regardless of age, appreciating family dynamics within different cultural frameworks is particularly crucial. Pertinent questions include

- How do your family, extended family, family friends, and peers view issues concerning physical appearance, dieting behaviors, and weight?
- In what ways do your family and community routinely incorporate meals and food into daily life and celebrations?
- What sorts of pressures, if any, do you feel from your friends and relatives regarding your eating, shape, weight, and eating-related behaviors?

These themes are especially important in cultures where being somewhat overweight has traditionally been valued. Such beliefs may be transgenerationally acceptable and even encouraged among family members. Identifying points of conflict between family and friends, peers, and the patient's own attitudes and beliefs regarding preferred appearance, eating patterns, and dieting behaviors may uncover important issues to be addressed in treatment.

Most of the widely used structured questionnaires and surveys for assessing eating disorders have been standardized on Caucasian female patient samples, and few have been standardized in non-Caucasian populations. Furthermore, as mentioned earlier, debate is ongoing concerning the cross-cultural validity of some of the criteria used to diagnose eating disorders. Pending further research, clinicians should remain alert to atypical presentations of eating disorders. Patients presenting with eating disorder syndromes that do not exactly fit formal DSM criteria for anorexia nervosa or bulimia nervosa may still suffer from considerable impairment and still merit fully appropriate treatment.

African Americans

Most African Americans represent a blend of many ethnic groups of both African and European origin. Although their culture as a group is clearly more closely identified to the dominant culture than to native African cultures, very distinct African American subcultures exist. Therefore, clinicians should appreciate some unique vulnerabilities among members of this group. For example, among those who buy into the European ideal of beauty, the self-esteem of African American women may be lower, in part because African American women may experience negative portrayals of their physical attributes and body types.

Since clinicians have traditionally assumed that African Americans are far less likely to exhibit eating disorders than are Caucasians, they may be less likely to screen African American patients for such disorders. As a result, many cases may be missed because of poor detection. Given the elevated rates of obesity and overweight among African American women, clinicians working with these patients should especially maintain high suspicion for binge eating and BED in this population.

Latin Americans

As described in the section "Body Image and Eating and Dieting Behaviors in Non-Caucasian Women," since elements of traditional Latin American female roles, as well as influences associated with assimilating into the dominant Western culture, may contribute to vulnerability to eating disorders, it is important that the nuanced complexities of ethnic identity that may contribute to the appearance and maintenance of eating disorders be appreciated and assessed in Latin American patients. As with any patient with an eating disorder, family involvement may be an integral part of treatment. For many, even when the patient herself is fluent in English, having Spanish-speaking clinicians will often make a considerable difference for assessing the family.

Asian Americans

Many of the issues described with regard to Latin American women apply to Asian American women as well. Particular awareness that atypical presentations of anorexia nervosa may be more prevalent among Asian Americans than among other populations, perhaps with less expressed fat phobia and greater degrees of somatic complaints manifesting as stomach discomfort or bloating, may be important. Among less assimilated Asian American populations, frank and open discussions of emotional issues may be culturally shameful and be discouraged by family and friends, and predominant cultural values such as "rigid emotional and moral self-control," described by Sing Lee (1995), may contribute to minimization or denial of eating disorder symptoms. With this in mind, clinicians should not interpret apparent stoicism, minimization, or frank denial primarily as resistance or uncooperativeness. Rather, clinicians should be empathetic and create a safe and nonjudgmental environment in which the patient may be encouraged to reveal information that she may never have previously been permitted to share with anyone.

Native Americans

Cultural considerations will vary with the individual's particular tribal culture and identification with traditional ways, the individual's degree of assimilation into the dominant culture and "two culture" thinking, and openness to Western values and medical beliefs. With the increase in obesity among certain Native American populations, reports of BED and of bulimia nervosa have emerged. For Native American populations residing on reservations and in pueblos, information about eating disorders may not be as available as elsewhere. Because of the stigma associated with psychiatric difficulties and distrust of Western ways regarding psychiatric care, Native American patients who adhere to traditional beliefs and practices may be reluctant to seek help. In such instances, mental health clinicians often learn about a patient's eating disorder symptoms and receive requests for consultation and assistance from school officials and primary care providers rather than from the patient herself. Helping these frontline caregivers understand the nature and treatment of eating disorders so that they can better work directly with the patients may be the best strategy for these patients.

The severe shortage of trained Native American mental health providers who are knowledgeable about eating disorders hampers access to care for these populations. When Native American patients who adhere to traditional beliefs are willing to be seen by Western practitioners, a respectful exploration of their health beliefs and those of their family and community regarding the eating disorder symptoms is essential. This exploration should sensitively include if and how spiritual beliefs concerning the eating disorder symptoms play a role in the patient's understanding.

Treatment of Eating Disorders in Non-Caucasian Patients

In general, although no data are available to suggest that race and ethnicity per se factor in treatment outcomes for eating disorders, they certainly do matter greatly with regard to access to care and health services utilization. While help seeking and treatment utilization seem to be inadequate for all segments of the eating disorder population, access and utilization are worse for minority populations. For example, Striegel-Moore et al. (2003) found low treatment rates among white and black women in their study. Another study assessing treatment barriers in an ethnically diverse population by Cachelin et al. (2001) found that although 85.2% of the sample wanted treatment, only 57% had ever sought treatment. In Cachelin et al.'s study, reasons cited for not seeking treatment included financial difficulties, lack of insurance, fear of being labeled, not knowing about resources, feelings of shame, turning instead to other sources, not thinking there was a problem, and counselors not of the same ethnic background.

Overall, treatment planning for eating disorders in non-Caucasian populations should be modeled after the treatment in dominant-culture populations, described at length in other chapters in this volume. However, the following points regarding treatment in ethnically diverse populations may be helpful. For many patients in ethnic minority communities, much more so than for Caucasian populations in the United States, care is much more likely to be provided by primary care clinicians than by mental health specialists, an example of only one of the many health care disparities that exist. Many of the communities are self-contained, and patients are often reluctant to seek care outside of their own communities. In this regard, ensuring the availability of trained professionals from the communities from which these patients emanate and in which they reside, and providing professionals who are fluent in the native language of non-English-speaking patients, are key ingredients for culturally sensitive health services. As illustrated in several of the vignettes presented earlier (see section "Body Image and Eating and Dieting Behaviors in Non-Caucasian Women"), disparities in access to care affect many minority group patients and families and may contribute to poor outcomes in many patients (Cachelin and Striegel-Moore 2006). In addition, where patients hold to health beliefs that include the use of traditional healers, such beliefs should be respected. Until proven otherwise, integrating traditional practices with evidence-based treatment seems the wisest course for ensuring that patients will adhere to treatment, and perhaps for increasing their likelihood of recovery.

In each instance, clinicians will have to consider how eating disorder–related attitudes and behaviors stem from the degree to which the individual's personal identifications, beliefs, and practices adhere to her traditional group's values; the extent to which her allegiances to the group of origin conflict with her desires to assimilate and identify with the dominant Western group; and the degree to which associated supports and/or conflicts stemming from family, friends, and peers might facilitate or compromise therapeutic interventions.

Conclusion

Although recognition of eating disorders in ethnic minorities in the United States and in international communities elsewhere has lagged behind such recognition in dominant Western populations, the emergence of eating disorders, and their apparently increasing prevalence, in these populations bears note. Applying general principles of cultural sensitivity to the assessment and treatment of eating disorders requires clinicians who are competent not only in understanding and managing these disorders but also in dealing with the specific cultural considerations of the individuals and families for whom they are providing care. We trust that the future will bring more culturally refined and validated eating disorder diagnostic criteria and assessment tools. We anticipate that larger numbers of culturally sensitive providers who are expert in treating eating disorders will be trained. We can only hope that the formidable barriers to care for many ethnic minority patients will be reduced so that these populations will enjoy a higher likelihood of receiving the competent and effective care that is increasingly available to other populations.

References

Atkinson DR: Counseling American Minorities, 6th Edition. New York, McGraw-Hill, 2004, pp 39–47

Becker AE: Television disordered eating, and young women in Fiji: negotiating body image and identity during rapid social change. Cult Med Psychiatry 20:533–559, 2004

Becker AE, Keel P, Anderson-Fye E, et al: Genes and/or jeans? Genetic and sociocultural contributions to risk for eating disorders. J Addict Dis 23:81–103, 2004

Bemporad JR: Self-starvation through the ages: reflections on the pre-history of anorexia. Int J Eat Disord 19:217–237, 1996

Bisaga K, Whitaker A, Davies M, et al: Eating disorders and depressive symptoms in urban high school girls from different ethnic backgrounds. J Dev Behav Pediatr 26:257–266, 2005

Cachelin FM, Striegel-Moore RH: Help seeking and barriers to treatment in a community sample of Mexican American and European American women with eating disorders. Int J Eat Disord 39:154–161, 2006

Cachelin FM, Rebeck R, Veisel C, et al: Barriers to treatment for eating disorders among ethnically diverse women. Int J Eat Disord 30:269–278, 2001

Croll J, Neumark-Sztainer D, Story M, et al: Prevalence and risk and protective factors related to disordered eating behaviors among adolescents: relationship to gender and ethnicity. J Adolesc Health 31:166–175, 2002

Davis C, Katzman MA: Perfection as acculturation: psychological correlates of eating problems in Chinese male and female students living in the United States. Int J Eat Disord 25:65–70, 1999

Gordon R, Katzman M, Nasser M (eds): Eating Disorders and Cultures in Transition. New York, Routledge, 2001

Hall CC: Beauty is in the soul of the beholder: psychological implications of beauty and African American women. Cult Divers Ment Health 1:125–137, 1995

Keel PK, Klump KL: Are eating disorders culture-bound syndromes? Implications for conceptualizing their etiology. Psychol Bull 129:747–769, 2003

Kempa ML, Thomas AJ: Culturally sensitive assessment and treatment of eating disorders. Eat Disord 8:17–30, 2000

Lee S: Self-starvation in context: towards a culturally sensitive understanding of anorexia nervosa. Soc Sci Med 41:25–36, 1995

Lee S, Lee AM, Leung T: Cross cultural validity of the Eating Disorder Inventory: a study of Chinese patients with eating disorders in Hong Kong. Int J Eat Disord 22:1–12, 1996

Neumark-Sztainer D, Croll J, Story M, et al: Ethnic/racial differences in weight-related concerns and behaviors among adolescent girls and boys: findings from Project EAT. J Psychosom Res 53:963–974, 2002

Pearce JMS: Richard Morton: origins of anorexia nervosa. Eur Neurol 52:191–192, 2004

Pernick Y, Nichols JF, Rauh MJ, et al: Disordered eating among a multi-racial/ethnic sample of female high-school athletes. J Adolesc Health 38:689–695, 2006

Phinney JS: Ethnic identity in adolescents and adults: review of research. Psychol Bull 108:499–514, 1990

Pike KM, Borovoy A: The rise of eating disorders in Japan: issues of culture and limitations of the model of "Westernization." Cult Med Psychiatry 28:493–531, 2004

Pike KM, Walsh BT: Ethnicity and eating disorders: implications for incidence and treatment. Psychopharmacol Bull 32:265–274, 1996

Pike KM, Dohm FA, Striegel-Moore RH, et al: A comparison of black and white women with binge eating disorder. Am J Psychiatry 158:1455–1460, 2001

Popkin BM: The nutrition transition and obesity in the developing world. J Nutr 131(3):871S–873S, 2001

Popkin BM, Gordon-Larsen P: The nutrition transition: worldwide obesity dynamics and their determinants. Int J Obes Relat Metab Disord 28 (suppl 3):S2–S9, 2004

Regan PC, Cachelin FM: Binge eating and purging in a multi-ethnic community sample. Int J Eat Disord 39:1–4, 2006

Regan P, Hersch J: Influence of race, gender and socioeconomic status on binge eating frequency in a population-based sample. Int J Eat Disord 38:252–256, 2005

Shisslak CM, Mays MZ, Crago M, et al: Eating and weight control behaviors among middle school girls in relationship to body weight and ethnicity. J Adolesc Health 38:631–633, 2006

Smith JE, Krejci J: Minorities join the majority: eating disturbances among Hispanic and Native American youth. Int J Eat Disord 10:179–186, 1991

Striegel-Moore RH, Dohm FA, Kraemer HC, et al: Eating disorders in white and black women. Am J Psychiatry 160:1326–1331, 2003

Warren CS, Gleaves DH, Cepeda-Benito A, et al: Ethnicity as a protective factor against internalization of a thin ideal and body dissatisfaction. Int J Eat Disord 37:241–249, 2005

White MA, Grilo CM: Ethnic differences in the prediction of eating and body image disturbances among female adolescent psychiatric inpatients. Int J Eat Disord 38:78–84, 2005

Wilfley DE, Schreiber GB, Pike KM, et al: Eating disturbance and body image: a comparison of a community sample of adult black and white women. Int J Eat Disord 20:377–387, 1996

Management of Patients With Chronic, Intractable Eating Disorders

Joel Yager, M.D.

Despite considerable recent research in the treatment of eating disorders, large numbers of patients with these conditions do not improve, and the course of their illness is seemingly intractable. Focusing on anorexia nervosa and bulimia nervosa, I review in this chapter clinical features associated with poor outcome, factors that contribute to intractability associated with lack of treatment response, and strategies for dealing with patients who do not improve with usual treatment programs. Difficulties associated with the management of binge-eating disorder and associated obesity are considered in Chapter 8 ("Management of Eating Disorders Not Otherwise Specified"), Chapter 9 ("Psychiatric

Aspects of Bariatric Surgery"), and Chapter 10 ("Medication-Related Weight Changes: Impact on Treatment of Eating Disorder Patients") in this volume.

Chronicity of Illness

Anorexia Nervosa

Unfortunately, chronicity of anorexia nervosa is all too common. In a review of 119 research studies reporting case series of outcomes covering 5,590 patients, mortality was significantly high. Among the surviving patients, on average, fewer than one-half recovered, one-third improved, and one-fifth remained chronically ill, and the presence of other psychiatric disorders at follow-up was very common, leading the authors to conclude that little had changed regarding the outcome of anorexia nervosa in the twentieth century (Steinhausen 2002). In a follow-up study of 242 adolescents followed for 6.4 years, only 50% met all three criteria for recovery, which included freedom from eating disorders, good or fair psychosocial functioning, and no other psychiatric disorder (Steinhausen et al. 2003). Although full recovery may take 5–7 years even among those who fully recover from anorexia nervosa (Strober et al. 1997), evidence from several studies suggests that after 7 (Dally 1969) to 12 (Ratnasuriya et al. 1991) years, patients with anorexia nervosa are unlikely to have improved. However, there is always hope, since even long-standing chronicity does not predict an inevitably poor outcome. In one study a small group of patients who had previously been categorized as showing poor outcome after 4 years nevertheless showed good outcome after 20 years (Ratnasuriya et al. 1991).

Although evidence is mixed, and some research has failed to uncover distinctively unfavorable prognostic features, many studies have reported specific clinical features associated with poor outcomes. Table 16–1 lists features, culled from the literature, that are thought to be predictive of chronicity. Individuals with combination syndromes, in which both anorexia nervosa and bulimia nervosa are present, are thought to be particularly unlikely to improve (G. F. M. Russell 1979). Also associated with adolescent eating disorders, the increased risk of longer-term medical and psychiatric consequences (Table 16–2) adds to the chronic impairments that patients face and that are likely to require ongoing attention (Johnson et al. 2002).

Table 16–1.   Clinical features associated with poor outcomes

Lower initial weight

Binge eating

Vomiting

Purgative abuse

Long duration and chronicity of illness

Long duration of inpatient hospitalizations

Prior treatment failure

Obsessive-compulsive personality symptoms

Impulsivity

Older age at onset (postadolescent)

Possibly very young age (e.g., preadolescent onset)

Premorbid asociality

Sexual problems

Disturbances in family relationships[a]

[a]Includes features such as poor communication; high levels of overcontrol, conflict, hostility, and negative expressed emotion; psychological, physical, and/or sexual abuse; parental neglect; and severe parental psychopathology.

Source.   Fichter et al. 2006; Steinhausen 2002; Strober et al. 1997.

Table 16–2.   Medical and psychiatric conditions associated with eating disorders that contribute to chronic course

Anxiety disorders

Cardiovascular symptoms

Chronic fatigue

Chronic pain

Depressive disorders

Infectious diseases

Insomnia

Neurological symptoms

Suicide attempts

Note.   Adolescent eating disorders increase the risk for other disorders during early adulthood.

Source.   Compiled from Fichter et al. 2006; Johnson et al. 2002; and Steinhausen 2002, among others.

Chronic courses vary along a number of clinical dimensions:

1. *Stability versus instability of clinical course.* Some patients remain at a chronically low weight and adhere to the same compulsive eating and exercise rituals day after day, year after year. Some patients who maintain their weight at 60%–70% of their recommended healthy weight have rarely missed work over a period of decades. Some live a socially isolated existence, whereas others enjoy seemingly satisfying relationships with families. Still other patients show more volatile and unpredictable courses, with surges in self-destructive behaviors and emotions, and rollercoaster weights— patterns that are not mutually exclusive. After years of chronically low weight and invariable ritual, for reasons that are hard to discern, some patients' patterns suddenly shift, for better or worse, with some showing real improvement, and others experiencing emergence of self-damaging behaviors for the first time (e.g., binge-purge cycles or laxative abuse manifesting after many years of pure restrictive eating). Some patients alternate among periods of restrictive eating, binge eating with purging, and binge eating without purging. As with other complex biological phenomena, more or less predictable patterns of behavior may suddenly and inexplicably reach a tipping point and become chaotic.

2. *Determination of which impairments contribute to chronicity.* Patients vary considerably with respect to which impairments debilitate them the most. For some, physical and behavioral impairments may be most troubling, whereas for others psychological and social impairments may be of greater consequence. Some patients capably conduct professional careers in spite of low weight and daily episodes of binge eating and purging, whereas others are utterly disabled by shame, negative self-image, obsessions, and compulsions regarding food despite maintaining relatively normal weights and reporting only infrequent episodes of binge eating or purging. For the first group, eating disorder–related behaviors and thoughts appear to be partitioned off from the rest of a productive life. To illustrate, I have followed patients with anorexia nervosa for 10–20 years, now in their 40s, who chronically weigh about 60%–70% of expected weight and who maintain unbroken successful careers as stockbrokers, nurses, psychiatric social workers, physicians, attorneys, and entrepreneurial businesswomen. In the second group are large numbers of patients whose concurrent avoidance, timidity,

anxieties, dysphorias, and other comorbid features render them nonfunctional to a degree that cannot be solely attributed to having an eating disorder.

Marked differences in debility occur within specific physical complications. For example, multiple genetic and environmental factors undoubtedly contribute to why some patients are particularly vulnerable to osteoporosis, others severe dental deterioration, and still others marked pancreatic and salivary gland inflammation, whereas other patients with comparable eating disordered behavior experience fewer difficulties.

Of course, some patients are totally disabled, unable to function independently or without supervision. To illustrate, I have seen a 48-year-old woman, ill since her teens, who has never been employable, who abuses laxatives (often taking hundreds of tablets each week), and who requires constant observation and frequent hospitalization for medical complications; a 35-year-old nurse whose few periods of sporadic employment over the past 15 years have alternated with debilitating periods of severe weight loss; a 28-year-old woman, ill since age 16, who has been unable to finish school or to work, who has been living in halfway houses on handouts from her parents, sometimes eating exclusively out of garbage cans; and a 40-year-old professional who has been entirely dependent on her mother and unable to recover weight since dropping out of a postdoctoral program as a consequence of chronic emaciation and weakness in her late 20s. It may seem remarkable that some of these patients go on living for as long as they do—a testimony to the adaptive capacities and resilience of the human body.

The presence of accepting and nurturing family and friends, especially those who can provide emotional as well as practical financial and domiciliary support, makes a real difference—if not in effecting a good versus bad outcome per se, at least in ameliorating the quality of the bad outcome with regard to the daily conveniences of life and availability of medical care.

Bulimia Nervosa

Poor outcome is not uncommon in bulimia nervosa, especially among patients who have required hospitalization, up to 80% of whom are reported to have poor outcome (Swift et al. 1987). Although earlier help seeking may have been fostered in recent years by increasing public awareness of bulimia nervosa in teenagers and their parents, at least up to several decades ago a chronic course in those seeking help for bulimia nervosa appeared to be the rule rather than the exception. University clinics observed that patients initially presenting had, on average, been bulimic for 6–7 years (Hamburg et al. 1989). In longer-term studies in which patients with bulimia nervosa were followed for more than a decade, the most prominent predictors for poor outcome were psychiatric comorbidity (Fichter and Quadflieg 2004; Fichter et al. 2006), duration of the disorder at presentation, and a history of substance abuse problems (Keel et al. 1999, 2002). Reports from clinicians in practice suggest that personality features associated with poor prognosis in their eating disorder patients include rigid overcontrol on the one hand, and emotional dysregulation with multi-impulsivity on the other (Westen and Harnden-Fischer 2001).

Treatment Nonresponse and Treatment Reluctance

Whereas *chronicity* refers to ongoing signs, symptoms, and impairments resulting from the ongoing nature of the disorder, *intractability* implies lack of response in the face of therapeutic efforts. With regard to anorexia nervosa, most contemporary treatments involve supervised refeeding in the context of an assortment of psychosocial and psychotherapeutic individual and family interventions, with little specificity established as yet for the psychotherapies or medication regimens. Furthermore, treatments in the community vary considerably from site to site. Therefore, it may be prudent to reserve the term *treatment resistance* for those patients who fail to recover substantially over time despite receiving care consistent with current established practice guidelines. From this perspective, many patients with chronic anorexia nervosa may never have received consistent care based on adequate guidelines to begin with and, consequently, may have been "undertreated." At the same time, although we would like to believe that adequate initial and early treatment might actually avert chronicity in anorexia nervosa, this appealing hypothesis has never been adequately tested.

With these caveats in mind, the term *intractable* may be a better overall term to describe two groups of patients: those who fully engage but nevertheless fail to respond to optimal treatment, and those who fail to engage or adhere to treatments available to them.

Nonresponse in Fully Engaged Patients

Some patients may be extremely treatment adherent and fully engaged in therapy but may not be able to improve in spite of their best efforts and the best therapeutic efforts of the staff (Hamburg et al. 1989). Their nonresponse is due not to a lack of desire or will on their part but instead possibly to a lack of effective therapies in today's limited cache to address their specific psychobiological deficiencies.

Nonadherence in Treatment-Reluctant Patients

Patients (and their families) may be reluctant to engage in treatment for reasons that may be either judicious or seemingly capricious. Judiciously nonadherent patients thoughtfully reject the treatments that are offered based on factors such as repeatedly bad previous experiences with professionals or treatment programs, adverse effects of treatments, financial or other social considerations, and a variety of idiosyncratic reasons that might not ordinarily occur to their health professionals. As a result of previous treatment failures, some may truly believe that they are hopeless and, consequently, have given up trying to get better. Some of these individuals, occasionally seen arguing for "pro-ana" lifestyles on Web sites, may come to embrace their diseases in what appears to be a "Stockholm syndrome"–like process of identifying with the aggressor. These objections have to be explored and considered responsibly so that acceptable negotiated treatment plans can be developed.

Conversely, capriciously nonadherent patients may be temperamentally impulsive, unable to overcome deep shame and humiliation, unable to trust, and/or suffering from other personality factors inhibiting secure attachment to their health professionals and health systems (Bulik et al. 1999; Fassino et al. 2002). Some patients who deeply intuit that they are incapable of mastering and changing the overriding obsessional and compulsive aspects of their eating disorders may try, alternatively, to gain a sense of mastery over their symptoms by convincing themselves that they actually desire the symptoms. In the face of perceived inalterable behavioral compulsions, they endeavor to reduce cognitive dissonance by attempting to render the disorder and its symptoms as "ego-syntonic," convincing themselves to believe that the eating disorder–related cognitions and behaviors are actually consistent with their own will, desires, and identity.

Some patients may feel so shamed by the disorders that they refuse to consider treatment for extended periods of time, at least initially (Hamburg et al. 1989). Such treatment reluctance may be abetted by patients' feelings of pessimism and humiliation about being sick and/or anxieties with regard to surrendering symptoms and causing difficulties for their families, relinquishing control and self-determination that may result from accepting treatment through surrendering decision making to caregivers, and being vulnerable in the face of unwanted "objective" appraisals of medical authorities (Goldner 1989).

Similarly, families may be reluctant to acknowledge a patient's serious impairments because of social shame and stigma, anger at the patient, concern that acknowledging problems in the patient might bring guilt and blame, fear of treatment costs, and other reasons.

The following case vignette underscores some frequently encountered features in patients with long-standing eating disorders and illustrates some of the intense clinical and existential challenges imposed by these heart-wrenching conditions:

> Teresa, a 44-year-old woman who had never married, had struggled with anorexia nervosa since her early teens. She had left a family in which her father and a brother had sexually molested her since she was 12, and her sympathetic but ineffective mother had been unable to protect her. In addition to having anorexia nervosa, binge-purge subtype, she began to abuse alcohol in her mid-teens and was alcohol-dependent by age 18. In her teens she also engaged in several years of heavy cocaine and methamphetamine abuse, in part, she said, to keep her weight down. She had been a chronic, heavy cigarette smoker for several decades and had never been able to quit. She had been hospitalized for suicide attempts at ages 16, 18, 21, and 28, each time taking overdoses of prescription medications, and twice requiring treatment in medical intensive care units. Remarkably, she had been able to graduate from college with good grades, but she had never been able to keep a job for any period of time. Although Teresa had received sporadic psychiatric care, including treatment for depression with selective serotonin reuptake inhibitors (SSRIs) over the years, and had participated in 1 month of a residential alcohol and substance abuse program a decade earlier, she had never been in a sustained treatment program for any of her several diagnosable mood, anxiety, personality, or eating disorders. Her

siblings saw her as "weak" and "flaky," and barely tolerated her marginal contacts with them, but they provided her with just enough financial support to keep her from being homeless, at least until she started receiving Social Security disability, at which time they became even more distant. Over the years, Teresa suffered from chronic malnutrition, fatigue, gastrointestinal distress, chronic pain, and a chronic hacking cough. Recently, she had been living on friends' sofas and had been unable to sustain a stable domicile. She was admitted to a psychiatric unit when a friend dragged her to an emergency room, fearful that she was just "wasting away." Teresa indicated that she had decided to stop eating in order to die within a few months, emphasizing that "going on the way I've been going is just too hard. I've tried and tried, but I've had enough."

Therapeutic Goals

Safety

As for any clinical situation, a fundamental goal concerns ensuring patient safety. For patients with intractable eating disorders this means sufficiently frequent monitoring and intervention to avert physical harm resulting from medical deterioration or suicidal behavior, in order to achieve maximum medical benefit consistent with available care. Treatment goals are relatively easy to establish for an acute deterioration (e.g., suddenly precipitous weight loss or medical complications in a habitually marginal patient); here the short-term goals will consist of instituting lifesaving interventions, with or without the patient's cooperation. Clinicians working with patients with intractable eating disorders are advised to set out clear expectations regarding circumstances that will require hospitalization or other safety-oriented interventions, and regarding consequences that may follow if the patient refuses to go along with these plans. As further discussed below (see section "Compassionate Clinical Decision Making for Intractable Patients"), clinical decision making may become more complicated for patients who have exhausted the medical system's likely ability to provide meaningful help.

Longer-Term Goals

For patients with chronic and intractable eating disorders, the clinician must establish therapeutic goals that neither grossly overestimate what can realistically be achieved nor underestimate the patient's potential. Since potential goals are multifaceted, as with other chronic psychiatric disorders, goals should be specified along discrete dimensions such as increasing (or at least maintaining) weight; reducing hospitalizations and psychopathological features such as obsessional thinking, ritualistic behaviors, depression, self-harming behaviors, and anxiety and panic attacks; and improving particular physical symptoms, social and vocational functioning, and so forth. Although improvement in one area may foster improvement in others, there are no assurances that across-the-board improvement will occur even when some of the seemingly central problems, such as malnutrition and anorectic attitudes toward food, abate.

Clinicians can be roughly subdivided into those who, when faced with intractable problems, become therapeutically aggressive and those who become unduly passive. Differences in therapeutic stance may be tied more closely to central personality features of the clinician rather than to objective situational factors. Clinicians must therefore monitor their own therapeutic biases to assess their propensities for undue therapeutic zeal on the one hand and therapeutic nihilism on the other (Kaplan and Garfinkel 1999; Strober 2004).

When clinicians first see patients suffering from truly chronic and intractable disorders, they sometimes fall into the trap of too readily attributing the patient's poor course to previously inept treatment, and they may set therapeutic goals too high. The problems potentially generated by such errors are considerable.

First, unrealistically high expectations on the part of the clinician may generate even greater internal performance pressures in patients than already exist, leading patients to feel additionally disappointed with themselves, shameful and guilty for failing to perform, and resentful of the clinician for setting excessive expectations in the first place. The resulting sense of failure and demoralization, added to the considerable burden already carried by these patients, may lead them to "give up" and occasionally contribute to a patient's suicide. This set of events has been well described among young patients with schizophrenia.

Second, for the clinician, having a patient who fails to meet expectations may result in a sense of professional failure, therapeutic nihilism, and self-criticism and in angry, resentful feelings toward the patient. These reactions may result in unkind nontherapeutic remarks that take the form of "blaming the victim" (i.e., the patient) and relative therapeutic neglect.

On the other hand, setting therapeutic expectations too low (i.e., expecting virtually no change) may lead the clinician to inadequately attend to the possibility of change, put insufficient emotional energy into the patient, and, perhaps unconsciously, squelch patient behavior that might actually represent positive transformation.

The task for the clinician is to work with the patient, to permit the patient to steer between these two poles by steadily setting and resetting explicit but very modest goals in a stepwise fashion. Small degrees of improvement can be objectified and additional improvements can be built onto prior steps. If no further improvement seems achievable, efforts may be directed toward ensuring that all the prior small gains are retained and consolidated.

When the patient's goals clearly differ from those of the clinician and/or her family, negotiating treatment becomes considerably more difficult. Some patients with intractable disorders simply want to be left alone and to avoid contact with health care professionals, a stance often at odds with the family's wishes for aggressive interventions. Assuming that the patient meets legal criteria for competency, in these instances clinicians must respect the patient's wishes and help family members understand the legal and ethical ramifications. If the patient is not at risk of imminently dying and has come to accept herself as a chronically dysfunctional individual who is at a plateau where she is unlikely to improve, the most humane, as well as practical, act is to accept the patient's wishes but to keep an open dialogue in the manner of motivational interviewing as described below (see section "Psychiatric Management"). In truly inalterable situations, as in the case of terminally ill cancer patients who are ready to die but whose families cannot bear thoughts of death and who demand all possible life-sustaining measures regardless of the cost, quality of life, or the patient's own wishes, the clinician's best intervention may be to help families accept the sad realities of the situation without forcing patients to endure a great deal of unwanted and ultimately ineffective and punishing treatment.

On the other hand, clinicians should remain alert to previously untried treatments that may be justified if they might rationally help yet not unduly harm and have potential advantages that far outweigh foreseeable risks, and bring these to the patient's attention. In such situations, when both the patient and her family are willing to try the treatment and proper informed consent is obtained, such interventions can be attempted. We return to the case example introduced earlier describing the care of Teresa, the 44-year-old woman who had struggled with anorexia nervosa, restricting subtype, since her teens:

After the hospital staff offered Teresa the opportunity to receive some treatment and aftercare aimed at treating her depression and eating disorder, without making unreasonable or unrealistic promises about what the public system in which she was being treated had to offer over the long term, she relented and agreed to a "trial" of inpatient psychiatric care on a unit that offered an eating disorder treatment program. For the next several weeks she cooperated with the program, including the weight-gain goals that she had negotiated with the staff. She also agreed to take olanzapine 2.5 mg/day plus fluoxetine 40 mg/day. However, when she reached a body mass index (BMI) of 16, she "hit a wall" and found that the idea of tolerating additional weight gain was impossible and unacceptable to her and despite the best attempts of the clinicians to convince her to stay for additional treatment she demanded discharge from the unit. She attended aftercare sporadically.

Several months later her friends again brought her to the hospital, in an even more severe state of malnutrition, and she reluctantly accepted a brief inpatient medical hospitalization for rehydration and to stabilize her vital signs. However, she declined further psychiatric inpatient care and stated that she would fight involuntary hospitalization. After long discussions among medical and psychiatric staff, a plan was devised to provide her with "safety" care when she and her friends thought she was in imminent medical danger. Psychiatric staff also offered regularly scheduled sessions for compassionate supportive care, but she declined continued involvement.

Psychiatric Management

The general principles applied to psychiatric management of all eating disorder patients apply to patients with intractable disorders as well. The clinician should coordinate care and collaborate with the other health professionals caring for the patient, to ensure that patient safety, general medical and psychiatric concerns, nutritional and dietary questions, and the patient's and family's psychological and psychosocial issues are appropriately assessed, monitored, and attended to sufficiently. The members of this team, who set up what Hamburg et al. (1989) refer to as a "safety envelope," should communicate frequently to ensure that all involved know one another's observations and activities.

Intervention and Care Models

In the treatment of patients with chronic, intractable eating disorders, several intervention and care models have been proposed in addition to the nutritional rehabilitation, cognitive-behavioral, interpersonal, psychodynamic, and family therapies used to treat more acute conditions. Three specific approaches advocated for these patients are harm reduction, motivational interviewing, and psychosocial rehabilitation, and these three have been employed concurrently in a comprehensive Community Outreach Partnership Program developed at the University of British Columbia (http://www.stpaulseating disorders.ca/treatrec.htm) for patients with chronic intractable eating disorders. It will be evident from what follows that these are slow but sustaining improvement–oriented strategies; they are not palliative care.

Harm Reduction

The harm reduction model has been used extensively in treating substance abuse patients (MacMaster 2004). The basic precepts of the model are to "meet people where they're at," to help patients understand the consequences of their behaviors on themselves, family, and community, and to help patients make harm-reducing decisions.

Motivational Interviewing

Motivational interviewing, like the harm reduction model, has been developed in conjunction with treating patients with substance abuse problems, and the approach has shown efficacy in randomized clinical trials with substance-abusing populations (Miller et al. 2003). Taking as a given the fact that ambivalence about recovery is common, motivational interviewing focuses on concepts of readiness and motivation, the patient's ambivalent attitudes, and the patient's perspective on the pros and cons of retaining the disorders. The clinician explicitly accepts that the eating disorder exists for a reason, that the patient herself knows when change is possible, that the patient's beliefs and values are important and worthy of full exploration, and that meaningful change takes time and is difficult to achieve. The clinician avoids debates and strives always to be on the same side as the patient, being curious about what is going on, reviewing options without judging, and assisting the patient to understand how the eating disorder has been helpful. The overall effort is to foster a trusting relationship that promotes self-awareness, self-acceptance, and responsibility for change. In the language of motivational interviewing, the goal of these discussions is to help patients increasingly shift from the motivational stages of *precontemplation* through *contemplation* to *action*.

Psychosocial Rehabilitation

The model of psychosocial rehabilitation (Sullivan et al. 2005) may enable clinicians to help patients develop an increasingly positive sense of identity and well-being through individualized plans that exploit patients' strengths and focus on sustainable goals and small successes. The goal here is to foster autonomy through productive activities and life-management skills that help restore patients' sense of realistic hope and belief in the possibility of change. Team members assist patients with such practical matters as housing, transportation, social networks, paid work, volunteer work, and educational programs. When the focus is on life skills and social skills, a variety of approaches, including dialectical behavior therapy, may be employed to help patients develop better self-management abilities with regard to their nutrition and psychiatric symptoms.

Specific Management Strategies

Within these frameworks, the following guidelines, drawn from considerable clinical experience and consensus, may be helpful in managing the care of patients with chronic, intractable eating disorders (Goldner 1989; Hamburg et al. 1989; Kaplan and Garfinkel 1999; Strober 2004; Yager 1992):

1. *Make every effort to establish a heartfelt connection with the patient to secure a durable and effective working alliance.* An inability to make this link—and such a connection may sometimes be quite difficult to achieve if the patient's personality is uninviting or unresponsive—will further complicate any therapeutic attempts. If the patient lacks a sense of working alliance with the clinician, the clinician's efforts may be experienced as controlling and coercive. Most observers believe that it is important to establish at least some areas of alliance and agreement (e.g., "At least we can both agree that you aren't very happy in your present condition"), and that it is generally counterproductive to argue or struggle with or to attempt to scare a chronically resistant low-weight patient. The principles of motivational interviewing described in the previous subsection are helpful at this point.

2. *Review as fully as possible the nature of previous psychological, psychosocial, and medical (including psychopharmacological) treatment attempts, and seek both the patient's and previous health professionals' perceptions of what worked and what failed, and the likely reasons for the successes and failures. If*

the clinician has been working with an intractable patient for a long period of time and perceives that she has reached a therapeutic impasse, a
similar fresh and thorough case review may be helpful.

3. *Assess the patient's current true goals for herself.* Listen carefully to statements that include the determination to maintain the status quo, and try
   to assess the degree to which such goals are based on depressive distortions
   or more realistic appraisals.

4. *Assess the patient's own beliefs about what future treatments might work or
   not work, and why.* If the patient's desires for specific treatments are based
   on a reasonable rationale, plan treatment around the patient's desires for
   modality-specific intervention.

5. *Encourage the patient to develop a detailed behavioral program* based on lifesaving nutritional and medical needs and/or on small steps directed to
   psychological, social, and vocational issues.

6. *Establish basic limits regarding weight and medical severity, beyond which the
   treatment team will insist that the patient be hospitalized at least for medical
   stabilization.* Similar expectations should be established for other self-
   harming behaviors. When medical interventions are required, in no instance should a program be inherently punitive. Such programs, if they
   work at all, work only for the time they are sustained, and over the long
   run they generally yield minimal symptomatic improvement with a large
   residue of frustration, resentment, and feelings of impotence in patient
   and staff alike.

7. *Reconsider the patient's program of psychotherapeutic interventions.* Even if the
   patient has previously received psychotherapy, reassessment regarding the
   potential utility of a specific psychotherapeutic approach and/or therapist is warranted. The patient may benefit from a change in psychotherapeutic strategy and/or psychotherapist. Many varieties of psychodynamic,
   cognitive-behavioral, experiential, and other forms of psychotherapy
   have been used for patients with eating disorders, and conceivably a novel
   approach may help a given patient when others have failed.

8. *Do not put the patient through expensive and time-consuming treatment or
   psychotherapy programs that are unlikely to effect any sustained improvement,
   and do not instill false hopes that are very likely to be dashed.* Although se-
   rially offering different therapeutic trials may be justified, the point here
   is not to overenthusiastically convince the patient and family into think-

ing that the next intervention will work magic. At the same time, even late-occuring, newfound motivation and hopefulness should be encouraged and not dashed. In each instance, in ongoing conversations the patient should understand that the clinician has her deep interests at heart, will continue to explore all therapeutic possibilities, and is not abandoning hope for improving the patient's clinical condition and quality of life.

Family Assessment and Treatment

Family assessment, education, and counseling should be offered in every case where feasible, and specific family therapy should be considered as a treatment option. In certain instances, the patient will refuse to have her family involved, and in these cases clinicians should carefully assess the patient's reasons for these wishes. Leaving the family out of treatment may make sense when the patient's reasons are based on objective concerns regarding a family member's abuse, malignant narcissism, or psychosis or in other situations likely to make matters worse. But when including the family might be of real benefit, the clinician might continue to discuss pros and cons to see if the patient might alter her views and ultimately invite the family to participate.

In dealing with patients with chronic and intractable disorders, family members are often uncertain as to how actively they should become involved in physically helping the patient eat and abstain from purging or exercise. They desire advice regarding what stance they should adopt regarding emotional, physical, and financial support; experience difficulties controlling their own rage and sadness regarding the patient's behaviors; feel guilty regarding their own potential contributions to the disorder's appearance and maintenance; harbor their own questions, suggestions, and expectations for the patient's goals and treatments; and worry that the patient will die as a result of medical complications or suicide. All these issues bear discussion and should be addressed so that family members are heard and are included as part of the treatment team, thereby contributing to solutions rather than problems.

Choice of a Treatment Site

In general, patients should be treated in the least restrictive setting likely to foster optimal recovery and quality of life. Since patients with chronic, intractable conditions usually have limited financial means and medical insurance benefits due to exhausting benefits during prior hospitalizations, being ineligible for insurance coverage under a parent's insurance policy after reaching a certain age, or relying on limited-benefit Medicaid and/or Medicare, financial realities always influence treatment options in substantial ways.

Hospitalization for such patients should occur to ensure basic safety. However, in contrast to younger patients with anorexia nervosa manifesting severe weight loss in an initial or second episode, in which restoration of weight to a near-optimum level sufficient to restore menses and ovulation may be the goal of hospitalization, restoring weight to a theoretically optimal level may be unrealistic and impractical for patients with long-term malnutrition. For these patients, the goals of hospitalization may be 1) to restore weight to a realistic and sustainable weight level that the patient may be able to maintain without immediate decline to dangerous levels, 2) to interrupt self-harming behavior patterns, and 3) to restore physical and psychic energy and morale sufficiently to permit the patient to return to a somewhat stable posthospital equilibrium. A realistic weight level for a given patient may be estimated on the basis of her sustainable-weight history over the preceding several years.

Depending on the patient's goals, the negotiated treatment plan, and the availability of clinical and financial resources, less intensive settings may vary from intermittent to long-term full-time residential treatment, partial hospitalization programs, organized intensive outpatient programs, to working with one or more clinicians in individual or group settings in private or public settings and facilities.

Several innovative activities in Canada, funded through provincial funds and private donations, have established organized community-based programs that offer clinician contact in the home or other nonclinic settings (see, e.g., the St. Paul's Hospital Eating Disorders Program at the University of British Columbia [http://www.stpaulseatingdisorders.ca/treatrec.htm]), including physical places where patients with chronic eating disorders may gather for contact, succor, and assistance (see, e.g., Sheena's Place in Toronto, Ontario [http://www.sheenasplace.org]).

Depending on family relationships, communication styles, and resources, patients with chronic, intractable disorders may find sustained and helpful practical and emotional support living at home with their parents, or they may do better living with other relatives or friends, or on their own. Difficult situations arise when financial and/or residential supports provided by families exact a considerable emotional cost on the patient. In these circumstances, a careful psychofinancial "cost-benefit" analysis may determine the least-worst situation available to the patient.

Medications and Other Somatic Treatments

Patients with chronic eating disorders vary considerably regarding their experiences with and willingness to consider medications. They may for the first time, after many years of illness, reluctantly accept that medications, including SSRIs and even atypical antipsychotic medications, may offer some assistance. The potential contributions of medications should be presented realistically, and not be oversold, in a spirit of collaboration. Reluctant patients should be given all information available and pointed to useful Web sites and journal articles, and expect a detailed, informed discussion with their clinicians regarding the possible benefits and possible adverse effects of any medication from which they are likely to benefit.

Negotiations about taking certain medications (e.g., very low-dose atypical antipsychotic medications) may take weeks or months before a patient may be willing to try even a single tablet. Since patients with previously intractable disorders are occasionally known to grudgingly confess that the medication regimens they have been so averse to even trying have ultimately been helpful, many clinicians habitually seek opportunities to offer medications as a resource, even in the absence of strong evidence from randomized controlled trials. The guidelines presented in the following subsections, offered here to supplement information in other chapters that thoroughly review medications used to treat eating disorders, may help clinicians struggling with the limited evidence-base.

Selective Serotonin Reuptake Inhibitors

Occasional patients with intractable anorexia nervosa are known to respond to high-dose SSRIs (Kaye et al. 2001; Kim 2003). In such patients, the almost delusion-like quality and intensity of obsessional thinking, and associated compulsive behaviors, may be ameliorated. The effective response may parallel that occasionally seen with high-dose SSRIs in the treatment of delusional depression and of body dysmorphic disorder. In case series fluoxetine 40–60 mg/ day or its equivalents have sometimes been helpful (Gwirtsman et al. 1990). In one open-label study, venlafaxine was reported to be as useful as fluoxetine for patients with atypical anorexia nervosa (Ricca et al. 1999).

Other Antidepressant Medications

The sparse literature regarding the use of monoamine oxidase inhibitors (MAOIs) in anorexia nervosa is not encouraging (Kennedy and Goldbloom 1991), but occasional patients with unremitting anorexia nervosa have responded dramatically to the judicious use of tranylcypromine or phenelzine, and MAOIs may be useful for treating bulimia nervosa (Kennedy et al. 1993). However, cautions regarding diet and blood pressure are in order.

Although some clinicians have anecdotally been reported to use mirtazapine to treat anorexia nervosa, because of its propensity to cause weight gain, its use in eating disorders has not been evaluated. Of course, some patients are often reluctant to take any medication that specifies weight gain as a side effect.

Bupropion is not advised for the treatment of patients with eating disorders, because of an increased risk of seizures. A black box warning has been issued by the U.S. Food and Drug Administration (FDA) regarding the use of this medication in eating disorder patients.

In a small open-label study, reboxetine, a selective noradrenergic inhibitor, was useful in the treatment of bulimia nervosa (Fassino et al. 2004), and it has also been suggested for possible use in anorexia nervosa. However, although this medication is now available in 50 countries, in May 2005 the FDA declined to authorize its use in the United States.

Atypical and Typical Antipsychotic Medications

Although many patients are reluctant to take atypical antipsychotic medications because of their known propensities to enhance weight, clinicians are increasingly using olanzapine and risperidone in the treatment of patients with anorexia nervosa who are willing to accept the medications. They may not only enhance weight but also reduce anorectic preoccupations, anxiety, quasipsychotic symptoms, and hyperactivity, even at very small doses (Powers et al. 2002; J. Russell 2004). Some clinicians have found that scoring the smallest tablets and building up the dose increases acceptability and helps patients and clinicians find the lowest doses with fewest adverse effects at which effectiveness is encountered. Of note, in an open-label study, low-dose haloperidol was, similarly, found to be effective in alleviating symptoms of anorexia nervosa and increasing weight in a group of treatment-resistant outpatients (Cassano et al. 2003).

Opiate-Related Medications

On the basis of observations that endogenous opioids may be elevated in patients with anorexia nervosa of the binge-eating/purging subtype and bulimia nervosa, narcotic antagonists have been used to treat these conditions with some success in randomized, double-blind, placebo-controlled trials (Marrazzi et al. 1995). Dosages of 25–75 mg/day of naltrexone have been used in patients with chronic anorexia nervosa (Luby et al. 1987). Hepatic enzyme elevations require close observation in these cases. An interesting single case report (Mendelson 2001) suggested that the synthetic opiate tramadol, which binds μ-opioid receptors and weakly inhibits the reuptake of norepinephrine and serotonin, was helpful for a patient with otherwise intractable anorexia nervosa, but this report has not yet been followed by systematic trials. However, contemplating its use for chronic anorexia nervosa is complicated by the fact that tramadol has been used as a drug of abuse.

Other Medications

Medications previously mentioned in the literature that receive little contemporary attention because of concerns about adverse effects and/or limited effectiveness in randomized clinical trials may, nevertheless, prove helpful for individual patients and may still be considered as less popular options for certain patients with intractable conditions. This group includes agents such as the histamine and serotonin antagonist cyproheptadine, which showed some efficacy for patients with anorexia nervosa, restricting type, in a double-blind, placebo-controlled trial (Halmi et al. 1986); lithium (Gross et al. 1981); benzodiazepines and other antianxiety agents if used very judiciously for anorexia nervosa (G.F.M. Russell 2001), and, for patients with bulimia nervosa, anticonvulsants such as topiramate (Hedges et al. 2003; Hoopes et al. 2003). Treating underlying bipolar disorders may help alleviate eating disorder symptoms in some patients (Kaplan et al. 1983). But clinicians should understand the hazards associated with the use of lithium in eating disorder patients, since dehydration and electrolyte shifts resulting from excessive exercise and purging increase the risk of lithium toxicity. For patients with comorbid attention-deficit disorder and bulimia nervosa, case reports indicate that treatment of the attention-deficit disorder with stimulant medication such as methylphenidate or amphetamines may alleviate eating disorder symptoms (Drimmer 2003; Schweickert et al. 1997; Sokol et al. 1999). Of course, since these stimulants often suppress appetite and weight, careful patient selection and close monitoring of patients in whom such interventions are attempted are required. Clearly, any of the medications mentioned above should be used only when medically safe and under close supervision. Finally, in several small randomized controlled trials, the antiemetic ondansetron was effective for the treatment of some patients with intractable bulimia nervosa (Faris et al. 2000).

Enteral and Parenteral Feedings

In life-threatening circumstances, nasogastric or other enteral forms of feeding may be lifesaving (Alvin et al. 1993) . In a nonrandomized study of 155 patients who voluntarily accepted nasogastric feeding in addition to oral feeding versus 226 who received oral refeeding alone, patients who received tube feeding for at least one-half their length of stay gained 1 kg per week, versus 0.77 kg per week for patients receiving oral refeeding alone. The authors reported that patients evidenced no differences in recovery from anorexia's psychological aspects, satisfaction with treatment, or medical complication frequency (Zuercher et al. 2003). Some patients are willing to accept enteral or liquid formula feedings when they are psychologically unable to take food orally on their own. For occasional patients, the psychological relief of having long-term parenteral feeding, particularly feedings directly into the small intestine to avoid gastric discomfort, may be preferable to having to obsess about consuming food orally. I consulted on a patient who, following six admissions to general hospitals for severe malnutrition and electrolyte imbalance in a 2-year period, took it upon herself to convince a surgeon to insert an in-dwelling line for total parenteral nutrition. She kept the line anti-coagulated and, to supplement the no more than approximately 300 kcal per day she was able to permit herself to take as food by mouth, intermittently administered total parenteral nutrition to herself. When I first saw her, she had maintained this arrangement for more than 4 years with the assistance of her internist. After the catheter was placed, the patient required no further medical hospitalizations. Forcing enteral feeding on unwilling patients is fraught with ethical and legal complications and presents nightmare situations clinically. These situations are discussed at greater length in the next section ("Legal, Ethical, and Humanistic Considerations").

Other Somatic Interventions

Although the literature is sparse, case reports suggest that in some patients with intractable anorexia nervosa and comorbid major depressive disorder, both disorders improve following electroconvulsive therapy (Ferguson 1993; Hill et al. 2001). Open trials (Lam et al. 2001) and one randomized, double-blind, placebo-controlled trial (Braun et al. 1999) have shown both mood and binge-eating symptoms to improve in response to bright light therapy in patients with bulimia nervosa and comorbid seasonal affective disorder. However, in one double-blind, placebo-controlled study, only mood symptoms, but not the eating disorder symptoms, improved in response to bright light (Blouin et al. 1996).

Legal, Ethical, and Humanistic Considerations

Every experienced clinician will encounter some eating disorder patients who, in spite of everyone's good intentions and the best currently available treatments, remain prisoners of the attendant obsessions, compulsions, rituals, and impulses. Some are content to remain in their diminished state, not wanting to beat a dead horse but attempting to adapt and resign themselves to their condition; others are willing to do anything, including psychosurgery, to alter their symptoms; and some are so fatigued, debilitated, and demoralized that they would just as soon die. Some simply want to be left alone, even if in dire social straits, because they feel that both their families and their caregivers are making them feel worse, not better. Clinicians must ask themselves, morally and legally, just when to agree with these patients, offering them an open door should they ever want to return, and asking permission to keep in touch simply to remain informed regarding the patient's condition and course.

As the complex and conflicting legal and ethical literature on the treatment of patients with intractable eating disorders who refuse treatment illustrate, no one opinion prevails. Working on a case-by-case basis with patients, families, ethicists, and local legal authorities, health providers have in some cases opted to pursue aggressive interventions despite the patient's expressed wishes, or have acceded to the patient's wishes and abstained from pushing aggressive involuntary interventions. These matters have been the subject of vivid debates in the literature (Birmingham 2003; Draper 1998, 2000, 2003; Giordano 2003; Oliver 1997). While courts may accede to involuntary treatment of patients with anorexia nervosa (Brahams 1997; Grubb 1994), they may not agree to force-feedings (Dyer 1993). Generally speaking, authorities favor intervening despite a patient's wishes when the patient is deemed incompetent or has a serious mental disorder. The clear difficulty arises in how to assess patients with anorexia nervosa along these lines. To what extent do patients with chronic and severe anorexia nervosa refuse further treatment as a result of their serious mental disorders, and to what extent might they be refusing treatment "rationally" following years of efforts to combat an exhausting and implacable condition?

Patients Who Refuse Treatment

When the clinician is working with patients who refuse treatment, Goldner's (1989) excellent perspectives are worth noting. Goldner emphasizes, among others, several points alluded to earlier, including the following:

- Identifying the patient's reasons for refusal
- Providing careful explanation of treatment recommendations
- Being prepared for negotiation
- Allowing the patient to retain autonomy
- Weighing risks versus benefits of treatment imposition, taking into consideration, for example, degree of physical compromise, vulnerability of the treatment alliance, previous outcomes of intervention and of nonintervention, available resources and supports, duration of illness, accuracy of the patient's judgments and perceptions, and any other prognostic indicators
- Avoiding battles and scare tactics (which ordinarily result in an escalation of symptoms and an erosion of the therapeutic alliance)

- Involving the family
- Obtaining legal clarification and support
- Considering legal means of treatment imposition only when refusal is judged to constitute a serious risk
- Conceptualizing refusal or resistance as an evolutionary process in which individuals who initially refuse treatment may alter their emotional and cognitive responses with the passage of time, particularly when they are aided by supportive individuals

Patients Who Are in Danger of Imminent Collapse but Who Refuse Treatment

For the more intransigent patient who is in danger of imminent collapse, other measures may be necessary. If a patient is unable to bring herself to eat a regular diet and the clinical staff views the situation as urgently life-threatening, the patient should be offered alternatives to regular food by mouth, such as liquid supplements, nasogastric feedings, or total parenteral nutrition.

In the event of acute, imminently life-threatening starvation with food refusal, depending on the patient's prior history and other psychiatric factors, the staff may opt to institute nasogastric feedings in the short run on a Good Samaritan basis while seeking emergency legal conservatorship for ongoing treatment. Here, the acute intervention, with treatment of both malnutrition and depression with or without conscious suicidality, may reverse the imminence of threatened death and is therefore warranted and justified. But without the patient's willing cooperation, plans based on enteral feeding are usually short-lived and are very likely to fail. Patients have been known to rip out surgically placed cannulas that were put in place against their will for total parenteral nutrition. However, there have also been cases in which patients who absolutely refused to eat were forced to accept one or two nasogastric tube feedings and, subsequently, acquiesced to take food by mouth.

In treating chronically food-refusing patients who seem to be constantly flirting with death—walking on the edge—the legal situation parallels murky areas that exist in the treatment of chronically suicidal patients. In this regard, several realities intrude: First, few facilities are able to keep such patients hospitalized indefinitely, and few patients and families have the means to pay for such prolonged care. Second, for these patients the only benefit one can expect from such aggressive and sometimes increasingly assaultive treatments is to prolong life, but certainly not to keep its quality from deteriorating. How long can or should such drawn-out suicides or dying processes continue?

Chronically Suicidal and Parasuicidal Patients

Clinicians should not actively assist suicidal behavior, but compassionate clinicians can understand that for some patients the pain of continuing life is more than they can bear, and that the ordeal of struggling against all odds is too terrible a price to pay for continuing a miserable existence. As with patients with terminal cancer or AIDS, it is often the treating staff and the family who are unable to accept the "rational" nature of the patient's desires to die. In these instances, the clinician's therapeutic tasks may include preparing the staff and family for the possibility or even likelihood of a fatal outcome, increasing their compassion and understanding of the patient's perspective, and, when death occurs, helping the staff and family in postvention around the same issues.

In some ways the more difficult situations are those in which patients who are ambivalent about suicide repetitively engage in suicidal or subsuicidal self-destructive acts, made in such a manner that they are obvious to the staff, so that the staff must continually rescue the patient. To make matters worse, in such situations the rescued patients are often petulant and ungrateful for having been saved, and as a result, treating staff members often become enraged at these patients. Therapeutic strategies require helping the patient understand the underlying causes for her angry acts, helping her to achieve alternative ways of coping to better express her emotions and meet her needs, and developing behavioral plans and constructing behavioral interventions that reduce counterproductive secondary gains for these activities. These pathological repetitive games sometimes result in fatalities, on occasion due to patient miscalculations, as when staff members inadvertently fail to recognize that a patient has taken a lethal overdose in plain sight.

Countertransference Issues and Their Management

Intractability among eating disorder patients, whatever its causes, can generate frustration and burnout among treating clinicians (Goldner 1989; Hamburg et al. 1989; Kaplan and Garfinkel 1999; Strober 2004; Yager 1992).

Several of the common countertransference problems have already been mentioned. Clinicians may feel narcissistically challenged by a bedeviling clinical problem, frustrated and angered by the patient's seemingly obstinate and oppositional behavior and failure to progress, blameful of the patient for not getting better (blaming the victim), and progressively therapeutically impotent and disengaged.

Management of countertransference requires that clinicians constantly assess their attitudes toward these patients and seek frequent consultation and supervision in their care. Clinicians involved in the patient's care must also communicate regularly to air their opinions of and experiences with these difficult-to-treat patients and to obtain validation and/or redirection regarding their feelings and attitudes.

Compassionate Clinical Decision Making for Intractable Patients

Mary, a 50-year-old former health professional, had been diagnosed with anorexia nervosa, restricting subtype, at the age of 14. During her teens and 20s she underwent several long inpatient hospitalizations and additional months-long episodes of care at several residential treatment programs, but she was never able to sustain any of the weight gain or behavioral improvements obtained during these stays. She was able to complete school and to work in a restricted role for about 15 years before her fatigue prevented her from continuing. Her shy, constricted, and rigid personality prevented her from developing many friendships or relationships outside those with her family, and she lived a quiet life in semi-seclusion with her highly protective mother. At a point when her elderly mother's health started to fail, Mary's weight dropped from a usual BMI of 17 to 15. Concerned about what might happen in the future when she was no longer able to provide care, her mother insisted that Mary once again involve herself in outpatient therapy.

Mary's therapist, who saw her diligently each week, and who also met with her mother and with the two of them from time to time, kept gently attempting to motivate her regarding her eating behaviors and other aspects of her social functioning. The therapist reported that Mary would sweetly and compliantly attend weekly meetings without fail, offer little in the way of spontaneous speech, and always agree with the therapist's questions, urgings, and mild admonitions. Despite this degree of participation, Mary's actual rigid, limited patterns of eating and social behavior remained unchanged. However, Mary constantly reassured the therapist that these weekly sessions were meaningful and

valuable for her, and she resisted any movements on the therapist's part to reduce the frequency of meetings. The therapist acknowledged that the existential
connection and "witnessing" that she offered provided Mary with a small but
significant degree of enrichment to an impoverished life.

Guidelines for treating these patients parallel those for treating other patients with chronic, unremitting illnesses that may lead to premature death:

1. *Do no harm* (primum non nocere). In the face of intractability, clinicians
   should avoid therapeutic overzealousness and should not succumb to the
   temptation of either orthodox or unorthodox interventions that may put
   the patients at undue risk. Patients and families should be fully informed
   of both obvious and hidden risks and costs, the odds of achieving potential benefits, and the pros and cons of doing nothing further. Patients
   should not be coerced into accepting ill-conceived treatment plans that
   are unlikely to ultimately be to their benefit.
2. *Base decisions about treatment on clinical effectiveness rather than on finances,
   to whatever extent possible.* Although ability to pay and payment sources un-
   avoidably dictate access to medical and psychiatric inpatient, residential,
   and outpatient care, decisions about treatment should ideally be based on
   clinical effectiveness rather than on finances. In practice, these issues are
   inevitably linked, but the costs and benefits of various choices should be
   made explicit to patients and their families, who may opt to involve extended families, attorneys, and other potential stakeholders in ultimate
   decisions about treatment.
3. *Avoid communicating undue optimism or self-protective nihilism.* It is clinically unsound and humanistically untenable to offer either undue optimism or harsh, unfiltered pessimism. For example, as a defense against
   the frustrations of therapeutic impotence, clinicians may opt for a self-
   protective going-in position of therapeutic hopelessness and nihilism.
   One self-protective strategy clinicians sometimes use in these situations
   has been called "hanging crepe" (a reference to the black crepe hung over
   coffins in years gone by), essentially a strategy in which the clinician opts to
   tell the patient and family the worst likely scenario—that the patient will
   die. In this way the physician is seen as a wise prognosticator if the patient
   does not improve, and as a magical healer if the patient does miraculously
   improve. Some clinicians have justified presenting patients and their fam-

ilies with bluntly described worst-case scenarios as the most likely outcome by suggesting that this presentation occasionally provokes paradoxical oppositional reactions in patients, in which the patient refuses to do badly just because the physician predicts that is what is going to happen. However, proof that such an approach has ever been successful with chronic patients is entirely lacking. The danger of hanging crepe lies in potentially depriving the patient and her family of any shreds of hope that might facilitate improvement.

4. *Realize that ongoing contact with a caring, involved clinician conveys meaning and hope.* When a patient appears to have achieved and exhausted maximum expectable tangible therapeutic benefit from all treatment options available to her, the patient may still derive substantial psychological benefit from ongoing contact with the clinician. In these circumstances, the clinician, patient, and family should explicitly discuss what the anticipated contacts are likely and unlikely to accomplish. For example, although significant cognitive or behavioral changes may be unlikely to occur, the clinician can always offer close, existential human companionship and contact with someone who will compassionately listen to the patient without rejecting, taunting, or belittling her, to witness what she is going through, and to be hopeful but candid. The clinician should always maintain and sustain hope based on the assurance that he or she will be informed of (and hopefully availed of) promising new treatments that may appear come up, and, in any event, assure the patient that the clinician will do what is possible (short of euthanasia) to relieve suffering. Such a relationship may provide an important human touchstone for the patient and family, in which she can be brutally honest with herself and another person about what is transpiring in her life and thoughts, and which diminishes her sense of human isolation. Clinicians must ask themselves if they feel personally equipped to honestly and unresentfully provide such services. Some clinicians feel that such work wastes their time or find that their negative countertransference toward such patients, whom they see as unmotivated, is so overwhelming that they cannot in good faith work constructively with such patients. Other clinicians approach these therapeutic tasks in the same spirit as working with dying patients who need close alliances and comforting. Certainly within the large tradition of medicine there is room and much precedent for such work.

5. *Obtain extensive consultation and institutional review, as for a research protocol, if any unorthodox treatment is contemplated.* Extensive documentation should be recorded in the medical record, and patients and their families should be asked to sign consents.

6. *Ensure that the patient is kept comfortable without undue restriction (except that necessary to sustain life) or imposition.* The basic necessities of life (i.e., food, clothing, shelter) should always be available.

7. *Keep the long view.* For as yet inexplicable reasons, the symptoms and resistances in patients with even very chronic disorders may change or evolve over time. If the clinician maintains a good relationship with the patient throughout, without alienating the patient by countertransference anger, derision, denigration, or other subtle attacks on the patient's self-esteem, these changes may be slowly guided in a positive direction. Prognostications should always contain broad statements that include the possibility of change. To support these statements, the clinician can point to cases of patients who changed for the better even after years of chronic intractability and poor functioning, for reasons that we do not understand (such as those described by Ratnasuriya et al. [1991]). The clinician can also emphasize that for reasons that still elude us, many patients with chronic eating disorders manage to survive for years on incredibly meager intakes, and note that rapid advances in scientific understanding have been producing more effective treatments not only for eating disorders but for associated symptoms such as depression, anxiety, obsessions, and compulsions. Families in particular also have to know that it may not be the worst thing in the world for a patient not to be in treatment, at least for a while.

8. *Make patients and families aware of the potential benefits of meeting with other patients and families who have been struggling with chronic eating disorders.* Patients and families may benefit from meeting with other patients and families who have been struggling with chronic eating disorders. Such support can be sought through, for example, family-involved local and national eating disorder–focused self-help organizations such as those listed in Table 16–3 and family-oriented self-help organizations such as the National Alliance on Mental Illness (formerly National Alliance for the Mentally Ill) that deal with chronic and severe mental illness. By resetting their expectations, patients and their families may be able to establish more realistic plans and psychological accommodations, and live

Table 16–3. Resources for patients with chronic, intractable eating disorders and their families

National Eating Disorders Association (NEDA)	http://www.nationaleatingdisorders.org/p.asp?WebPage_ID=337
National Association of Anorexia Nervosa and Associated Disorders (ANAD)	http://www.anad.org/site/anadweb/
Academy for Eating Disorders (for professionals, patients, and families)	http://www.aedweb.org
Something Fishy (pro-recovery Web site)	http://www.something-fishy.org/
Gürze Books (specializing in eating disorders)	http://www.Gurze.com

together with less tension and frustration, than would otherwise be the case. In the face of severe, chronic disabling symptoms, we as clinicians should do whatever we can under the circumstances to help the patient sustain the highest quality of life possible.

References

Alvin P, Zogheib J, Rey C, et al: Severe complications and mortality in mental eating disorders in adolescence: on 99 hospitalized patients [in French]. Arch Fr Pediatr 50:755–762, 1993

Birmingham CL: Clinical decision analysis and anorexia nervosa. Int J Law Psychiatry 26:719–723, 2003

Blouin AG, Blouin JH, Iversen H, et al: Light therapy in bulimia nervosa: a double-blind, placebo-controlled study. Psychiatry Res 60:1–9, 1996

Brahams D: UK compulsory detention for anorexia makes legal history. Lancet 349:860, 1997

Braun DL, Sunday SR, Fornari VM, et al: Bright light therapy decreases winter binge frequency in women with bulimia nervosa: a double-blind, placebo-controlled study. Compr Psychiatry 40:442–448, 1999

Bulik CM, Sullivan PF, Carter FA, et al: Predictors of rapid and sustained response to cognitive-behavioral therapy for bulimia nervosa. Int J Eat Disord 26:137–144, 1999

Cassano GB, Miniati M, Pini S, et al: Six-month open trial of haloperidol as an adjunctive treatment for anorexia nervosa: a preliminary report. Int J Eat Disord 33:172–177, 2003

Dally P: Anorexia Nervosa. New York, Grune & Stratton, 1969, pp 139–147

Draper H: Treating anorexics without consent: some reservations. J Med Ethics 24:5–7, 1998

Draper H: Anorexia nervosa and respecting a refusal of life-prolonging therapy: a limited justification. Bioethics 14:120–133, 2000

Draper H: Anorexia nervosa and refusal of naso-gastric treatment: a reply to Simona Giordano. Bioethics 17:279–289, 2003

Drimmer EJ: Stimulant treatment of bulimia nervosa with and without attention-deficit disorder: three case reports. Nutrition 19:76–77, 2003

Dyer C: Court rules against force feeding. BMJ 307:1164–1165, 1993

Faris PL, Kim SW, Meller WH, et al: Effect of decreasing afferent vagal activity with ondansetron on symptoms of bulimia nervosa: a randomised, double-blind trial. Lancet 355:792–797, 2000

Fassino S, Daga GA, Piero A, et al: Dropout from brief psychotherapy in anorexia nervosa. Psychother Psychosom 71:200–206, 2002

Fassino S, Daga GA, Boggio S, et al: Use of reboxetine in bulimia nervosa: a pilot study. J Psychopharmacol 18:423–428, 2004

Ferguson JM: The use of electroconvulsive therapy in patients with intractable anorexia nervosa. Int J Eat Disord 13:195–201, 1993

Fichter MM, Quadflieg N: Twelve-year course and outcome of bulimia nervosa. Psychol Med 34:1395–1406, 2004

Fichter MM, Quadflieg N, Hedlund S: Twelve-year course and outcome predictors of anorexia nervosa. Int J Eat Disord 39:87–100, 2006

Giordano S: Anorexia nervosa and refusal of naso-gastric treatment: a response to Heather Draper. Bioethics 17:261–278, 2003

Goldner E: Treatment refusal in anorexia nervosa. Int J Eat Disord 8:297–306, 1989

Gross HA, Ebert MH, Faden VB, et al: A double-blind controlled trial of lithium carbonate primary anorexia nervosa. J Clin Psychopharmacol 1:376–381, 1981

Grubb A: Treatment without consent (anorexia nervosa): adult—Riverside Mental Health Trust v Fox. Med Law Rev 2:95–99, 1994

Gwirtsman HE, Guze BH, Yager J, et al: Fluoxetine treatment of anorexia nervosa: an open clinical trial. J Clin Psychiatry 51:378–382, 1990

Halmi KA, Eckert E, LaDu TJ, et al: Anorexia nervosa: treatment efficacy of cyproheptadine and amitriptyline. Arch Gen Psychiatry 43:177–181, 1986

Hamburg P, Herzog DB, Brotman AN, et al: The treatment-resistant eating disordered patient. Psychiatr Annals 19:494–499, 1989

Hedges DW, Reimherr FW, Hoopes SP, et al: Treatment of bulimia nervosa with topiramate in a randomized, double-blind, placebo-controlled trial, Part 2: improvement in psychiatric measures. J Clin Psychiatry 64:1449–1454, 2003

Hill R, Haslett C, Kumar S: Anorexia nervosa in an elderly woman. Aust N Z J Psychiatry 35:246–248, 2001

Hoopes SP, Reimherr FW, Hedges DW, et al: Treatment of bulimia nervosa with topiramate in a randomized, double-blind, placebo-controlled trial, Part 1: improvement in binge and purge measures. J Clin Psychiatry 64:1335–1341, 2003

Johnson JG, Cohen P, Kasen S, et al: Eating disorders during adolescence and the risk for physical and mental disorders during early adulthood. Arch Gen Psychiatry 59:545–552, 2002

Kaplan AS, Garfinkel PE: Difficulties in treating patients with eating disorders: a review of patient and clinician variables. Can J Psychiatry 44:665–670, 1999

Kaplan AS, Garfinkel PE, Darby PL, et al: Carbamazepine in the treatment of bulimia. Am J Psychiatry 140:1225–1226, 1983

Kaye WH, Nagata T, Weltzin TE, et al: Double-blind placebo-controlled administration of fluoxetine in restricting- and restricting-purging-type anorexia nervosa. Biol Psychiatry 49:644–652, 2001

Keel PK, Mitchell JE, Miller KB, et al: Long-term outcome of bulimia nervosa. Arch Gen Psychiatry 56:63–69, 1999

Keel PK, Mitchell JE, Davis TL, et al: Long-term impact of treatment in women diagnosed with bulimia nervosa. Int J Eat Disord 31:151–158, 2002

Kennedy SH, Goldbloom DS: Current perspectives on drug therapies for anorexia nervosa and bulimia nervosa. Drugs 41:367–377, 1991

Kennedy SH, Goldbloom DS, Ralevski E, et al: Is there a role for selective monoamine oxidase inhibitor therapy in bulimia nervosa? A placebo-controlled trial of brofaromine. J Clin Psychopharmacol 13:415–422, 1993

Kim SS: Role of fluoxetine in anorexia nervosa. Ann Pharmacother 37:890–892, 2003

Lam RW, Lee SK, Tam EM, et al: An open trial of light therapy for women with seasonal affective disorder and comorbid bulimia nervosa. J Clin Psychiatry 62:164–168, 2001

Luby ED, Marrazzi MA, Kinzie J: Treatment of chronic anorexia nervosa with opiate blockade. J Clin Psychopharmacol 7:52–53, 1987

MacMaster SA: Harm reduction: a new perspective on substance abuse services. Soc Work 49:356–363, 2004

Marrazzi MA, Bacon JP, Kinzie J, et al: Naltrexone use in the treatment of anorexia nervosa and bulimia nervosa. Int Clin Psychopharmacol 10:163–172, 1995

Mendelson SD: Treatment of anorexia nervosa with tramadol. Am J Psychiatry 158:963–964, 2001

Miller WR, Yahne CE, Tonigan JS: Motivational interviewing in drug abuse services: a randomized trial. J Consult Clin Psychol 71:754–763, 2003

Oliver J: Anorexia and the refusal of medical treatment. Law Rev 27:621–647, 1997

Powers PS, Santana CA, Bannon YS: Olanzapine in the treatment of anorexia nervosa: an open label trial. Int J Eat Disord 32:146–154, 2002

Ratnasuriya RH, Eisler I, Szmukler GI, et al: Anorexia nervosa: outcome and prognostic factors after 20 years. Br J Psychiatry 158:495–502, 1991

Ricca V, Mannucci E, Paionni A, et al: Venlafaxine versus fluoxetine in the treatment of atypical anorectic outpatients: a preliminary study. Eat Weight Disord 4:10–14, 1999

Russell GFM: Bulimia nervosa: an ominous variant of anorexia nervosa. Psychol Med 9:429–448, 1979

Russell GFM: Involuntary treatment in anorexia nervosa. Psychiatr Clin North Am 24:337–349, 2001

Russell J: Management of anorexia nervosa revisited. BMJ 328:479–480, 2004

Schweickert LA, Strober M, Moskowitz A: Efficacy of methylphenidate in bulimia nervosa comorbid with attention-deficit hyperactivity disorder: a case report. Int J Eat Disord 21:299–301, 1997

Sokol MS, Gray NS, Goldstein A, et al: Methylphenidate treatment for bulimia nervosa associated with a cluster B personality disorder. Int J Eat Disord 25:233–237, 1999

Steinhausen HC: The outcome of anorexia nervosa in the 20th century. Am J Psychiatry 159:1284–1293, 2002

Steinhausen HC, Boyadjieva S, Griogoroiu-Serbanescu M, et al: The outcome of adolescent eating disorders: findings from an international collaborative study. Eur Child Adolesc Psychiatry 12 (suppl 1):I91–I98, 2003

Strober M: Managing the chronic, treatment-resistant patient with anorexia nervosa. Int J Eat Disord 36:245–255, 2004

Strober M, Freeman R, Morrell W: The long-term course of severe anorexia nervosa in adolescents: survival analysis of recovery, relapse, and outcome predictors over 10–15 years in a prospective study. Int J Eat Disord 22:339–360, 1997

Sullivan MJ, Feuerstein M, Gatchel R, et al: Integrating psychosocial and behavioral interventions to achieve optimal rehabilitation outcomes. J Occup Rehabil 15: 475–489, 2005

Swift WJ, Ritholz M, Kalin NH, et al: A follow-up study of thirty hospitalized bulimics. Psychosom Med 49:45–55, 1987

Westen D, Harnden-Fischer J: Personality profiles in eating disorders: rethinking the distinction between axis I and axis II. Am J Psychiatry 158:547–562, 2001

Yager J: Patients with chronic, recalcitrant eating disorders, in Special Problems in Managing Eating Disorders. Edited by Yager J, Gwirtsman HE, Edelstein CK. Washington, DC, American Psychiatric Press, 1992, pp 205–232

Zuercher JN, Cumella EJ, Woods BK, et al: Efficacy of voluntary nasogastric tube feeding in female inpatients with anorexia nervosa. JPEN J Parenter Enteral Nutr 27:268–276, 2003

Index

Page numbers printed in **boldface** *type refer to tables or figures.*

Acamprosate, 97
Acarbose, 268, **270**
Acculturation, and ethnic identity,
  390–391, 395
ACT model, 144
Adjustment disorders, 235
Adolescents. *See also* Age
  age-adjusted body mass index
    (BMI) for, 35
  eating disturbances in absence of
    diagnostic criteria in, 3
  family therapy for anorexia nervosa
    in, 152–161
  inpatient treatment for, 49
  psychosocial approaches to anorexia
    nervosa in, 132–133
  psychotherapy for, 374
Affective disorders, and comorbidity,
  80, 235
African Americans
  body image and eating behavior in,
    391–392
  culturally sensitive assessment for,
    399
  prevalence of anorexia nervosa in,
    7

Age. *See also* Adolescents; Age at onset;
    Children; Older patients
  physical presentation of anorexia
    nervosa and, 4
  psychotherapy and, 374
Age at onset, of eating disorders, 6, 11,
  15–16
Alcohol abuse or dependence, 82, 83,
  97. *See also* Substance use
    disorders
"All or none" thinking, 289
Amenorrhea, as diagnostic criteria for
    anorexia nervosa, 2–3. *See also*
    Menstruation
Amitriptyline, **178**
Amphetamine, **270**
Androgen antagonists, 183
Anorexia nervosa
  athletes and, 372–374
  chronicity and, 10, 143–144, 408–
    411
  clinical features of, 4–6
  comorbidity and, 80, 81–83, 84,
    85, 86, 88
  diagnostic criteria for, 2–3,
    350–351, 353–354

Anorexia nervosa *(continued)*
  differential diagnosis of, 6
  epidemiology of, 6–7, **8**
  etiology of, 7–9
  family therapy for, 119–120, 132,
    134, 136, 152–162
  gender and, 350–351
  hospitalization for, 114–116, **117**,
    143–144
  inpatient treatment of, 116–122
  outcome of, 9–11, **12**, 408, **409**
  partial hospitalization for, 122–124
  pharmacology for outpatient
    treatment of, 138–142, 274
  pregnancy and, 341
  psychosocial approaches to,
    119–120, 132–138
  relapse and, 9–10, 139, 143
  target symptoms and treatment
    goals in outpatient
    management of, 129–132
Anticonvulsants
  binge-eating disorder and, **206**
  bipolar disorder and, 92
  borderline personality disorder and,
    104
  weight regulation and, 264, 267,
    270
Antidepressants. *See also* Selective
    serotonin reuptake inhibitors;
    Tricyclic antidepressants
  anorexia nervosa and, 138–139
  bulimia nervosa and, 175–176,
    178–181
  chronic disorders and, 425
  weight regulation and, 261–264,
    267, **270**
Antidiabetic agents, and weight
    regulation, 265, 268, **270**

Antihypertensive medications, and
    weight regulation, 265–266,
    270
Antipsychotics, and weight regulation,
    259, **260**, 267, **270**. *See also*
    Atypical antipsychotics
Anxiety disorders, and comorbidity,
    81–82, 94–95, 235
Aripiprazole, 93, **94**, 259
Asian Americans, and cultural issues,
    394–395, 400
Assessment. *See also* Diagnosis and
    diagnostic criteria
  in athletes, 361–366
  bariatric surgery and, 241–246
  chronic cases and, 420–421,
    422
  comprehensive process for patient,
    32–43
  comorbidity and, 88–89, 90–91,
    94, 96, 99–100, 105
  cultural issues in, 398–401
  of family, 43–44, 119–120, 422
ATHENA (Athletes Targeting Healthy
    Exercise and Nutrition
    Alternatives) program, 376
Athletes, and eating disorders
  identification and assessment of,
    361–366
  prevention of, 376–378
  risk of disordered eating in, 357
  sports environments and
    predisposition to, 358–361
  sports participation for
    symptomatic patients,
    366–371
  treatment for, 371–376
Athletic Milieu Direct Questionnaire,
    366

Attachment
  psychodynamic therapy and
    patterns of, 327
  sports participation and, 367
Attention-deficit/hyperactivity disorder
    (ADHD), 275
Attitudes, and assessment, 40–42, 44.
    See also Beliefs
Atypical antipsychotics. *See also*
    Antipsychotics
  anorexia nervosa and, 121, 139–140
  chronic disorders and, 425–426
  comorbidity and, 90, 93, **94**, 96,
    104
  weight gain and, 259, 274
Avoidant personality disorder, 84

"Bad object," in psychodynamic
    therapy, 323–324
Bariatric surgery
  binge-eating disorder and, 200, 235,
    237, 239–240, 248, 249
  increase in use of, 225–226
  night-eating syndrome and, 237,
    240
  overview of procedures, 226–234
  psychiatric issues in candidates and
    patients, 235–238
  psychological assessment for,
    241–246
  psychological management and,
    246–250
  psychosocial outcomes of, 238–241
Basal metabolic rate, and weight
    regulation, 257
Beck Depression Inventory (BDI),
    243
BED. *See* Binge-eating disorder

Behavior. *See also* Behavioral
    interventions; Compensatory
    behaviors; Eating patterns;
    Feeding behaviors; Purging
    behaviors; Self-destructive
    behavior
  assessment of patient, 36–37, 39–40
  distorted cognitions and
    maladaptive, 288–291
Behavioral interventions. *See also*
    Cognitive-behavioral therapy
  for bariatric surgery patients, 246–247
  for chronic eating disorders, 421
Beliefs. *See also* Attitudes; Culture;
    Religion
  assessment and, 40–42
  chronic disorders and, 421
  cultural issues and traditional, 400,
    401, 402
Benzodiazepines, 95, 426
Beta-blockers, **270**
Biliopancreatic diversion, 232, **234**
Binge eating, and assessment, 37
Binge-eating disorder (BED)
  athletes and, 375–376
  bariatric surgery and, 200, 235,
    237, 239–240, 248, 249
  bulimia nervosa compared with, 20
  clinical features of, 21–23
  diagnostic criteria for, 20, **22**, 196
  differential diagnosis of, 23
  epidemiology of, 23–24, **25**
  etiology of, 24–25
  night-eating syndrome and, 209
  outcome of, 25, **26**
  treatment of, 197–207
Binge-eating/purging subtype, of
    anorexia nervosa, 2

Biological factors. *See also* Genetics
in anorexia nervosa, 7–8
in bulimia nervosa, 16
Bipolar disorder, and comorbidity with
eating disorders, 80, 90–94
Bisphosphonates, 142
Blame, and family assessment, 44
Blood chemistry studies, and
assessment, **38**
BMI. *See* Body mass index
Body image. *See also* Weight
binge-eating disorder and, 22
eating behaviors in non-Caucasian
women and, 389–396
perceptual distortions and, 288–289
Body mass index (BMI)
anorexia nervosa and, 34–35, 119,
130, 370
for African American women,
391
Bone density, and anorexia nervosa, 4,
36, 118, 372. *See also* Osteopenia
and osteoporosis
Borderline personality disorder (BPD),
and comorbidity, 84, 91, 96, 99–
105
Boston Interview for Gastric Bypass,
244, 245–246
Brief hospitalization, for anorexia
nervosa, 115
Bright light therapy, 428
Brofaromine, **180**
Bruch, Hilde, 318, 351
Bulimia nervosa
athletes and, 375
binge-eating disorder compared
with, 20
chronic cases of, 411–412
clinical features of, 12–15

cognitive-behavioral therapy for,
173–174, 184, **185–186**, 293,
294–297, 375
combined therapy for, 184,
185–186
comorbidity and, 80, 81, 82, 83,
87, 88–89
diagnostic criteria for, 11–12, **13**,
350
differential diagnosis of, 15
epidemiology of, 15–16, **17**
etiology of, 16–18
family therapy for, 162–163, 164,
166
gender and, 350
hospitalization for, 49–50
monitoring and follow-up of
treatment for, 188
nutritional issues in, 173
outcome of, 18–19, **20**
pregnancy and, 341
psychopharmacology for, 174–188
psychosocial approaches to
treatment of, 173–174
relapse and, 18–19, 175, 188
target symptoms and treatment
goals in, 173
Bulimia Test—Revised, 365
Bupropion
anorexia nervosa and, 139
bulimia nervosa and, 177, **179**
chronic disorders and, 425
weight regulation and, 263, 267,
270
Buspirone, 95, 97, 106

Canada, and programs for chronic
eating disorders, 423
Cannabis abuse, 82

Carbamazepine
  bipolar disorder and, 92, **93**
  weight gain and, 261, **270**
Cardiac abnormalities
  of anorexia nervosa, 4, **5**, 11
  assessment and, 36
  athletes and, 362–363, **364**
  of bulimia nervosa, **14**
  pregnant patients with eating
    disorders and, 344
Careers, of patients with anorexia
  nervosa, 410
Care models, for chronic eating
  disorders, 418–420
Catastrophizing, and cognitive
  distortions, 289
Centers for Disease Control and
  Prevention, 34
Cerebral atrophy, 347, 349
Charcot, Jean-Martin, 149
Children. *See also* Age
  age-adjusted BMI for, 35
  eating disturbances in absence of
    diagnostic criteria in, 3
  inpatient treatment for, 49
  of mothers with eating disorders,
    343–344
  psychotherapy and, 374
China, and international trends in
  eating and dieting behavior, 397
Chlorpromazine, 121, **260**
Cholecystokinin, 16
Chronicity, of eating disorders
  choice of treatment site for, 422–424
  clinical dimensions of anorexia
    nervosa and, 410–411
  compassionate clinical decision
    making for, 432–436
  countertransference and, 431–432

disability and 411
  family assessment and treatment, 422
  legal, ethical, and humanistic issues
    in, 428–431
  management strategies for, 418–422
  monitoring and follow-up for
    anorexia nervosa and, 143–144
  outcome in anorexia nervosa and,
    408, **409**
  outcome in bulimia nervosa and,
    411–412
  psychopharmacology and, 424–428
  relapse of anorexia nervosa and, 10
  resources for patients with, **436**
  therapeutic goals and, 415–418
  treatment nonresponse and
    reluctance, 412–415
Circadian pattern, and night-eating
  syndrome, 209
Cisapride, 141
Citalopram, 183, **206**
Clinical examples
  of bariatric surgery, 227, 229–230,
    232
  of chronic disorders, 418, 432–433
  of cognitive-behavioral therapy,
    291–292, 298–299
  of cultural influences, 391,
    392–393, 394, 396
  of diabetes, 336–339
  of family therapy for anorexia
    nervosa, 155, 157–158, 160
  of hospitalization for anorexia
    nervosa, 114–116
  of male patients, 349
  of night-eating syndrome, 207–208
  of older patients, 346
  of outpatient management of
    anorexia nervosa, 127–129

Clinical examples *(continued)*
   of pregnancy, 340
   of psychodynamic therapy,
      319–320, 321, 322, 323–324,
      325–326
   of sports participation, 370–371
   of treatment for binge-eating
      disorder, 197
   of treatment for bulimia nervosa, 172
   of treatment modifications for
      comorbidity, 84, 88, 98–99
   of treatment nonresponse and
      reluctance, 414–415
   of weight effects of medications,
      271–272, 274
Clinical features
   of anorexia nervosa, 4–6, 410–411
   of binge-eating disorder, 21–23
   of bulimia nervosa, 12–15
Clinical Global Impression of
   Improvement Scale (CGI-I), 217
Clinical interview, and assessment for
   bariatric surgery, 242, 244–246
Clinical recommendations, on weight-
   altering medications, 276–278.
   See also Guidelines
Clomipramine, 96
Clozapine
   clinical characteristics of, **94**
   weight gain and, 259, **260, 270,** 275
Coaches, and eating disorders in
   athletes, 360–361, 376–377
Cocaine addiction, 97
Cognitive analytic therapy, 134–135,
   303
Cognitive-behavioral therapy. *See also*
   Behavioral interventions
   anorexia nervosa and, 120, 131,
      133, 135–136

binge-eating disorder and, 201–205
bulimia nervosa and, 173–174, 184,
   185–186, 293, **294–297,** 375
comorbidity and, 89
manuals for, **300–301**
night-eating syndrome and, 213,
   214–215, 216
patient selection for, 291–292
treatment resistance and, 299, 301,
   303
Cognitive distortions. *See also* Beliefs;
   Thinking and thoughts
   anorexia nervosa and, 119
   applications of, 292–299
   assessment and, 40–42
   maladaptive behaviors in eating
      disorders and, 288–291
Cognitive restructuring, and bariatric
   surgery, 249–250
Combined therapy
   for binge-eating disorder, 205
   for bulimia nervosa, 184, **185–186**
Community Outreach Partnership
   Program (COPP), 419
Comorbidity
   assessment and, 42–43
   bariatric surgery and, 235–236, 241
   binge-eating disorder and, 198
   older patients and, 349
   prevalence of, 80–84, **85, 86, 87,**
      257
   site of treatment and, **54,** 131
   treatment modifications for, 84,
      88–96
Compensatory behaviors
   assessment and, 40
   in binge-eating disorder, 23
   in bulimia nervosa, 11
Compliance. *See* Non-adherence

Compulsive behaviors, 290
Conflict, role of in psychodynamic
    therapy, 318–320
Conflict avoidance, and family therapy,
    152
Coping strategies
    in bulimia nervosa, 17
    psychodynamic therapy and, 314
Corticosteroids, and weight gain, 264,
    270
Counseling, nutritional, 119, 123, 374
Countertransference, and chronic
    eating disorders, 431, 435. *See also*
    Transference
Culture
    assessment and, 398–401
    bariatric surgery and, 236
    body image and eating behaviors in
        non-Caucasians and, 389–396,
        397
    epidemiology in non-Caucasians
        and, 389
    etiology of anorexia nervosa and, 9
    etiology of bulimia nervosa and, 18
    international trends in eating
        behavior and, 397
    male patients and, 351, 397
    overvaluation of thinness and, 388
    prevalence of anorexia nervosa and,
        6–7
    sports environments and, 359–360
    treatment and, 401–402
Cyproheptadine
    anorexia nervosa and, 121, 426
    weight effects of, 264, **270**

Daniels, Lucy, 307, 308–309, 310,
    311, 312, 315, 316, 317–318,
    326, 328, 329

Dare, Christopher, 153
Death. *See also* Mortality
    anorexia nervosa and causes of, 11
    postvention for staff and family, 431
Denmark, and study of night-eating
    syndrome, 212
Dental complications, of bulimia
    nervosa, 13, **14**
Dependent personality disorder, 84
Depression. *See also* Major depression
    in diabetes patients with eating
        disorders, 337, 339
    loss of appetite in elderly patients
        and, 349
Desipramine
    binge-eating disorder and, **206**
    bulimia nervosa and, **178, 179,**
        185, 186
Development issues, in assessment,
    33–34. *See also* Adolescents;
    Children
Dexfenfluramine, **206**, 207
Diabetes mellitus, and eating disorders,
    336–339
Diagnosis and diagnostic criteria.
    See also Assessment; Diagnostic
    migration; Differential diagnosis
    anorexia nervosa and, 2–3,
        350–351, 353–354
    binge-eating disorder and, 20, **22,**
        196
    bulimia nervosa and, 11–12, **13,**
        350
    eating disorder not otherwise
        specified and, 19–20, **21,** 196,
        353, 372
    gender and, 350, 352
    night-eating syndrome and, 208, 209
    sports participation and, 368

Diagnostic Interview for Borderlines
  (DIB), 100
Diagnostic migration
  anorexia nervosa and, 10
  binge-eating disorder and, 25
  bulimia nervosa and, 19
Dialectical behavior therapy (DBT),
  103, 204, 299
Diaries
  cognitive-behavioral therapy, 298, **302**
  night-eating syndrome and,
    208–209, 213
Dietary restraint model, of bulimia
  nervosa, 16
Dieting. *See also* Eating patterns
  binge-eating disorder and, 24–25,
    198, 199–200
  body image in non-Caucasian
    women and, 389–396
  mood assessment and, 88–89
Differential diagnosis
  of anorexia nervosa, 6
  of binge-eating disorder, 23
  of bulimia nervosa, 15
  of weight loss in older patients, **348**
Disability, and chronic eating disorders,
  411
Discharge, from inpatient settings for
  anorexia nervosa, 120–121, 123
Disulfiram, 97
Documentation, of treatment of
  patients with intractable
  eating disorders, 435
Domaperidone, 141
Drop out rates
  for inpatient treatment of anorexia
    nervosa, 116, 134
  from partial hospitalization for
    anorexia nervosa, 122

DSM-IV, and binge-eating disorder, 20
DSM-IV-TR
  diagnostic criteria for anorexia
    nervosa in, **3**, 350, 353–354,
    372
  diagnostic criteria for binge-eating
    disorder in, **22**
  diagnostic criteria for eating
    disorder not otherwise
    specified in, **21**, 372
  gender bias and, 350, 352
  subtypes of anorexia nervosa in, 2
  subtypes of bulimia nervosa in, 11
Dual-energy X-ray absorptiometry
  (DEXA), 36, **38**, 372
Dysthymia, 80

Eating Attitudes Test, 352, 394
Eating disorder assertive community
  treatment (ED ACT), 144
Eating disorder not otherwise specified
  (EDNOS)
  diagnosis of, 19–20, **21**, 196, 353,
    372
  prevalence of, 19, 195
  treatment of, 218–219
Eating disorders. *See also* Anorexia
  nervosa; Binge-eating disorder;
  Bulimia nervosa; Eating disorder
  not otherwise specified; Night-
  eating syndrome; Sleep-related
  eating disorder
  applications of cognitive-behavioral
    therapy in, 292–299
  athletes and, 357–385
  characteristics of, 1–2
  cognitive distortions and
    maladaptive behaviors in,
    288–291

comorbidity of psychiatric disorders in, 42–43
comprehensive assessment of, 31–34
core beliefs and attitudes associated with, 40–42
cultural factors in, 387–403
diabetes mellitus and, 366–339
eating behavior and assessment of, 36–37, 39–40
family assessment and, 43–44
history of concept, 2, 149
laboratory assessment for, 36, **38–39**
level of care guidelines for patients with, **51–56**
male patients and, 349–353
older patients and, 346–349, **350, 351**
physical status and assessment of, 34–36
pregnancy and, 340–344, **345**
self-help books and Internet resources on, **45–46, 300–301, 436**
weight-altering medications and, 256, 269–278
Eating Disorder Inventory, 352, 365, 395, 396
Eating Disorders Questionnaire (EDQ), 32–33, 60–77, 242, **243,** 366, 391
Eating patterns. *See also* Dieting; Nutritional issues
assessment for bariatric surgery and, 244–245
body image in non-Caucasian women and, 389–396
family and, 150

international trends in, 397
night-eating syndrome and, 209
patient assessment and, 37
Education. *See also* Self-help books; Self-help organizations
for anorexia nervosa patients, 120, 134
bariatric surgery and, 246, 248
for binge-eating disorder patients, 201
cognitive-behavioral therapy and, 89, 298
for prevention of eating disorders in athletes, 376–377
Eisler, Ivan, 153
Electrocardiograms, 4, 36, **38,** 372
Electroconvulsive therapy, 428
Electrolyte abnormalities, in anorexia nervosa, 4
Empowerment, and family therapy, 153–154
Endocrine sequelae, of anorexia nervosa, 4, **5**
Energy balance, and weight regulation, 256, **258**
Enmeshment
family therapy and, 152
psychodynamic therapy and, 318
Enteral and parenteral feedings, 427–428
Epidemiology. *See also* Prevalence
of anorexia nervosa, 6–7, **8**
of binge-eating disorder, 23–24, **25**
of bulimia nervosa, 15–16, **17**
of eating disorders in non-Caucasian populations, 389
Estrogen, 141–142

Ethical issues, in chronic cases of eating
disorders, 144, 428–431
Ethnicity, and epidemiology of eating
disorders, 389. *See also* Culture
Etiology
of anorexia nervosa, 7–9
of binge-eating disorder, 24–25
of bulimia nervosa, 16–18
European Collaborative Longitudinal
Study on Eating Disorders, 327
Evening hyperphagia, 208, 209
Exenatide, 265, 268, **270**
Exercise
anorexia nervosa and, 130
athletes as patients and, 372–374
bariatric surgery and, 248
patient assessment and, 37
site of treatment and, **54**
Exercise bulimia, 375
Expectations
bariatric surgery and, 245–246
treatment of chronic disorders and,
416–417
Exposure and response prevention
techniques, 120

Family. *See also* Family therapy;
Parenting
assessment of, 43–44, 119–120
athletes with eating disorders and,
377–378
etiology of bulimia nervosa and, 17
as targets for treatment, 150
treatment of patients with
intractable eating disorders
and, 435–436
treatment reluctance and, 414
Family-based treatment (FBT),
155–161, 162–163, 164

Family dynamic history, 43–44
Family systems theory, and anorexia
nervosa, 8–9
Family therapy
anorexia nervosa and, 119–120,
132, 134, 136, 152–162
athletes with eating disorders and,
374
bulimia nervosa and, 162–163, 164,
166
chronic disorders and, 422
empirical support for effectiveness
of, 163–166
future directions in, 166–167
types of, **151**
Famotidine, 268
Feeding behaviors, in children of
parents with eating disorders,
343–344
Felbamate, **270**
Female athlete triad, 372–374
Fenfluramine, 207
Fiji, and cultural shifts, 388–389
Financial resources, and treatment of
chronic disorders, 423–424,
433
Fluoxetine
anorexia nervosa and, 139
binge-eating disorder and, **206**
bulimia nervosa and, 176, **181, 185,
186,** 375
chronic disorders and, 425
weight regulation and, 262–263,
267, 271
Fluoxetine Bulimia Nervosa
Collaborative Study Group, 176
Fluphenazine, **260**
Flutamide, 183
Fluvoxamine, **206,** 262

Focal hypothesis, in psychodynamic therapy, 326

Focal psychotherapy treatment, for anorexia nervosa, 134

Follow-up. *See also* Outcome
in chronic cases of anorexia nervosa, 143–144
treatment of binge-eating disorder and, 207
treatment of bulimia nervosa and, 188
treatment of night-eating syndrome and, 217–218

Gabapentin
anxiety disorders and, 95
clinical characteristics of, **93**
weight effects of, 264, **270**

Gastric banding, 232, **233**

Gastric bypass, 226–227, 229–230, **231**, 232

Gastrointestinal system. *See also* Bariatric surgery
anorexia nervosa and, 4, **5**
bulimia nervosa and, 13, **14**, 15
normal anatomy of, **227**

Gender. *See also* Males
diagnostic criteria for eating disorders and, 350, 352
role conflicts and etiology of anorexia nervosa, 9
treatment modification and, 352–353

Generalized anxiety disorder, 81

Genetics
of anorexia nervosa, 7
athletic performance and, 362
of binge-eating disorder, 24
of bulimia nervosa, 16

Globalization, and cultural shifts, 388–389, 397

Group therapy, for anorexia nervosa, 120, 136

Growth chart, 34. *See also* Weight chart

Guidelines. *See also* Clinical recommendations
for level of care, **51–56**
for treatment of patients with intractable eating disorders, 433–436

Gull, William, 149

Haloperidol, **260**, 426

Harm reduction model, 419

Health care. *See* Medical care and medical status

Health maintenance criteria, for sports participation, 370–371

Health-Related Quality of Life (HRQOL), 183, 238, 240–241

Hematological abnormalities, in anorexia nervosa, 5

Herbal preparations, and bariatric surgery, 244

Histrionic personality disorder, 84

Homework assignments, and anorexia nervosa, 120

Horizontal gastroplasty, 226, **229**

Hormone replacement therapy, for osteoporosis, 141–142

Horse racing, and eating disorders in jockeys, 359

Hospitalization. *See also* Inpatient treatment
for anorexia nervosa, 114–116, **117**, 143–144
for bulimia nervosa, 49–50

Hospitalization *(continued)*
    comorbidity and, 90, 93–94, 95,
        98, 104–105
    factors suggesting choice of, 48–49,
        423
Hyperemesis gravidarum, 341, 344
Hyperglycemia, 338
Hypocalcemia, 344
Hypoglycemia, 337

ICD-10, and diagnostic criteria for
    anorexia nervosa, 350
Identity. *See also* Culture; Self
    core beliefs and, 42
    ethnicity and, 390–391
    sports participation and, 367
Imipramine
    binge-eating disorder and, **206**
    bulimia nervosa and, **178, 185**
    weight gain and, 262
Impact of Weight on Quality of Life—
    Lite (IWQOL-Lite), 238, **243**
Individually estimated healthy weights,
    48
Infertility, and impact of eating
    disorders, 340–341
Inflammatory bowel disease, 272
Inpatient treatment. *See also*
        Hospitalization
    of anorexia nervosa, 116–122
    of eating disorders in athletes, 373
Insulin
    eating disorders in diabetes patients
        and, 337
    weight gain and, 264–265, **270,**
        271–272
Interdisciplinary team management, 47
Integrative cognitive therapy (ICT),
    103

Internet resources, on eating disorders,
    46, 301
Interpersonal psychotherapy
    acute loss and, 311
    anorexia nervosa and, 135
    for binge-eating disorder, 203–204
    depression and, 89
Intractability, and treatment non-
        response or reluctance, 412–415
Involuntary admission, and anorexia
    nervosa, 116
Isocarboxazid, **180,** 264, **270**

Jejunoileal bypass (JIB), 226, **228**

Kentucky Derby Museum, 359

Laboratory tests
    anorexia nervosa and, 4–5, 118
    assessment and, 36, **38–39**
    athletes with eating disorders and,
        372
    older patients and, **351**
    pregnant patients with eating
        disorders and, **345**
Lamotrigine, 92, **93,** 261
Language, and non-English speaking
    patients, 402
Laseque, Charles, 149
Latin Americans, and cultural issues in
    eating disorders, 392–394,
        399–400
LEARN program, 199
Legal issues
    chronic eating disorders and,
        428–431
    safety of patient and, 50
Life stage theory, in psychodynamic
    therapy, 327

Liquid formulas, for nutritional
  rehabilitation, 118
Listening, and psychodynamic therapy,
  312–313
Lithium
  anorexia nervosa and, 141
  bipolar disorder and, 91, 92
  chronic disorders and, 426–427
  clinical characteristics of, **93**
  weight regulation and, 259, 261, **270**
Living arrangements, for patients with
  eating disorders, 161
Loss, and psychodynamic therapy,
  310–312

Magnification, and cognitive
  distortions, 289
Major depression, and comorbidity, 80,
  198, 235. *See also* Depression
Males. *See also* Gender
  binge-eating disorder in, 23
  eating disorders in non-Caucasian,
    397
  prevalence of anorexia nervosa in, 6
  as special population in eating
    disorders, 349–353
Marriage and marital therapy,
  161–162, 249
Maudsley Hospital (London), 153,
  164, 326
McLean Screening Instrument for
  Borderline Personality Disorder
  (MSI-BPD), 100
Meal plans, for anorexia nervosa, 119,
  123, 131. *See also* Nutritional issues
Media
  cultural influences on eating and,
    388, 389
  eating disorders in athletes and, 360

sociocultural factors in etiology of
  bulimia nervosa and, 18
Medical care and medical status. *See
  also* Medical complications;
  Medical disorders
  for anorexia nervosa, 117–119
  assessment for bariatric surgery and,
    245
  chronic eating disorders and, 421
  hospitalization for anorexia nervosa
    and, **117**
  levels of care guidelines and, 51–52
  outpatient care for anorexia nervosa
    and, 129–130
  for pregnant women with eating
    disorders, 344, **345**
Medical complications. *See also* Cardiac
  abnormalities; Gastrointestinal
  system; Medical care and medical
  status; Medical disorders;
  Neurological abnormalities;
  Reproductive system
  of anorexia nervosa, 4–5
  of bariatric surgery, 232
  of binge-eating disorder, 21–22
  of bulimia nervosa, 12–14
  of comorbid eating disorders and
    diabetes, 337, **339**
  of eating disorders in older patients,
    347–349, **350**
  of obesity, 225
  of pregnant women with eating
    disorders, 341, **343**, 344
Medical disorders. *See also* Medical
  complications; Medical care and
  medical status
  assessment and, 43
  differential diagnosis of anorexia
    nervosa, 6

Medical disorders *(continued)*
  differential diagnosis of binge-eating
    disorder and, 23
  differential diagnosis of bulimia
    nervosa and, 15
Medications. *See* Antidiabetic agents;
    Antihypertensive medications;
    Oral contraceptives;
    Psychopharmacology; Stimulant
    medications
Menstruation, and assessment, 34.
    See also Amenorrhea
Mesoridazine, **260**
Metformin, 265, 268, **270**
Methylphenidate, **270**
Metoclopramide, 266, **270**, 275
Mianserin, **179**
Miglitol, 268, **270**
Minuchin, Salvador, 149, 152–153
Mirtazapine
  anorexia nervosa and, 139
  anxiety disorders and, 96
  chronic disorders and, 425
  weight effects of, 263, **270**
Moclobemide, **180**
Modafinil, 266, **270**
Modell, Arnold, 317
Molindone, **260**, 267, **270**
MONICA study (Denmark), 212
Monitoring. *See also* Self-monitoring
  chronic anorexia nervosa and
    long-term, 143–144
  outpatient treatment of anorexia
    nervosa and, 50
  sports participation and, 367
  treatment of binge-eating disorder
    and, 207
  treatment of bulimia nervosa and,
    188

treatment of night-eating syndrome
    and, 217–218
Monoamine oxidase inhibitors
    (MAOIs)
  bulimia nervosa and, 175–176
  chronic disorders and, 425
  comorbid mood disorders and, 90
  weight regulation and, 264
Mood disorders, and comorbidity, 80,
    88–90
Mood stabilizers. *See also* Lithium
  anorexia nervosa and, 140–141
  weight gain and, 259, 261, **270**
Mortality. *See also* Death
  in anorexia nervosa, 10–11, 408
  in bulimia nervosa, 19
Motivation
  assessment and, 42, 245
  bariatric surgery and, 245
  site of treatment and, **53**
  sports participation and, 368, 369
Motivational enhancement therapy
    (MET), 136–138, 299
Motivational interviewing, 419
Multiple family groups, 167
Muscle dysmorphia, 352

Naltrexone
  alcohol abuse and, 97
  binge-eating disorder and, **206**
  bulimia nervosa and, **178**, 184
  chronic disorders and, 426
Nasal gastric tube feeding, 116, 427,
    430
Nateglinide, 265
National Alliance on Mental Illness,
    272–273, 435
National Collegiate Athletic
    Association, 376

National Comorbidity Survey
Replication Study, 15, 24
National Institute of Mental Health,
140
Native Americans, and cultural issues,
396, 397, 400–401
Nefazodone, 263
Neurochemistry, and etiology of eating
disorders, 7–8, 16
Neurological abnormalities, in anorexia
nervosa, 5
Neurological disorders
differential diagnosis of binge-eating
disorder and, 23
differential diagnosis of bulimia
nervosa and, 15
Neutrality, and psychodynamic therapy,
313
Night Eating Symptom Scale (NESS),
213
Night-eating syndrome (NES)
bariatric surgery and, 237, 240
obesity and, 196
treatment of, 207–218
Nizatidine, 268
Nocturnal eating and drinking
syndrome (NEDS), 210
Nonadherence, with medication regimens, 271–273, 339, 413–415
Nonexercise adaptive thermogenesis,
257, **258**
Nonpurging subtype, of bulimia
nervosa, 11
Nonresponse, to treatment in chronic
cases, 412–415
Nonspecific factors, in cognitive-
behavioral therapy, 292–293
Nonspecific supportive clinical
management (NSCM), 135

Nortriptyline, 272
Nutritional issues. *See also* Dieting;
Eating patterns; Meal plans
in binge-eating disorder, 199–201
in bulimia nervosa, 173
counseling on, 119, 123, 374
in night-eating syndrome, 212
rehabilitation for anorexia nervosa
and, 117–119, 130

Obesity
binge-eating disorder and, 25,
197–198
genetics of, 24
increase in rates of, 225, 388
medical complications of, 21–22,
225
night-eating syndrome and, 196
quality of life and, 238
Obligate energy expenditure, 256–257,
258
Obsessive-compulsive disorder
comorbidity and, 81–82, 95–96,
105–106
eating disorders in athletes and, 365
outpatient management of anorexia
nervosa and, 131
Obsessive-compulsive personality
disorder, 84, 365
Olanzapine
anorexia nervosa and, 140
chronic disorders and, 425
clinical characteristics of, **94**
weight gain and, 93, 259, **260, 270,**
274, 275
Older patients, and special issues in
eating disorders, 346–349, **350,**
351
Ondansetron, 177, 182, 427

Opiate-related medications, and
    chronic eating disorders, 426
Oral complications, of bulimia nervosa,
    13–14
Oral contraceptives, 92, 142, 265
Oral feeding and refeeding, 427
Orlistat, 205, **206**, 271
Osteopenia and osteoporosis, and
    anorexia nervosa, 4, 141–142,
    363. *See also* Bone density
Outcome
    for anorexia nervosa, 9–11, **12**, 408,
        409
    bariatric surgery and psychosocial,
        238–241
    for binge-eating disorder, 25, **26**
    for bulimia nervosa, 18–19, **20**
    for eating disorders in pregnancy,
        342
Outpatient settings
    eating disorders in athletes and, 373
    as initial choice for treatment, 50,
        57
    pharmacological approaches to
        anorexia nervosa and, 138–142
    psychosocial approaches to anorexia
        nervosa and, 132–138
    target symptoms and goals of in
        anorexia nervosa, 129–132
Overgeneralization, and cognitive
    distortions, 289
Overprotectiveness, and families of
    anorexia nervosa patients, 152

Panic disorder, 81
Parenting, and mothers with eating
    disorders, 343–344
Paroxetine, 262, 263, **270**
Partial hospital programs, 50, 122–124

Patient history, and assessment, 33,
    420–421
Perceptual distortions, about body size,
    288–289
Perfectionism, 33, 41, 289. *See also*
    Personality
Performance, and eating disorders in
    athletes, 362, 377
Personality. *See also* Perfectionism
    anorexia nervosa and, 5, 8
    bariatric surgery patients and, 236
    bulimia nervosa and, 14–15
    eating disorders in athletes and,
        363, 365
Personality Diagnostic Questionnaire–4
    (PDQ-4), 100
Personality disorders, and comorbidity,
    84, **85**, **86**, **87**, 236
Personal relationships, and assessment
    for bariatric surgery, 246, 249.
    See also Family; Marriage and
    marital therapy; Support systems
Phenelzine
    bulimia nervosa and, **180**
    weight effects of, 264, **270**, 425
Philadelphia Child Guidance Center,
    152
Physical activity, and weight regulation,
    257, **258**
Physical presentation
    of anorexia nervosa, 4
    of binge-eating disorder, 21
    of bulimia nervosa, 12
Physical status, and assessment, 34–36.
    See also Weight
Physiology
    screening for eating disorders in
        athletes and, 366
    of weight regulation, 256–257

Pioglitazone, 265
PISIA criteria, for borderline
    personality disorder, 100, **101**
Postpartum depression, 341, 343
Posttraumatic stress disorder, 83, 104
"Practice Guideline for the Treatment
    of Patients with Borderline
    Personality Disorder" (American
    Psychiatric Association 2001),
    100, 104
Practice network approach, to
    psychodynamic therapy, 328
Pramlintide, 265, 268, **270**
Pregabalin, 264, **270**
Pregnancy, and eating disorders,
    340–344, **345**
Presurgical interventions, and bariatric
    surgery, 247–250
Prevalence
    of anorexia nervosa, 6, **8**
    of binge-eating disorder, 24, **25**
    of bulimia nervosa, 15, **17**
    of comorbidity in bariatric surgery
        patients, 235, 241
    of comorbidity in eating disorders
        patients, 80–84, **85, 86, 87,**
        257
    of eating disorder not otherwise
        specified, 19, 195
    of eating disorders in African
        American women, 392
    of eating disorders in diabetes
        patients, 337
    of eating disorders in male patients,
        351–352
    of psychopathology in bariatric
        surgery patients, 236–237
Prevention, of eating disorders in
    athletes, 376–378

Problem-solving strategies
    binge-eating disorder and, 201
    family of anorexia nervosa patient
        and, 152
Progressive muscle relaxation (PMR),
    and night-eating syndrome,
    213
Project EAT, 391, 394, 395
Prokinetic agents, and anorexia nervosa,
    141
Psychodynamic therapy
    conflict and, 318–320
    growth of self and, 317–318
    key aspects of, 309
    perceived weakness and, 315–316
    repetition of themes in, 322
    research on, 326–328
    self-destructive behavior and,
        313–315
    self-punishment and, 320–322
    sense of being listened to, 312–313
    sensory data in, 324–326
    support and working through
        separation and loss,
        310–312
    transference and, 323–324
Psychological factors
    in etiology of anorexia nervosa,
        8–9
    in etiology of bulimia nervosa,
        16–17
Psychological presentation
    of anorexia nervosa, 5–6
    of binge-eating disorder, 22–23
    of bulimia nervosa, 14–15
Psychological Screening Test for Eating
    Disorders/Disordered Eating
    among Female Collegiate
    Athletes, 366

Psychopharmacology. *See also*
  Anticonvulsants; Antidepressants;
  Antipsychotics; Beta-blockers;
  Combined therapy; Monoamine
  oxidase inhibitors; Mood
  stabilizers; Selective serotonin
  reuptake inhibitors; Stimulant
  medications; Treatment
  anorexia nervosa and, 121,
    138–142, 274
  binge-eating disorder and, 204–207
  bulimia nervosa and, 174–188
  chronic eating disorders and,
    424–428
  comorbidity and, 90, 91–93,
    95–96, 97–98, 104, 106
  night-eating syndrome and, 215,
    217–218
  nonadherence and, 271–273, 339,
    413–415
  weight-affecting medications and,
    259–278
Psychosocial approaches, to treatment
  of anorexia nervosa, 119–120,
    131–138
  bariatric surgery patients and,
    237–238
  of binge-eating disorder, 201–204
  of bulimia nervosa, 173–174
  of chronic eating disorders, 420
  of night-eating syndrome,
    212–213
Psychosocial outcomes, of bariatric
  surgery, 238–241
Psychosocial variables, in binge-eating
  disorder, 24
*Psychosomatic Families: Anorexia
  Nervosa in Context* (Minuchin et
  al. 1978), 153

Psychostimulants, 97. *See also*
  Stimulant medications
Psychotherapy. *See also* Cognitive-
  behavioral therapy; Family
  therapy; Group therapy;
  Interpersonal psychotherapy;
  Psychodynamic therapy;
  Treatment
  athletes with eating disorders and,
    374
  chronic eating disorders and, 421
  comorbidity and modification of,
    90, 91, 94–95, 96–97,
    100–101, 103–104, 105–106
  male patients and, 353
Purging behaviors
  assessment and, 37, 39
  site of treatment and, 55
Purging subtype, of bulimia nervosa, 11

QT interval, prolonged, 363, **364**
Quality of life
  bariatric surgery and, 240–241
  obesity and, 238
Questionnaire on Eating and Weight
  Patterns—Revised (QEWP-R),
  243
Quetiapine, **94, 270,** 274

Reboxetine, 183, 425
Recombinant human IGF, 142
Refusal, of treatment, 429–431
Relapse
  in anorexia nervosa, 9–10, 139, 143
  bariatric surgery patients and, 250
  in binge-eating disorder, 25, 203
  in bulimia nervosa, 18–19, 175, 188
  psychodynamic therapy and,
    315–316

Religion, and "holy anorexia,"
387–388. *See also* Zen Buddhism
Reluctance, and treatment of chronic
disorders, 412–415
Renal abnormalities, in anorexia
nervosa, 4–5
Repaglinide, 265
Repetition, of themes in
psychodynamic therapy, 322
Repetitive behaviors, 290
Reproductive system. *See also*
Amenorrhea; Oral contraceptives;
Pregnancy
anorexia nervosa and, 4, **5**
bulimia nervosa and, 14
fertility rates and infertility
treatment, 340–341
Restricting subtype, of anorexia
nervosa, 2
Reverse anorexia nervosa, 352
Risidronate, 142
Risperidone
bipolar disorders and, 93
chronic disorders and, 425
clinical characteristics of, **94**
weight regulation and, 259, **260**,
270, 274, 275
Russell, Gerald, 153

Safety
assessment and, 34
chronic eating disorders and, 415,
423
legal interventions and, 50
sports participation and, 367
St. Paul's Hospital Eating Disorders
Program, 423
Schema-focused CBT (SFCBT),
301

Screening
for eating disorders in athletes,
365–366
for eating disorders in pregnant
women, **345**
Seasonal affective disorder, 428
Selective abstraction, 289
Selective serotonin reuptake inhibitors
(SSRIs)
binge-eating disorder and, 204, **206**
bulimia nervosa and, 176
chronic disorders and, 424–425
comorbidity and, 90, 95–96, 104,
106
diabetes and, 338–339
night-eating syndrome and, 215
outpatient management of anorexia
nervosa and, 131, 138–139
weight regulation and, 262–263,
267
Self. *See also* Identity; Self-esteem
core beliefs and, 41, 42
psychodynamic therapy and, 317–318
Self-destructive behavior, and
psychodynamic therapy, 313–315
Self-esteem
bariatric surgery patients and,
237–238
cognitive distortions and, 290
sports participation and, 367
Self-Harm Inventory (SHI), 100,
102–103
Self-help books, 45–46, 300–301
Self-help organizations, and chronic
eating disorders, 435, **436**
Self-monitoring, and cognitive-
behavioral therapy, 298, **302**
Self-punishment, and psychodynamic
therapy, 320–322

Self-referential personalization, 289
Self-Regulatory Approach (SRA), for
   borderline personality disorder,
   101
Self-report questionnaires, 100,
   241–242, **243**
Sensory data, in psychodynamic
   therapy, 324–326
Separation/individuation, and psycho-
   dynamic therapy, 310–312, 327
Serotonin levels, in anorexia nervosa, 7–8
Sertindole, **260**
Sertraline
   binge-eating disorder and, **206**
   night-eating syndrome and, 215,
      217–218
   weight regulation and, 262–263
Session-by-session schedule, for
   cognitive-behavioral therapy, 298
Sexuality, and psychotherapy for male
   patients, 353
Shame, and treatment reluctance, 414
Sibutramine, 205, **206**
Site, of treatment. *See also*
   Hospitalization; Outpatient
   settings
   chronic eating disorders and,
      422–424
   initial choice of, 47–57
Skills training, sport-related, 373
Sleep-related eating disorder (SRED), 210
Social Function–36 (SF-36), **243**
Sociocultural factors, in etiology of
   eating disorders, 9, 18. *See also*
   Culture
Socioeconomic status, and prevalence
   of anorexia nervosa, 7
Specialized inpatient eating disorder
   setting, 116

Special populations, and eating
   disorders. *See also* Athletes
   diabetes mellitus and, 336–339
   older patients and, 346–349
   pregnancy and, 340–344, **345**
Split management, 47
Sports. *See also* Athletes
   environments for and risk of eating
      disorders, 358–361
   participation in for symptomatic
      patients, 366–371
Stability, in clinical course of anorexia
   nervosa, 410
Stimulant medications. *See also*
   Psychostimulants
   chronic disorders and, 427
   weight loss and, 266, 275
Strength training, 352
Stress
   diabetes and, 337
   family assessment and, 44
   patient assessment and, 34
   etiology of anorexia nervosa and, 8
   site of treatment and, **55**
Substance use disorders. *See also*
   Alcohol abuse or dependence
   bariatric surgery patients and, 235
   bulimia nervosa and, 14
   comorbidity in eating disorder
      patients, 82–83, 96–98
Subthreshold variants, of anorexia
   nervosa, 3
Subtypes
   of anorexia nervosa, 2
   of bulimia nervosa, 11
Sudden cardiac death, 362–363
Suicide and suicidality
   anorexia nervosa and, 10–11
   assessment of, 34

chronic eating disorders and, 415,
430–431
hospitalization and, 104–105
level of care guidelines and, 52
Sulfasalazine, 272
Sulfonylureas, 265, **270**
Superstitious thinking, 289
Supportive psychotherapy, 89
Support systems. *See also* Family;
Personal relationships
assessment for bariatric surgery, 246
psychodynamic therapy, 310–312
sports participation and, 367
Surgery. *See* Bariatric surgery
*Systems Training for Emotional
Predictability and Problem Solving*
(STEPPS), 103

Tamoxifen, 265
Team approach, to treatment, 46, 47
Testosterone, 352–353
Therapeutic alliance. *See also* Transference
chronic eating disorders and, 420
family therapy and, 164
initial psychiatric management and
establishment of, 44
Therapeutic stance, and chronic eating
disorders, 416–417, 433–434
Therapist-patient relationship. *See also*
Transference
patients with intractable eating
disorders and, 434–435
in psychodynamic therapy, 327
Thiazolidinediones, 265, **270**
Thinking and thoughts, night-eating
syndrome and dysfunctional, 210,
211. *See also* Beliefs; Cognitive
distortions
Thioridazine, **260**

Third-generation psychotherapies, for
anorexia nervosa, 136–138
Thought-shape fusion, 289
Three Factor Eating Questionnaire
(TFEQ), **243**
Thyroid hormone abuse, 271
Tiagabine, **93**
Topiramate
alcohol abuse and, 97–98
binge-eating disorder and, 205, **206**
bipolar disorder and, 92, **93**
bulimia nervosa and, 182–183
night-eating syndrome and, 217
weight regulation and, 267, **270,**
271, 275
Tramadol, 426
Transdiagnostic model, 288
Transference, and psychodynamic
therapy, 314, 323–324. *See also*
Countertransference;
Therapeutic alliance
Trans-theoretical model of change, 137
Tranylcypromine, 264, 425
Trazodone, **179,** 264
Treatment, of eating disorders. *See also*
Family therapy; Hospitalization;
Inpatient treatment; Outpatient
settings; Psychopharmacology;
Psychosocial approaches;
Psychotherapy; Site; *specific
disorders*
for athletes with eating disorders,
371–376
bariatric surgery patients and,
246–250
chronicity and nonresponse or
reluctance in, 412–415
comorbidity and modifications of,
84, 88–98

Treatment, of eating disorders
    (continued)
    compassionate decision making for
        patients with intractable eating
        disorders, 432–436
    cultural issues in, 401–402
    gender-specific needs for, 352–353
    initial approach to psychiatric
        management, 44, 46–47
    initial choice of site for, 47–57
    management strategies for chronic
        cases, 418–422
    partial hospitalization for anorexia
        nervosa, 122–124
    refusal of, 429–431
    sports participation and progress in,
        370
    therapeutic goals in chronic cases
        and, 415–418
Treatment contract, and medications, 277
Treatment resistance, and cognitive-
    behavioral therapy, 299, 301, 303
Tricyclic antidepressants (TCAs)
    anorexia nervosa and, 138
    bulimia nervosa and, 175–176
    comorbid mood disorders and, 90
    weight gain and, 262, **270**, 272
Tustin, Francis, 324
Twelve-Step programs, 98
Two-track approach, to treatment of
    anorexia nervosa, 133

University of British Columbia, 419,
    423

Validity, of diagnostic criteria
    for anorexia nervosa, 2–3
    for binge-eating disorder, 196
    for bulimia nervosa, 11–12

Valproate, **93**, 261, **270**
Values. *See* Culture
Venlafaxine, 263, 425
Vertical-banded gastroplasty, 226, **230**
Vigabatrin, **270**

Weight. *See also* Body image; Body
        mass index; Weight chart
    anorexia nervosa and target, 118
    assessment and measurement of,
        34–35, 244
    athletes with eating disorders and
        restoration of, 372
    chronic eating disorders and, 421
    differential diagnosis of loss in older
        patients, **348, 351**
    hospitalization and acute versus
        chronic loss of, 143
    medications affecting, 259–276
    physiology of regulation, 256–257
    site of treatment and, 48, **53**
Weight chart, for family-based
        treatment of anorexia nervosa,
        159. *See also* Growth chart
Weight and Lifestyle Inventory
        (WALI), 242
*With a Women's Voice: A Writer's
        Struggle for Emotional Freedom*
        (Daniels 2001), 307, 308–309
Wrestling, and eating disorders in
        athletes, 360

Zen Buddhism, 204
Ziprasidone, 93, **94, 260**
Zolpidem, 275
Zonisamide, 205, 267, **270**